SCIENTIFIC AMERICAN

Introduction to

MOLECULAR
MEDICINE

SCIENTIFIC AMERICAN Introduction to Molecular Medicine

Edward Rubenstein, M.D., Series Editor

SCIENTIFIC AMERICAN Introduction to Molecular Medicine
*Edited by Philip Leder, M.D., David A. Clayton, Ph.D., and
Edward Rubenstein, M.D.*

Forthcoming Titles

SCIENTIFIC AMERICAN Molecular Cardiovascular Medicine
Edited by Edgar Haber, M.D.

SCIENTIFIC AMERICAN Molecular Oncology
Edited by J. Michael Bishop, M.D., and Robert A. Weinberg, Ph.D.

SCIENTIFIC AMERICAN

Introduction to
MOLECULAR MEDICINE

Edited by

Philip Leder, M.D.
John Amory Adrus Professor and Chairman
Department of Genetics,
Senior Investigator, Howard Hughes Medical Institute
Harvard Medical School

David A. Clayton, Ph.D.
Associate Director, Beckman Center
Professor of Developmental Biology
Stanford University School of Medicine

Edward Rubenstein, M.D.
Professor of Medicine Emeritus, Active
Stanford University School of Medicine

Scientific American, Inc., New York

Cover Illustration: Tom Moore

Library of Congress Cataloging-in-Publication Data

Scientific American introduction to molecular medicine / edited by Philip Leder, David A. Clayton, Edward Rubenstein.
p. cm.
Includes bibliographical references and index.
ISBN 0-89454-015-7
1. Medical genetics. 2. Molecular biology. 3. Pathology, Molecular. I. Leder, Philip. II. Clayton, David A. III. Rubenstein, Edward, 1924– . IV. Scientific American, Inc.
V. Title: Introduction to molecular medicine.
[DNLM: 1. Genetics, Biochemical. 2. Genetics, Medical. 3. Genetic Techniques.
QZ 50 S416 1994]
RB155.S36   1994
616'.042—dc20
DNLM/DLC
For Library of Congress   94-15489
                                                                                                           CIP

Publisher	Hilary Evans
Senior Project Editors	Richard P. Lindsey
	Maureen O'Sullivan
Development Editor	Armand Schwab
Art and Design	Elizabeth Klarfeld
	Talar Agasyan
Production	Mark Flanagan
Electronic Composition	Jennifer Smith

ISBN: 0-89454-015-7

Scientific American, Inc., 415 Madison Avenue, New York, NY 10017

Contributors

Paul Aebersold, Ph.D. Microbiologist, Division of Blood Applications, Center for Biologic Evaluation and Research, U.S. Food and Drug Administration, Bethesda, Maryland

Anne N. Baldwin, Ph.D. Department of Neurobiology, Stanford University School of Medicine

Gregory S. Barsh, M.D., Ph.D. Assistant Professor, Department of Pediatrics, Stanford University School of Medicine

Douglas L. Brutlag, Ph.D. Associate Professor of Biochemistry, Stanford University School of Medicine

David A. Clayton, Ph.D. Associate Director, Beckman Center, Professor of Developmental Biology, Stanford University School of Medicine

Charles Durfor, Ph.D. Scientific Reviewer, Hematologic Products Branch, Division of Biological IND, U.S. Food and Drug Administration, Bethesda, Maryland

Major Melissa Fries, M.D., USAF Clinical Geneticist and Obstetrician, Keesler Medical Center, Keesler Air Force Base, Mississippi

Mitchell S. Golbus, M.D. Professor of Obstetrics, Gynecology, and Reproductive Sciences, Professor of Pediatrics, University of California Medical Center, San Francisco

Dennis Klinman, M.D., Ph.D. Chief, Section of Retroviral Immunology, Division of Viral Products, Center for Biologic Evaluation and Research, U.S. Food and Drug Administration, Bethesda, Maryland

Robert Kozak, Ph.D.   Research Microbiologist, Laboratory of Cytokine Research, Division of Cytokine Biology, U.S. Food & Drug Administration, Bethesda, Maryland

Philip Leder, M.D.   John Amory Adrus Professor and Chairman, Department of Genetics, Senior Investigator, Howard Hughes Medical Institute, Harvard Medical School

Maynard V. Olson, Ph.D.   Department of Molecular Biotechnology, University of Washington, Seattle

John L.R. Rubenstein, M.D., Ph.D.   Center for Neurobiology and Psychiatry, Nina Ireland Laboratory for Developmental Neurobiology, University of California, San Francisco

Curtis L. Scribner, M.D.   Deputy Director, Division of Blood Applications, Center for Biologic Evaluation and Research, U.S. Food and Drug Administration, Bethesda, Maryland

Eric Shooter, Ph.D.   Professor, Department of Neurobiology, Stanford University School of Medicine

Robert A. Weinberg, Ph.D.   Whitehead Institute for Biomedical Research, Cambridge, Massachusetts

Huntington F. Willard, Ph.D.   Henry Willson Payne Professor and Chairman, Department of Genetics, and Director, Center for Human Genetics, Case Western Reserve University School of Medicine, Cleveland, Ohio

Preface

Molecular medicine, the newest and most advanced branch of medical science, began some 2,400 years ago, when Democritus proposed that the living organism is composed of arrangements of atoms that are continuously lost and faithfully replaced. Democritus, the father of the atomic theory, was to become a patient of Hippocrates, the father of western medical practice, who proposed that physicians assist nature in achieving a cure. These two ideas are the central concepts of molecular medicine today.

Although the goal of gaining a physical view of biologic systems at the level of their simplest constituents is more than 2,000 years old, only during the lifetimes—or, in many cases, the professional careers—of those now engaged in clinical and laboratory pursuits have we attained the ability to define the ultimate biologic structures with stunning precision. We are in the midst of revolutionary changes in basic science that will allow us to identify and to correct or circumvent molecular defects that give rise to some of the most prevalent afflictions of humanity, including many forms of atherosclerosis, hypertension, diabetes, neoplasia, autoimmune diseases, and disorders of mendelian inheritance. Henceforth, clinicians will increasingly employ diagnostic methods and therapeutic interventions made possible by the manipulation of the genes of microorganisms, plants, animals, and humans.

In short, we have entered the era of molecular medicine. Recent and current developments in this field are bestowing on physicians unprecedented powers to improve health, increase longevity, and ease suffering. Accordingly, clinicians are rapidly becoming aware of the need to master the principles of this field and to incorporate them into their daily work. This is not an easy task. New information about the fundamental bases of many diseases and about therapeutic interventions at the molecular level is being generated at a blinding rate that threatens to overtake our ability to remain current. What is more, new concepts and technologies have led to the creation of an ever-growing stock of new words and expressions. Thus, physicians will need to learn not only a new discipline but also a new language.

We are still at an early stage in the development of molecular medicine, a stage when almost everyone is a beginner. For this reason, the Editors have designed this book to be of practical use for those in clinical pursuits—practicing physicians and surgeons, house officers, medical students, and others involved in health care—as well as for biomedical scientists and educators. The goal has been twofold: to bring together a description of a new discipline and to provide a foundation for mastering the principles of that discipline.

The initial chapters outline some of the novel concepts that have evolved from the fusion of genetics and molecular biology. The book begins by reviewing how genes are organized and how their information is transmitted. The subsequent chapters provide basic information about DNA, RNA, and the ultimate building blocks of life, the proteins. In the field of protein chemistry, new, highly sophisticated concepts of protein structure are emerging that will ultimately explain biologic structure and disclose how structure determines function. For this reason, the discussion of this subject is detailed and introduces a number of advanced ideas. The next chapter explains the powerful evolutionary strategies that have given rise to the extraordinary diversity of nature, strategies that are intimately involved in immune response and disorders thereof.

The text then turns to the technique of gene cloning, which is fundamental to molecular biology and molecular medicine and has given rise to the field of genetic engineering. There follows a description of the Human Genome Project, an undertaking aimed at determining the complete genetic information of the human organism and, ultimately, at understanding how genes stipulate the structure and function of their products. This enterprise promises to yield enormous medical benefits.

The next group of chapters presents current information about practical problems in prenatal diagnosis and about the clinical and molecular aspects of important genetic diseases, including hereditary and acquired gene disorders that give rise to malignancies. The final chapters deal with bioengineered agents and the current status of gene therapy. The point is made that molecular medicine is now well established as a branch of medicine with which all physicians need to become familiar.

Molecular medicine is a burgeoning field that is expanding with breathtaking speed. To create a picture of such a fast-moving discipline, as we have attempted to do in this book, we have had to freeze its motion at a given point. The picture displayed here will inevitably be superseded by ever sharper and more complete representations, which the Editors plan to provide in future revisions of this book. Still in the full vigor of its youth, molecular medicine has already begun to spawn its descendants. We are now preparing a series of second-generation books dealing with offspring subspecialties, such as molecular cardiovascular medicine, molecular oncology, and molecular neuroscience and neurology.

Edward Rubenstein, M.D.
Stanford University School of Medicine
May 1994

Contents

CHAPTER 1

Human Genetics

Huntington F. Willard, Ph.D.

Just as an awareness of the role of microbial organisms in the etiology and pathogenesis of disease revolutionized the practice of medicine in the first decades of this century, so growing awareness of the role of genes and their products in etiology and pathogenesis is transforming the practice of modern medicine. Only 40 years ago the concept of a "gene" was ill-defined and its relevance to everyday medicine was questionable. Now, after years of stunning advances in the characterization and detailed molecular understanding of literally hundreds of genes, the role of genetics in medicine is clearly established; its relevance is undeniable in medical specialties ranging from perinatology to hematology to oncology, from obstetrics to cardiology to ophthalmology. Virtually every differential diagnosis can be facilitated by consideration of principles of human genetics. The physician must question and evaluate the role of a patient's genetic makeup as a cause of or contributor to symptoms, as a determinant of recurrence risks for the patient or family, and as a factor in designing appropriate management.

The modern view of genetics in medicine encompasses, in the first place, the individually rare conditions that follow quite simple rules of inheritance, such as the defects affecting enzymatic steps in intermediary metabolism that were recognized as genetic by the physician Sir Archibald Garrod in the first years of this century, even before the term genetic was coined; it also includes serious multisystem birth defects and syndromes. The modern view goes further, though: it takes into account the contribution of genes to relatively common medical conditions, such as pyloric stenosis, congenital heart defects, and neural tube defects in infants or hypertension, diabetes, breast cancer, and many forms of psychiatric illness in adults, to name but a few. In these conditions the role of genetics is less easily defined but is nonetheless undeniable. The physician who attempts to diagnose or deal with such patients without being aware of the possible role of genes in predisposing the patient to any such condition or without considering the effect of genetic factors on the possibility of the same condition in other family members, does so at a disadvantage.

This chapter focuses on the fundamental principles of human genetics as applied to medicine.[1-3] The basic organization of genetic material and its transmission from generation to generation will be reviewed as a foundation for considering defects involving chromosomes, their structure, and their inheritance. The composition and variability of individual genes will be examined, as will both simple and complex patterns of inheritance of genetic conditions; terms and concepts of genetics will be introduced that will figure not only in subsequent chapters, but also—increasingly—in the literature of clinical medicine. A theme of this chapter is that an understanding of genetic principles can make possible the formulation of new molecular and genetic paradigms for considering health and disease.

Genetics in Medicine

In clinical practice, the significance of genetics lies primarily in its contribution to the etiology of a large number of disorders. Although perhaps most directly involved in pediatrics, medical genetics is highly relevant to virtually all clinical specialties, most notably obstetrics, neurology, hematology, and oncology, and to adult medicine in general. In obstetrics, prenatal diagnosis of genetic defects is a standard part of prenatal care that is becoming increasingly important as more and more genetic disorders are recognized and delineated [see Chapter 8]. In adult medicine, many common diseases not generally recognized by practicing physicians as having a genetic basis, including diabetes mellitus, hypertension, and cancer, have important genetic components that are currently being defined. Appreciation of a genetically determined susceptibility to major illness in adulthood would have far-reaching consequences for the practice of medicine.

One of the lessons of the past decades is a growing realization that the influence of genetics on health and disease is widespread. Indeed, it is now estimated that more than five percent of live-born individuals younger than 25 years have a disease with a significant genetic component.[4] Several studies have estimated that from 20 to 30 percent of diseases among hospitalized children are genetic in origin[5]; at least one adult in 10 has a medical condition influenced by genetics. Clearly the common belief among many practitioners that genetic disease is rare and that consideration of genetic principles applies only to individually rare and bizarre disorders is untenable.

Three major types of disorders determined totally or partially by genetic factors are distinguished [see Table 1]. There are single-gene disorders, in which clinical manifestations are determined mainly by changes in individual genes, with regular and predictable patterns of transmission through families; there are chromosomal disorders, caused by defects

Table 1 Examples of Genetic Disorders

Disorder	Approximate Frequency
Single-gene defects	
Cystic fibrosis	1/2000 (in Caucasians)
Familial hypercholesterolemia	1/500
Fragile X mental retardation	1/1500 males
Duchenne's muscular dystrophy	1/3500 males
Neurofibromatosis type 1	1/3000
Sickle cell anemia	1/400 (in blacks)
Overall	**~1/100**
Chromosomal disorders	
Down syndrome	1/800
Klinefelter syndrome	1/1000 males
Turner syndrome	1/5000 females
Overall	**~1/160 live-borns**
Multifactorial diseases	
Cleft lip (with or without cleft palate)	~1/500
Neural tube defects	1/500
Diabetes mellitus	1/10 to 1/20 adults
Breast cancer	1/170 females < 50 years of age; 1/10 females, lifetime
Overall	**~1/10**

either in the number or structure of chromosomes; and there are multifactorial disorders, in which a combination of multiple factors (both genetic and environmental), rather than a defect in a single gene, generates or predisposes to a clinical disorder such as a congenital malformation or a common medical condition of adult life. Multifactorial traits tend to recur in families but without the characteristic patterns of transmission seen in single-gene disorders.

Organization and Expression of the Genetic Material

Before considering the nature and impact of genetic defects, it is necessary to review briefly the levels of organization and expression of human genetic material in its usual state. Additional details are provided in other chapters in this volume. The human genome comprises the complete genetic information of the species and is roughly estimated to contain about 50,000 to 100,000 different genes that control aspects of embryogenesis, development, growth, reproduction, and metabolism—essentially all biologic aspects of what makes a human a functional organism. A gene is a linear sequence of deoxyribonucleic acid (DNA) that is required to produce a functional product, usually a protein. DNA is a polymeric nucleic acid macromolecule consisting of four different nucleotides, each containing one of four informational bases. The specific linear arrangement of these four bases constitutes the chemical information encoded within genes, which is required for the exact transmission of genetic material from one cell to its progeny cells during cell division and from one generation to the next during reproduction. Long, linear DNA molecules (in a double helical form) containing up to hundreds of millions of bases and encoding many thousands of genes are packaged into rod-shaped organelles called chromosomes, which become visible under the light microscope during each cell division. The position of a gene along a chromosome is called its locus. Different copies of a particular chromosome normally have the same genes in the same linear organization, but the specific DNA sequence of those genes varies significantly among individuals. The multiple alternative forms of a gene are called alleles.

The expression of individual genes is rigorously orchestrated in a developmental and tissue-specific context. Some genes are expressed in abundance throughout life in all cells of the organism. Others are expressed in precisely controlled amounts, restricted spatially and temporally—specific to a particular cell type in the brain or liver or hematopoietic lineage, for example, or specific to a particular moment of early embryonic development. Only a small percent of the estimated total number of genes has been identified to date, and the role of only a few of these is currently understood. Nonetheless, given the fundamental role of genes in cellular processes, it is not surprising that defects in chromosome structure and gene function can lead to the panoply of clinical disorders seen in medical genetics.

Human Chromosomes

All normal nucleated human somatic cells contain 46 chromosomes—23 pairs, made up of one chromosome from each parent. Of these 23 pairs, 22 are alike in males and females and are called autosomes. The remaining pair comprises the two sex chromosomes: an X and a Y chromosome in males and two X chromosomes in females. The normal chromosome complement (called the karyotype), then, is 46,XY for males and 46,XX for females. Members of each chromosome pair are called homologues and carry corresponding (but not identical) genetic information.

Cytogenetics—the study of human chromosomes, their structure, and their transmission—has become an important diagnostic procedure in clinical medicine because chromosome anomalies are leading causes of reproductive loss and birth defects and are common in many forms of cancer. The ability to interpret a chromosome report and to understand the significance and limitations of chromosome studies are important skills for practicing physicians.

The chromosomes of a dividing human cell are readily observed at the metaphase (or prometaphase) stage of mitosis. Under the microscope, each of the 22 pairs of autosomes and the two sex chromosomes can be identified and distinguished on the basis of size, location of the primary constriction (centromere) that divides each chromosome into a long arm (q) and a short arm (p), and a unique pattern of transverse, alternating light and dark bands [*see Figure 1*]. The autosomes are numbered, essentially according to size, from 1 to 22. In most laboratory reports chromosomes are arranged in the form of a standard karyotype [*see Figure 2*], which facilitates analysis and interpretation. Particular banding patterns, which are generated by a number of standardized staining methods [*see Figure 2*], characterize each chromosome pair. These patterns are valuable not only for chromosome identification but also for assessment of chromosome structure. Individual chromosome bands are identified by a system of cytogenetic nomenclature [*see Figure 3*] that permits unambiguous reporting of abnormal karyotypes [*see Table 2*]. Even relatively minor alterations in chromosome structure can be diagnostic of major clinical problems, since individual chromosome bands typically contain some five to 10 million bases of DNA and on the order of hundreds of genes. More thorough accounts of chromosome structure and function and cytogenetic technology are available elsewhere.[1,6]

The Chromosomal Basis of Heredity

Somatic cell division, or mitosis [*see Figure 4a*], occurs throughout the organism and, in some cell lineages, dozens or hundreds of times. Cells in the germ line instead undergo meiosis [*see Figure 4b*], which occurs only once in each generation and results in the formation of gametes (ova or spermatozoa) containing only 23 chromosomes, one of each pair. Each gamete, then, contains one copy of each chromosome, so that new combinations of chromosomes are generated during fertilization, when an ovum and sperm unite to form a diploid zygote with 46 chromosomes.

The assortment of different chromosomes into gametes in meiosis is independent. That is, if the two members of each pair of homologues are designated A and B, one gamete may get either the A or the B copy of chromosome 1, either the A or the B copy of chromosome 2, and so on; which member of each pair the gamete receives is determined at random and independently. This generates an enormous amount of diversity

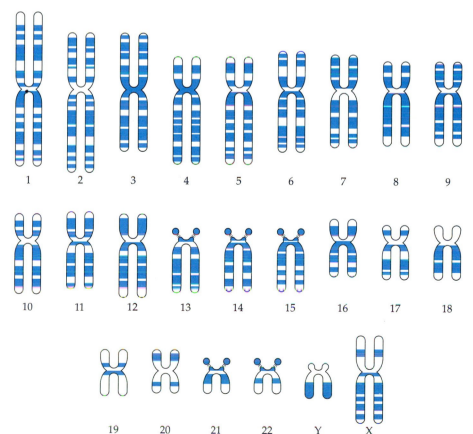

Figure 1 Shown are schematic drawings of one of each of the 23 human chromosomes, showing the bands seen with Giemsa staining.

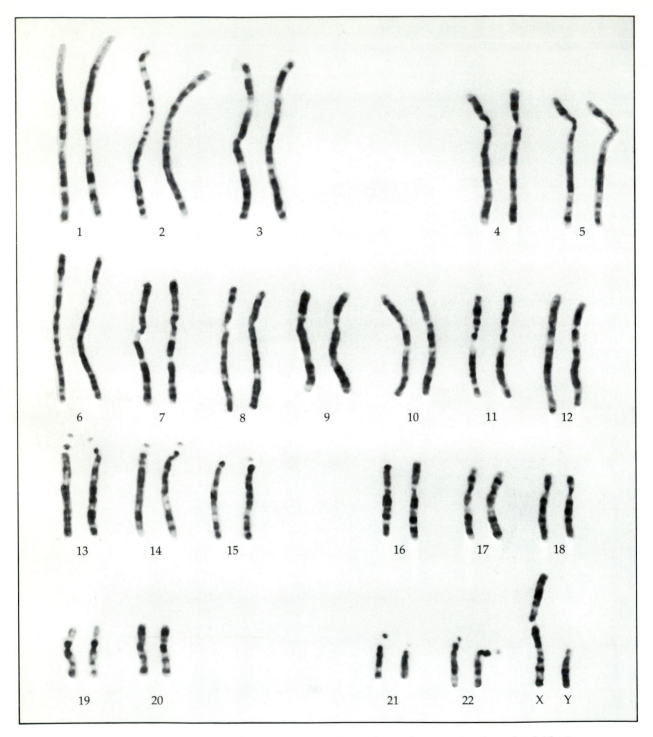

Figure 2 *Shown is a karyotype of a normal male. Giemsa staining shows about 850 bands per haploid set.*

among the possible combinations of chromosomes (and their particular set of encoded genes) observed in progeny: for 23 pairs of chromosomes, 2^{23} possible combinations can be present in any gamete.

The level of genetic diversity is increased even more by the process of meiotic recombination, in which pairs of homologous chromosomes normally exchange equivalent segments in meiosis. As a consequence of recombination, particular combinations of genes found on the two copies of a chromosome (one inherited from each parent) are shuffled in the next generation [*see Figure 4b*]. It is believed that approximately 50 or more recombination events occur in each meiosis; longer chromosomes can undergo three or more recombination events in each meiosis. Recombination together with random assortment of the recombined chromosomes ensures that each and every gamete, and so each and every individual except for identical twins, is truly genetically unique.

It follows from the linear organization of genes on each chromosome and the phenomenon of recombination that particular alleles of genes far apart on a chromosome are more likely to be separated by a recombination event than are alleles of genes that lie close to each other. This concept is called genetic linkage, which is defined as the tendency for alleles close together on the same chromosome to be transmitted together through meiosis. The strength of linkage can serve as a unit of measurement to distinguish how close genes are to each other. A centiMorgan (cM) is the genetic length over which recombination is observed during meiosis one percent of the time.

The significance of genetic linkage in medicine is that it allows one to predict transmission of a gene through a family by following the segregation of alleles at genes that are genetically linked. This helps the geneticist to identify genes responsible for inherited disease, assign these genes to a chromosome, and assess the likelihood of the presence or absence of a disease gene in family members. Following genes by linkage analysis allows one to identify medically relevant genes that have not yet yielded to biochemical or molecular analyses. If one knows that a specific disease gene is linked to a readily detectable DNA sequence, one can use allelic variation at the linked sequence to predict whether a particular individual has inherited a normal or abnormal copy of the disease gene.[1,7,8]

The Chromosomal Organization of Genes

The molecular structure of DNA and the organization and expression of genes are described in detail elsewhere in this volume [*see Chapter 2*]. What will be stressed here is the organization of genes on each chromosome and the aspects of gene structure and function that are most relevant to the understanding of genetic disease.

A human chromosome consisting of about 150 million bases of DNA (about the size of the X chromosome, for example) is believed to encode some 2,500 to 5,000 genes. Although there is no such thing as a typical gene, most genes are encoded over a linear segment of chromosomal DNA

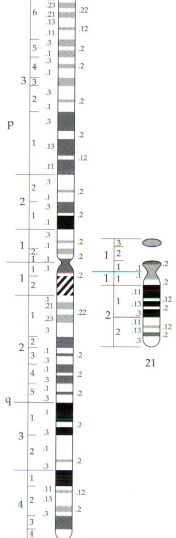

Figure 3 *The banding pattern and nomenclature are represented in this diagram of the haploid form of the normal human chromosomes 1 and 21. The chromosomes, shown at the 1,000-band stage, were prepared using Giemsa staining techniques. The differing shades of gray represent the gradations of color intensity observed, with black indicating the darkest-staining bands and white indicating the lightest-staining regions. The cross-hatched band on chromosome 1 designates a heterochromatic region.*

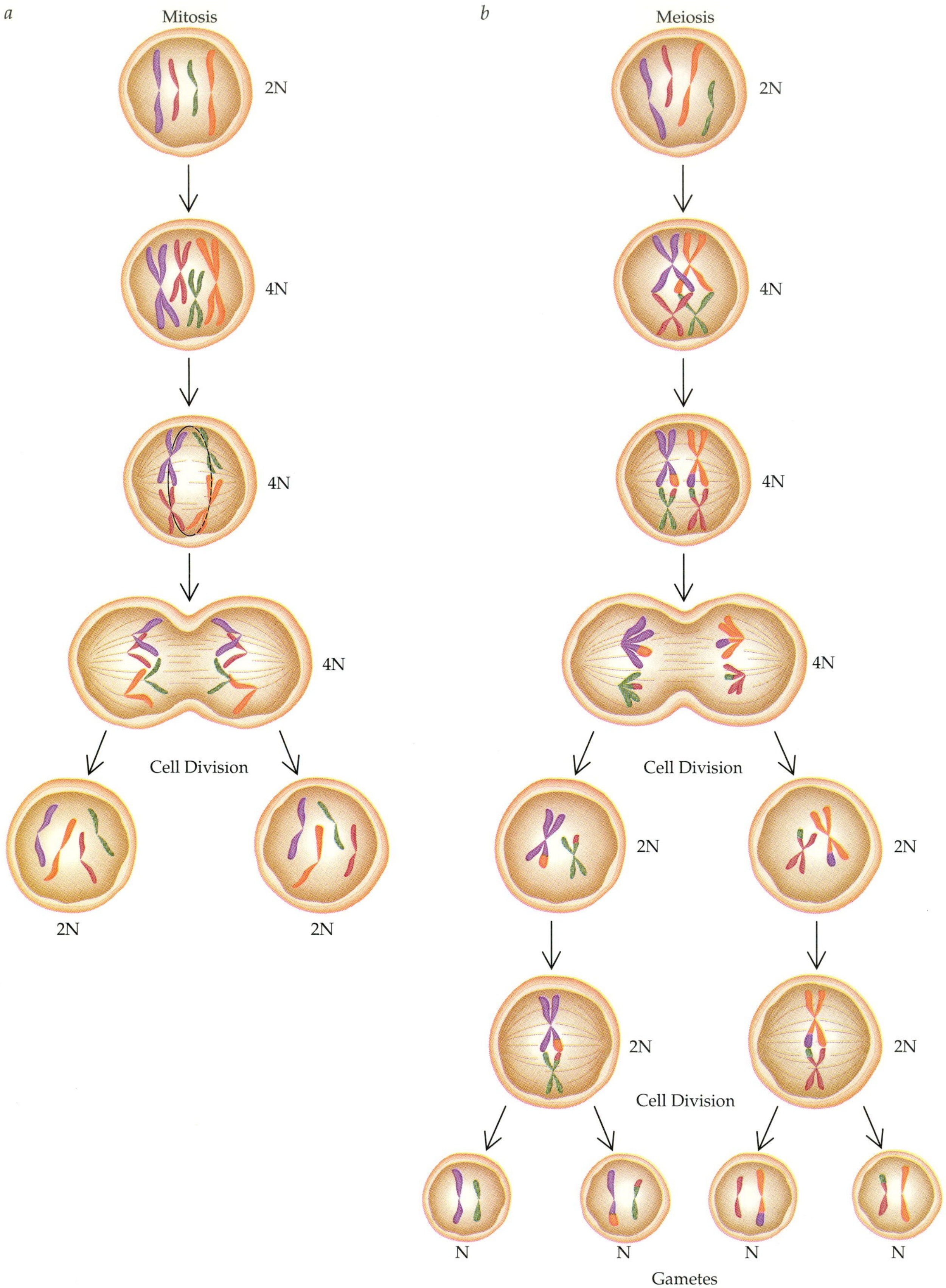

a
Mitosis
2N
4N
4N
4N
Cell Division
2N
2N
b
Meiosis
2N
4N
4N
4N
Cell Division
2N
2N
2N
2N
Cell Division
N
N
N
N
Gametes

Table 2 Examples of Karyotypes

Karyotype	Explanation
46,XY	Normal male
46,XX	Normal female
47,XX,+21	Female with trisomy 21 (Down syndrome)
46,XY,5p– or del(5p)	Male with deletion on short arm of one chromosome 5
46,XX,t(2;8)	Female with balanced translocation involving chromosomes 2 and 8
47,XY,+der(2)	Son of woman above; unbalanced with extra chromosome from t(2;8)
46,XY,t(9;22)(q34;q11)	Male with so-called Philadelphia chromosome, translocation characteristic of chronic myelogenous leukemia in bone marrow chromosome preparation

that stretches some 5,000 to 25,000 nucleotides. (Some long genes range up to about 300,000 nucleotides, and one exceptional gene—the gene responsible for Duchenne's muscular dystrophy—covers more than two and a half million nucleotides!) It is clear, then, that much of the DNA on a chromosome does not actually consist of genes but rather lies between the genes and is currently of unknown function. The spacing of genes is not constant along chromosomes; some chromosomes and some regions of each chromosome, generally those that are light-staining [*see Figure 1*], appear to have a higher density of genes than other regions. This point is highly relevant to understanding the medical significance of chromosomal abnormalities.

Very few genes exist as continuous coding sequences; most are interrupted by one or more noncoding regions called introns. Introns alternate with coding regions (exons) that ultimately encode the amino acid sequence of a protein [*see Chapter 2*]. In many genes, the cumulative length of the introns accounts for a far greater proportion of a gene's total length than the exons do. In total, it is estimated that less than five percent of the total DNA in the human genome corresponds to coding sequences. Nonetheless, cytogenetic studies show that very few regions of the genome can be altered or eliminated without major clinical consequences. The molecular basis for this observation and the potential functions of the noncoding DNA—whether the introns or the DNA between genes—remain unknown.

Many different alterations in the DNA sequence of a gene can lead to the absence of function or inadequate function that underlies genetic disease. Usually the spectrum of abnormalities detected in patients with a particular genetic disorder is highly informative with respect to learning the pathogenesis of the disorder or designing appropriate treatment; the

Figure 4 *(a) Mitosis, or somatic cell division, leads to two identical daughter cells that each have the same number of chromosomes at the parent cell (i.e., the diploid number). (b) Meiosis, or sex cell division, produces four gametes that each have half the number of chromosomes of the parent cell (i.e., the haploid number). In meiosis, the chromatids form junctions known as chiasmata, and segments of the chromatids cross over and exchange genetic material.*

molecular changes in gene structure can be the basis of specific diagnostic assays for use in clinical laboratories.

The proper expression of the estimated 50,000 to 100,000 genes encoded in the genome depends on complex relations among correct gene dosage (determined by the karyotype and controlled by mechanisms of chromosome replication and segregation), gene structure (determined by the DNA sequence), and gene action (controlled by mechanisms of gene and protein expression). The nature of inherited variation in the structure and function of chromosomes and genes—and the influence of this variation on the clinical expression of specific traits—is central to the field of medical genetics and to clinical medicine in general.

The Consequences of Genetic Variation and Mutation

One of the central concepts of genetics is that genetic disease is only the most obvious (and often most extreme) manifestation of genetic change, which is superimposed on a background of entirely normal genetic variability. Inherited disorders—as well as genetic influences on diseases that are not widely thought of as genetic—can be viewed conceptually as an extension of the normal, genetically based individuality that is obvious to even the most casual observer.

Many different proteins are synthesized in each cell, including enzymes, structural components, and signal-transducing agents responsible for all the developmental, metabolic, and communication requirements of a complex multicellular organism. Nucleotide changes (mutations) in the sequence of a gene may lead to formation of a variant (mutant) protein with altered properties stemming from its changed structure. It is now clear that a gene encoding a particular protein often exists in multiple, different forms in a population of clinically well individuals.[9] This normal protein variation—illustrated, for example, by well-known variants at the ABO blood-group locus or variants at the α_1-antitrypsin locus (some of which are associated with chronic obstructive lung disease, cirrhosis of the liver, and an increased risk of emphysema)—reflects even more widespread variation in the DNA sequence of the genome. The presence of multiple alleles at a gene locus in appreciable frequencies in a population is called genetic polymorphism.

The widespread occurrence of polymorphism implies that any individual is likely to carry in his or her genome different alleles at many gene loci, encoding different forms of, for example, a particular protein. This situation is called heterozygosity, and an individual (a heterozygote) carrying two distinguishable alleles at a locus is said to be heterozygous at that locus. In contrast, a homozygote carries two identical, indistinguishable alleles and is said to be homozygous at that locus. It can be estimated from population surveys for many different enzymes that individuals are likely to be heterozygous at as many as 15 to 20 percent of their loci. This estimate underscores the dramatic degree of biochemical individuality that exists within the human species.

What emerges from these findings is that genetic variation at a locus such as the ABO blood-group locus is simply the most visible and widely recognized example of genetic polymorphism. Variation in ABO blood groups was recognized nearly a century ago because of the availability of simple serological techniques. For many years it was not clear whether such examples represented special cases, but it now seems likely that it is genes that do *not* show obvious variation that are exceptional. Indeed, to the extent that every complex metabolic or developmental pathway can be thought of as the collective action of many different polymorphic gene products, each individual is truly unique in his or her genetically determined capacity to carry out certain cellular or organ functions. For each individual there is a particular genetically determined fulcrum for the seesaw representing the interplay of genes and their products with environmental influences [*see Figure 5*]; each individual has a particular genetically determined susceptibility to a variety of medical disorders.[10] Diseases widely recognized as genetic or inherited disorders are only the most extreme of all the clinical conditions that are influenced by genetic variation among individuals.

The Frequency and Origin of Mutation

A mutation can be defined as any permanent change in DNA involving a change in either the sequence or the arrangement of DNA in the genome. Mutations can occur in any cell, either in the germline or in somatic lineages; only germline mutations, however, can be perpetuated from one generation to the next. Gene mutations, such as substitutions of one base for another or insertions or deletions of one base or more, can originate as errors introduced during the normal process of DNA replication or as errors caused by exogenous mutagenic agents. Most changes introduced as errors during replication are corrected by DNA repair enzymes, so that the overall mutation rate for single-base changes is remarkably low, about one base change per genome per cell division. However, since there are so many cell divisions in the lifetime of an organism, this means that literally every base position in the genome has suffered thousands of mutations somewhere in the body; indeed, such somatic mutations are the most common cause of cancers when they introduce critical changes into genes controlling cell proliferation [*see Chapter 10*].

The frequency of mutations varies from gene to gene in the genome, from about 10^{-4} to 10^{-7} mutations per locus per generation (or per gamete). The average frequency appears to be about 10^{-6} mutations per locus per generation, suggesting that (given the estimated number of genes in the genome) at least one in 10 persons is likely to have received a newly mutated gene from one or the other parent. It is therefore not surprising that a significant proportion of cases of many types of genetic disease appears to be sporadic mutations never seen before in a family.

The frequency of mutations can be increased markedly by exposure to mutagens. Genes in epithelial cells exposed to ultraviolet rays of sunlight mutate at a higher rate; exposure to high doses is clearly correlated with an increased incidence of skin cancer. Exposure to other mutagenic agents is also correlated with the generation of new cancer-causing somatic mutations specific to a particular tissue and type of exposure.[11] Given the role that DNA replication and repair enzymes play in mutation surveillance and prevention, inherited defects that alter the function of such enzymes lead to dramatic increases in the frequency of mutations that predispose to various types of cancer. Individuals with ataxia telangiectasia, who are homozygous for a mutant DNA repair gene, show increased sensitivity to radiation and perhaps other potential mutagens and have a cancer risk more than 50 times that of the population in general.[12] It is a matter of current controversy (and of great medical significance) whether heterozygotes carrying one normal and one mutant allele for the DNA

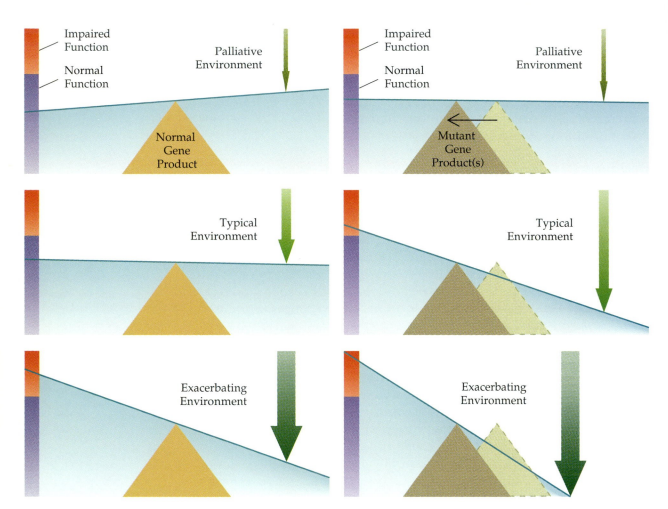

Figure 5 *Health can be viewed as a state of equilibrium between the organism, with an inborn functional capacity, and the environment, including dietary intake, exposure to microbes, and lifestyle. Disease can therefore be viewed as a state of disequilibrium. The "fulcrum" on which hinges interactions between biologic function and extrinsic environmental events is a normal or mutated gene product. Mutation in one or more genes can alter the position of the fulcrum, leading to disequilibrium. In some cases (left), a normal gene product will maintain equilibrium regardless of the environment (top, middle) or a particular environment will disturb the equilibrium, regardless of one's genotype (bottom). In other cases (right), an abnormal or variant gene product will maintain equilibrium under some environmental conditions (top), but will disturb the equilibrium under other conditions (middle, bottom). For example, an exacerbating environmental factor such as massive dietary intake of fat and cholesterol may eventually lead to coronary heart disease regardless of one's genotype (bottom); however, specific abnormal genotypes can lead to coronary heart disease even in individuals with a typical diet (middle), as in the case of a single-gene disorder affecting cholesterol metabolism, or may predispose to coronary heart disease only under certain excessive dietary conditions, as in the case of multifactorial disorders involving lipid metabolism. Similarly, the progression of emphysema in individuals with a mutant form of α_1-antitrypsin is greatly exacerbated by smoking, an example of the powerful effect of environmental factors on a particular genotype.*

repair gene are also genetically susceptible to such mutations. If they are, given the relatively high frequency of heterozygotes for this gene in the general population (about one or two percent), they could account for a significant proportion of all cases of certain cancers; their presymptomatic identification would represent a major medical advance.[13]

Chromosomal Disorders

Chromosomal disorders are quite common. Abnormalities of either chromosome number or structure are present in from 0.5 to one percent of live births, in about two percent of pregnancies in women older than 35 years of age, and in fully 50 percent of first-trimester spontaneous abortions. In all, at least 10 percent of all conceptions result in chromosomal abnormalities.[1] Such anomalies are responsible for a large number of well-recognized, identifiable syndromes and are associated with a wide spectrum of clinical problems, making cytogenetic analysis an important medical test, particularly in the newborn period. Chromosomal abnormalities are also associated with a number of other disorders of childhood or later life, such as developmental delay, short stature, ambiguous genitalia, absence of secondary sexual characteristics, mental retardation, fertility problems, multiple spontaneous abortions, or a variety of hematologic malignancies and solid tumors. Any of these findings, with or without a family history, would suggest a need for cytogenetic analysis.

Abnormalities of chromosomes may be either numerical or structural or both and may involve one or more autosomes, sex chromosomes, or both. The most common type of abnormality is aneuploidy, a gain or loss of one or more chromosomes, which occurs in at least three to four percent of recognized pregnancies. Most aneuploid patients have either one copy or three copies, rather than the normal two copies, of each chromosome. Such conditions are called monosomy or trisomy, respectively. The most common trisomy in live-born infants is trisomy 21 (Down syndrome), seen in about one in 800 live births in the general population and associated with mental retardation, characteristic dysmorphic facies, hypotonia, and other physical findings.[14] The most common group of aneuploidies involves the sex chromosomes: Klinefelter syndrome (47,XXY males), Turner syndrome (45,X females), 47,XXX females, and 47,XYY males. In total, numerical abnormalities of the sex chromosomes are found in about one in 500 live births. Generally, they are associated with less severe clinical symptoms than autosomal defects, for two reasons: the specialized and restricted genetic function of the Y chromosome in determining sex and the phenomenon of X chromosome inactivation (see below), which minimizes the functional imbalance of an extra or missing X chromosome. Patients with sex-chromosome abnormalities often go undetected until puberty, when absent or atypical sexual characteristics, infertility, or both bring them to clinical attention. Of the sex-chromosome abnormalities, only Turner syndrome is associated with significant physical findings that may be apparent at birth or before puberty, including short stature, gonadal dysgenesis, and neck webbing.

The most common mechanism of aneuploidy is nondisjunction, the failure of a pair of homologues to segregate in the normal way during one of the meiotic cell divisions [*see Figure 4b*]. Epidemiologic studies have indicated that the vast majority of trisomies, including trisomy 21, result from nondisjunction in meiosis I of oogenesis. The extra chromosome 21 in trisomy 21 is of maternal origin in 95 percent of cases. The frequency of nondisjunction of many chromosomes, but most notably chromosome 21, increases with maternal age[15]; the risk of Down syndrome increases from about one in 900 at age 30 to one in 350 at age 35 and one in 100 at age 40.[1] Accordingly, advanced maternal age is one of the leading indications for prenatal diagnosis [*see Chapter 8*].

A second class of chromosomal disorders includes structural rearrangements, such as translocations between two different chromosomes, or large deletions or duplications leading to monosomy or trisomy for a portion of a chromosome. Rearrangements are said to be balanced if the chromosome set contains the normal dose of genetic material and unbalanced if there is additional or missing genetic information. Balanced rearrangements are usually not associated with clinical findings, since all of the genetic information is present, even if rearranged. Carriers of balanced rearrangements such as translocations do produce a high frequency of unbalanced gametes, however, and so they are at increased risk of having abnormal offspring with unbalanced karyotypes. Indeed, balanced rearrangements often first come to clinical attention because of the birth of a child with an unbalanced rearrangement. In such cases it is important to evaluate the chromosomes of the clinically normal parents, because they may be balanced carriers who have a high risk of conceiving a child with an unbalanced rearrangement in subsequent pregnancies. In turn, if one of the parents is found to have a balanced rearrangement, that individual's primary relatives should also be karyotyped.

It is interesting to consider the pathogenesis of chromosomal disorders. In such conditions, with few exceptions, the individual genes on the relevant chromosome are normal; in most instances, clinical abnormalities are associated with abnormal gene dosage, not with abnormal gene structure or expression. The characteristic clinical signs of Down syndrome are caused by a triple dose of the estimated 1,000 to 2,000 genes encoded on chromosome 21, rather than by the lack of function or the abnormal function of a specific gene, as in the case of single-gene disorders. This finding emphasizes the importance for normal function of interactions among different gene products, each produced in correct amounts. Metabolic and developmental pathways may rely critically on the proper stoichiometry of particular pathway components that are involved in feedback regulation or rate-limiting steps. Genetic imbalance introduced by an extra or missing dose of a region of a chromosome or of an entire chromosome may disturb the genetic homeostasis normally reinforced and perpetuated by balanced karyotypes.[16]

Single-Gene Disorders

Single-gene traits are often called mendelian because, like the traits originally studied by Mendel, they segregate clearly within families and occur in predictable proportions among the offspring of certain types of matings. The genotype of an individual is his or her genetic makeup, either generally or specifically at one locus. Single-gene disorders are those in which inherited variation of the type described above results in a specific mutated allele at a single genetic locus on one or both members of a chromosome pair. The phenotype is the observable expression of a genotype as a morphological, biochemical, or molecular trait; in the context of medical genetics, genetic disorders are those in which the mutant phenotype is clearly definable in medical terms and results in one or more clinical symptoms.

Single-gene disorders are characterized by their patterns of transmission in families, usually summarized in the form of a pedigree. Patterns of inheritance for simple mendelian traits usually reflect the chromosomal location of the gene in question (autosomal or X-linked) and whether the mutant phenotype is dominant (expressed clinically in heterozygotes, who carry a mutated allele on only one chromosome of a pair) or recessive (expressed clinically only in homozygotes, who carry a mutated allele at both copies of a gene).

Although the distinction between dominant and recessive is quite useful for pedigree analysis and for providing genetic counseling, it is not absolute. Rather it is an arbitrary designation, based on clinical phenotypes, that does not necessarily hold significance at the level of gene action. For autosomal genes, both copies are typically expressed, and the phenotype is the consequence of their combined expression. In dominant disorders, even though a clinical phenotype is apparent in heterozygotes, homozygotes for a mutant allele will usually have much more severe symptoms. In recessive disorders, even though the phenotype is defined as being undetectable in heterozygotes, heterozygotes frequently show manifestations when examined at the cellular, biochemical, or molecular level. Overall, then, the distinction between dominant and recessive is a largely arbitrary one based on an accepted threshold of clinical symptoms. If all or most individuals recognized as affected are homozygotes, then clinical geneticists tend to refer to the disorder as recessive. If many affected individuals are heterozygotes, then the disorder is called dominant.

Both the genetic usefulness of the distinction and the overlap in terms of gene expression are illustrated in the case of sickle cell disease, the well-known disorder of hemoglobin. The disorder is inherited as an autosomal recessive trait. Affected individuals are homozygous for a mutated allele at the beta globin locus on chromosome 11 and produce an abnormal hemoglobin (Hb S) instead of the normal adult hemoglobin (Hb A) in their red cells. Heterozygotes express both Hb A and Hb S in their red cells. They also have a mild anemia and thus show both a biochemical and a hematologic phenotype. Although severe sickle cell disease is considered a recessive trait genetically, it can be thought of as dominant biochemically; molecularly, it behaves more as codominant, because the two alleles are coexpressed in the heterozygous state.

At least 3,000 different single-gene disorders have been recognized by geneticists.[17] As mentioned above, although most of these are individually rare, their collective incidence is about one per 100 live births [*see Table 1*] and their overall impact on health and medicine is significant. Most single-gene disorders are apparent by the time of puberty, and a significant proportion present in childhood, although there are others that characteristically do not give rise to clinical symptoms until well into adulthood. Many abnormal phenotypes involve multiple anatomic systems, but one or more disorders can affect virtually all organ systems. The nervous system, musculoskeletal system, eye, and skin are frequently involved.[17,18] Practitioners in every medical specialty may encounter patients with genetic disease, often before the disease is actually diagnosed as being genetic. Watchful primary care physicians and specialists are therefore critically important in the recognition of genetic disease. Physicians should routinely ask themselves whether the symptoms they encounter in a patient have—or could have—a genetic explanation.

Autosomal Dominant Disorders

Dominant disorders are those that lead to clinical symptoms in heterozygotes, who have a normal allele at the gene in question on one copy of an autosome and a mutated allele at that same gene on the other copy of the autosome. Among single-gene disorders, about half are autosomal dominant diseases.[17] A number of such disorders are relatively common, with an incidence ranging from one in 500 to about one in several thousand. The burden of autosomal dominant disorders is increased further because of their mode of inheritance: because only a single copy of a mutated allele is required for clinical expression of the disease phenotype, they can be transmitted through families for many generations.

In a typical autosomal dominant disorder, each affected individual in a pedigree has an affected parent and grandparent, as far back as the family history can be traced [*see Figure 6a*]. Because the gene responsible for the disease is on an autosome, both males and females are affected in equal numbers; the disease can be transmitted from a male parent to either male or female offspring and from a female parent to either male or female offspring. Most mutated alleles causing genetic disease are relatively rare in comparison with normal alleles, so that in most (but not all) cases, the affected parent is heterozygous for the mutated allele, whereas the other parent is homozygous for a normal allele. Because both alleles have an equal probability of being passed on to the next generation, there is a 50 percent risk that an offspring of an individual with an autosomal dominant disorder will inherit the same disorder. Statistically, then, one expects an equal number of affected and unaffected offspring and an equal number of affected males and females in a family. It is important to emphasize, however, that in today's typical small families deviations from this general statistical expectation are frequently observed; they do not necessarily indicate an unusual pattern of transmission, particularly if the phenotype is a well-known, previously characterized autosomal dominant condition.

Occasionally, either because the frequency of a particular mutated allele is high enough that two affected heterozygotes will marry by chance (for example, in familial hypercholesterolemia, an autosomal dominant condition with a frequency of one in 500) or because affected heterozygotes for a particular condition have a tendency to marry each other (for example, in achondroplasia, an autosomal dominant condition marked by short-limb dwarfism), one observes affected individuals who are homozygous for a mutant allele. In such families, homozygous affected offspring are typically more severely affected than are their two heterozygous parents. For example, in familial hypercholesterolemia, heterozygotes develop coronary artery disease in early middle age and represent about five percent of all heart attack victims younger than 50 years of age. Affected homozygotes, on the other hand, develop symptoms much earlier and usually succumb to coronary artery disease in childhood.

Although many pedigrees will show affected offspring to have one affected parent, one not infrequently encounters a family in which an affected individual has two clinically normal parents. Such pedigrees illustrate one of two important special cases noted in autosomal dominant conditions: (1) the occurrence of new mutations in the germline of an unaffected parent [*see Figure 6b*] and (2) reduced penetrance, that is, the absence of clinical manifestations of the disorder in an individual who must, according to the pedigree, carry the mutated allele [*see Figure 6c*].

New mutations, of course, have to occur at some time. Indeed, given the typical frequency of new mutations (about 10^{-5} to 10^{-6} mutations per gene per generation), one would predict that autosomal dominant disorders (requiring only a single mutated allele) would appear as a new, sporadic mutation at a given gene every 50,000 to 500,000 live births. In such a case, the parents, who are clinically normal, usually are not at

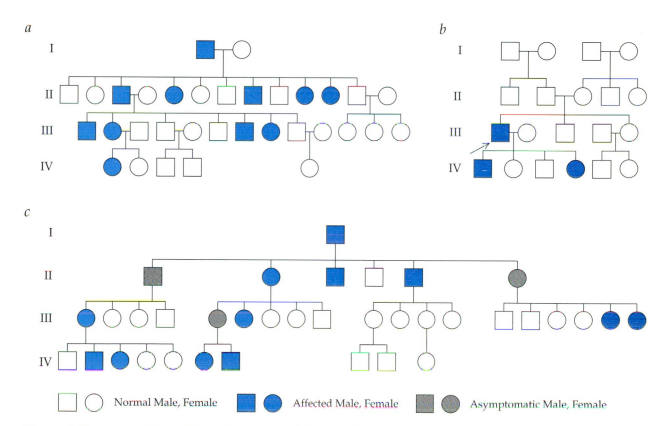

Figure 6 *Shown are pedigrees illustrating autosomal dominant inheritance. (a) A typical multigeneration pedigree is displayed. (b) Pedigree of a family with neurofibromatosis shows an apparent new mutation in one of the unaffected parents of the proband (arrow). (c) Pedigree shows reduced penetrance of a defect. Individuals marked in gray must carry the gene, in that they pass it on to one or more offspring, but they are themselves unaffected. Other unaffected individuals in the pedigree may also be carriers who do not express the defect, thus complicating risk assessment and genetic counselling.*

increased risk of having another affected child (except in exceptional cases in which the new mutation was in the primordial germline cells and will result in numerous gametes carrying the new mutated allele). The affected individual, however, carries the mutation in all of his or her cells and has a 50 percent risk of passing the disorder on to offspring [*see Figure 6b*].

The proportion of new mutations among all detected cases of an autosomal dominant disorder is characteristic of the particular condition. For example, most cases (80 percent) of achondroplasia are the result of a new mutation occurring in the germline of a clinically normal parent (usually the father because of the extremely large number of germline divisions during spermatogenesis). Pedigrees of familial achondroplasia in multiple generations are relatively uncommon. This finding does not reflect anything unusual about the achondroplasia gene. Rather it reflects the fact that affected individuals have fewer offspring (only about 20 percent of the number born to unaffected individuals), so that in any generation relatively few cases will be inherited from an affected parent and relatively more of the cases seen will be the result of the usual process of new mutations occurring in previously normal copies of the gene. Similarly, about 50 percent of cases of neurofibromatosis, a relatively common nervous system disorder, occur initially as sporadic cases. In contrast, other autosomal dominant conditions appear virtually always to be inherited from an affected parent.

Some autosomal dominant disorders are not expressed at all in some individuals known to carry the mutated allele. The gene is then said to demonstrate reduced penetrance [*see Figure 6c*], which can confound pedigree analysis and risk assessment in an individual or a family. In some cases, reduced penetrance may indicate that clinicians have identified (and therefore now are looking for) something that is not the primary defect, which may be present in all cases, but rather a secondary characteristic or disorder that is sometimes present and sometimes not. In other cases, the genetic defect in question may not be apparent, perhaps because the cells have exceeded a critical amount of the particular gene product during development of the relevant tissue or organ. In any case, it is important to stress that individuals carrying the mutated gene, whether they manifest a defect or not, are still at a 50 percent risk of transmitting the gene to their offspring.

Many autosomal dominant conditions are characterized by a high degree of phenotypic variability among affected individuals, even in the same family. Such a disorder is said to exhibit variable expressivity. In neurofibromatosis, for example, some affected family members may show severe symptoms, including multiple disfiguring neurofibromas, whereas other affected family members show only mild expression—perhaps only a few café-au-lait spots—even though they carry the identical mutated allele [*see Chapter 9*]. The basis for variable expressivity is not understood in most cases; it may reflect interactions with other genes, environmental factors, or stochastic effects.

A final concept important in autosomal dominant conditions is age of onset. Many disorders are apparent at birth, but patients with other conditions characteristically do not develop symptoms until later in life. For example, in Huntington disease, a disorder characterized by choreic

a

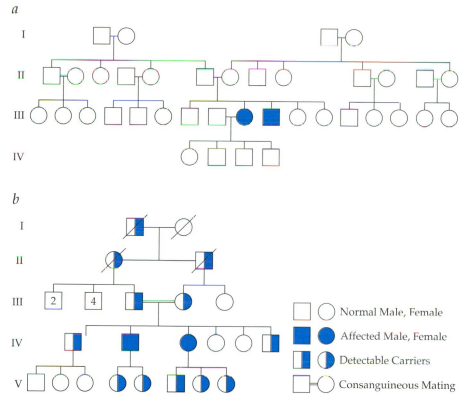

b

□ ○	Normal Male, Female
■ ●	Affected Male, Female
◧ ◑	Detectable Carriers
□─○	Consanguineous Mating

Figure 7   *Shown are pedigrees illustrating autosomal recessive inheritance. (a) In a typical pedigree, the only affected individuals are in the same sibship. Unaffected individuals may be homozygous for a normal allele or may be heterozygous, with one normal and one mutant allele. (b) Pedigree of family with a rare autosomal recessive condition demonstrates effect of consanguinity (in this case, the union of two first cousins).*

movements and progressive dementia, clinical symptoms are rare before the age of 25 and only about half of individuals who carry the mutant gene show symptoms by the age of 40. Without definitive molecular testing for the genetic defect responsible for Huntington disease, genetic counseling can be extremely difficult, since one cannot be sure whether an individual below the typical age of onset carries the gene. This is particularly tragic in Huntington disease: many individuals have already had a full family (with each offspring at a 50 percent risk of carrying the mutant gene) by the time they realize that they themselves are heterozygotes.

Autosomal Recessive Disorders

Autosomal recessive phenotypes are expressed only in individuals who are homozygous for a mutated allele, having inherited a mutated allele from each parent. In a pedigree typical of classical autosomal recessive inheritance [*see Figure 7a*], in contrast to an autosomal dominant pedigree, multiple affected individuals are usually found within the same sibship, rather than being found in multiple generations. Because the responsible genes are autosomal, both males and females are affected in equal proportions. Very typically, especially in small families, only a single child may be affected; however, if the disorder is a well-characterized and previously recognized autosomal recessive condition,[17] the diagnosis can be made with certainty even if the pedigree itself seems insufficient to establish the presence of an inherited disorder.

Unaffected parents of an affected child are heterozygotes and therefore carriers. Each has a 50 percent risk of transmitting the mutated allele to offspring, so that the chance of a homozygous offspring is one in four. In contrast to autosomal dominant inheritance, in which all copies of the mutated allele are found in affected individuals, most copies of mutated genes for autosomal recessive disorders are found in asymptomatic carriers in the general population, most of whom are unaware that they are carriers. For example, even for one of the most common autosomal recessive conditions, cystic fibrosis, 98 percent of mutated genes are found in heterozygotes. The likelihood that a heterozygote will have a child affected with the recessive disease in question is one quarter of the risk that he or she will marry, simply by chance, another heterozygote from the general population. This possibility can be calculated from the observed frequency of the disorder.[1] For example, one can estimate that about one in 25 Caucasians is heterozygous for cystic fibrosis and about one in 10 blacks is heterozygous for sickle cell disease.

For rare autosomal recessive conditions, the possibility of two heterozygotes marrying by chance is extremely unlikely. This chance is dramatically increased, however, if two individuals are related and have a common ancestor [see Figure 7b]. When one is taking a family history, it is therefore important to ask about possible consanguinity and family background. The less common a disorder is, the more likely it is that an affected individual may have come from a consanguineous mating. For common traits, however, that have a correspondingly high carrier frequency in certain populations, consanguinity is usually not evident.

Mutated alleles for autosomal recessive traits can be passed down for generations without ever appearing in homozygous form and without, therefore, ever coming to medical attention. Consequently, it is not surprising that new mutations leading to recessive disease are seen rarely, if ever—in dramatic contrast to what is observed with autosomal dominant disorders. This is not to say that such genes do not suffer mutations; they do, at approximately the same frequency as dominant disease genes. It is far more likely, however, that a new mutation will appear in heterozygous form (and thus escape detection) than that it will appear in an individual who also inherits a second mutated allele from a carrier parent. A new mutation leading to an autosomal recessive disorder is essentially not observed, and so the parents of any affected child can be assumed to be carriers, with a 25 percent risk of having additional affected offspring.

X-Linked Disorders

Genes on the X chromosome have a distinctive pattern of transmission. In contrast to autosomal genes, a male transmits his only X chromosome to all his daughters and none of his sons. A female, on the other hand, transmits one of her two X chromosomes to each offspring, regardless of sex; her male offspring are at a 50 percent risk of inheriting a mutated allele carried on one of her X chromosomes. X-linked recessive mutations are generally expressed phenotypically in all males who receive the affected X chromosome, since they have only a single X; such individuals are said to be hemizygous with respect to X-linked genes [see Figure 8a]. Females in such pedigrees who carry a mutated allele will be heterozygous. Except in unusual circumstances, they do not show clinical signs of X-linked recessive disease.

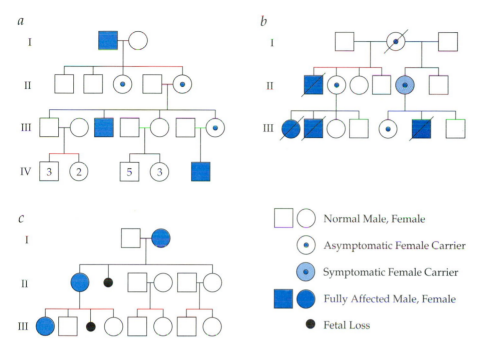

Figure 8 *Shown are pedigrees illustrating X-linked inheritance. (a) X-linked recessive inheritance for a disorder such as hemophilia A involves transmission from an affected male through his carrier daughters to an affected grandson and great-grandson. All affected individuals are male. (b) Illustrated is X-linked dominant inheritance for ornithine transcarbamylase deficiency. Some heterozygous females are asymptomatic, some show symptoms of protein intolerance only as adults, and some are as disabled as affected males, illustrating the variability of expression in females heterozygous for X-linked traits, as a result of X inactivation. (c) Pedigree demonstrates an X-linked dominant disorder that is lethal in males during the prenatal period.*

X-linked dominant disorders can exhibit more variable pedigrees. In some cases both males and females are affected, although hemizygous males are generally more severely affected than their heterozygous female relatives, because such males do not have any normal allele. One relatively common genetic disorder is X-linked ornithine transcarbamylase (OTC) deficiency. Complete OTC deficiency in the liver leads to neonatal hyperammonemia and death in affected males, whereas heterozygous females display variable features of protein intolerance, sometimes in childhood and sometimes not until adult life [*see Figure 8b*]. Other X-linked dominant traits appear to be lethal in males before birth and so are expressed exclusively in females [*see Figure 8c*]. In practice, it can be difficult to distinguish X-linked dominant inheritance from autosomal dominant inheritance in such cases, particularly in small families. However, in larger families, the absence of affected males, a deficit of male births overall, or a high incidence of fetal loss during pregnancy can be informative clues.

Expression of X-linked traits in heterozygous females is determined by the phenomenon of X chromosome inactivation.[1,19] Early in embryonic development, one of the two X chromosomes in female somatic cells is inactivated, thus achieving functional dosage equivalence with males who have only a single X. X inactivation is initially random: in any cell of the embryo at the time of X inactivation, each X has a 50/50 chance of being inactivated. Once inactivation occurs, however, the process is irreversible, so that during growth and differentiation discrete clones develop in which all cells contain the same active and inactive X chromosomes. After the time of X inactivation, then, females are mosaics, with some of their cells expressing the alleles on one X and others expressing the alleles on the other X. Although a few X-linked genes escape inactivation and continue to be expressed from both homologous chromosomes (like autosomal genes), it is generally believed that most X-linked genes do undergo inactivation on one member of the X chromosome pair.

Some of the cells in a female heterozygous for an X-linked mutation will express the normal allele (that X being active in those cells), whereas other cells will express the mutated allele (the X with the normal allele being inactive in those cells). The relative proportion of cells of the two types may vary either by chance or by preferential growth or survival of one type. Depending on the proportion of the two types of cell in each tissue, a heterozygous female may be asymptomatic or may show mild or severe clinical signs of the disease. In OTC deficiency, some carrier females are asymptomatic, some show only protein intolerance, and others develop severe neonatal hyperammonemia comparable to that seen in affected males. The variability introduced by X inactivation can complicate clinical or biochemical detection of heterozygotes, because as a consequence of random X inactivation, carriers characteristically show a much wider range of manifestations or biochemical activities than heterozygotes for autosomal traits.

As with autosomal dominant disorders, new mutation can play an important role in X-linked pedigrees, notably in disorders in which affected males show reduced (or absent) reproductive capacity. For example, in Duchenne muscular dystrophy, in which affected males do not reproduce, as many as one third of mutant alleles are a result of new mutations.[1] Assessment of the carrier status of females in such families is critical, because carrier women have a 50 percent chance of having an affected son, whereas mothers of a child affected by a new mutation are not at appreciable risk of having additional affected offspring. As in many such instances, molecular diagnostic approaches offer the best chance of making a definitive determination [*see Chapters 8 and 9*].

This section has focused on X-linked disorders and ignored any contribution to genetic disease by the Y chromosome. This is because (aside from its role in determining sex) the Y chromosome has very few identified genes, none of which has yet been implicated in any genetic disease. Such an inherited disorder would be expected to show strict male-to-male transmission, in contrast to autosomal or X-linked modes of inheritance.

Mitochondrial Disorders

Some exceptional pedigrees in human genetics cannot be explained by the principles of mendelian inheritance described in the above sections. A few genetic disorders have been found instead to exhibit mitochondrial inheritance, reflecting defects in genes encoded within the small circular chromosome of mitochondria in the cytoplasm of cells. Human cells have hundreds of copies of the mitochondrial chromosome, which encodes only 13 known structural genes. Mutations in mitochondrial genes have been demonstrated in several neuromuscular disorders as well as in one form of late-onset diabetes mellitus. The unusual feature of pedigrees of inherited mitochondrial disorders is their strict maternal inheritance. The offspring of affected males are never affected, whereas all offspring of affected females are affected, although they frequently exhibit considerable clinical variability.[20]

Genomic Imprinting

On the basis of mendelian principles, one expects autosomal genes to be equally likely to be transmitted from a parent of either sex to a child of either sex. It has recently become clear, however, that the level of expression of those genes can depend on their parent of origin. In several well-documented cases, the severity of a clinical phenotype has been shown to depend on whether a mutated allele was inherited from the mother or from the father, a situation called genomic imprinting.[21] The effect must reflect the alteration (or imprint) of gene sequences during the formation of either a sperm or an egg in such a way that the gene remembers its parental origin and its expression is permanently modified. Methylation of DNA is probably one of the biochemical mechanisms of embryonic modification of either paternal or maternal genes.[22] A number of imprinted conditions have now been described [see Chapter 9]. Many of these disorders bridge the gap between single-gene disorders and chromosomal disorders: the underlying mutation that revealed the imprinted nature of these conditions was, in some instances, a cytogenetically visible deletion of multiple genes within an imprinted region.

Multifactorial Disorders

Among genetic phenotypes, both chromosomal and single-gene disorders are vastly outnumbered by birth defects or chronic common diseases of adult life that appear to run in families but do not show any particular pedigree pattern.[23] These disorders are said to show multifactorial inheritance, indicating that they are caused by multiple factors, both genetic and nongenetic, that can vary in individual cases. In multifactorial disorders, multiple genes at independent loci can have additive effects. An individual inheriting a particular combination of alleles at these loci may be genetically susceptible to developing a clinical condition, perhaps in response to additional environmental triggers (such as an inappropriate diet in the case of coronary heart disease or chemical mutagens in the case of colon cancer). Multifactorial inheritance should be distinguished from genetic heterogeneity, which is often seen in single-gene disorders. This term refers to the observation that different individual genes can produce a particular condition in different families.

In multifactorial disorders, an assessment of the risk that the disorder will recur in another family member must be based on empirical risk figures obtained from previous families with the disorder, rather than on theoretical consideration of principles of inheritance. The empirical risk usually increases when there is more than one affected family member (in contrast to recurrence risks in single-gene disorders), because it then becomes more likely that the particular set of genes present in that family more strongly predisposes its members to the specific disorder. In the extreme case of a major susceptibility gene with a particularly deleterious (i.e., predisposing) allele, the empirical risk can approach 50 percent—similar to that of a simple autosomal dominant trait. Such families are generally characterized by an earlier age of onset of disease than more typical nonmendelian families that show multifactorial inheritance. These rare early-onset families are, however, tremendously significant: they provide an opportunity to apply genetic linkage analysis to attempt to map and identify the major susceptibility gene or genes involved. This has been done successfully for early-onset breast cancer and a form of early-onset non–insulin-dependent diabetes mellitus.[24,25] The presumption in such disorders is that the genes involved in the rare mendelian families will turn out to be the same ones that predispose some members of the general population to the condition.

Another approach to defining the genetic component of multifactorial disorders involves studies of monozygotic and dizygotic twins who are concordant or discordant for the trait in question. A trait determined entirely by a single gene would be expected to show complete concordance in monozygotic twins who are identical and have, therefore, 100 percent of their genetic material in common. Dizygotic twins (and other siblings), on the other hand, have, on average, only 50 percent of their genes in common, and so would be expected to show reduced concordance. A trait determined solely by nongenetic factors, however, would show equivalent concordance (significantly less than 100 percent) in monozygotic and dizygotic twins because their different genetic relationships would be irrelevant.

Although in practice it is sometimes difficult to control for environmental effects in such studies, the results are so compelling for some multifactorial disorders that the involvement of a major genetic component is undeniable.[23] For example, in the case of the congenital malformation cleft lip and palate, which has an incidence of about one in 1,000 births, monozygotic twins show a concordance rate of about 40 percent, 10 times that of dizygotic twins (and several hundred times that of two unrelated individuals). Similarly, for insulin-dependent diabetes mellitus, monozygotic twins show 50 percent concordance, five times that of dizygotic twins. In both cases, the data clearly support the existence of one or more major susceptibility genes.

One of the challenges in human genetics and medicine is to identify the genetic factors involved in multifactorial disorders. Major malformations such as neural-tube defects and cleft lip and palate constitute a significant proportion of birth defects; disorders such as hypertension, coronary artery disease, diabetes, and cancer account for most morbidity and mortality in adult life. Application of many of the lessons in genetic analysis learned from single-gene disorders should lead to the refinement of genetic models and permit more accurate assessment of risk, both in the general population and in obviously susceptible families. Given the frequency of many of these conditions (relative to chromosomal and single-gene disorders), human genetics can expect to have its strongest impact on the practice of medicine through improved diagnosis and management of the multifactorial disorders.

Genetics and the Prevention of Disease

Human genetics and the study of genetic disorders have never been more relevant or significant for the practice of medicine than they are today. Developments in molecular biology are rapidly introducing new tools for diagnosing, understanding, and ultimately treating genetic disease. Inherited diseases, many easily detected before birth or before clinical signs are evident, exact a terrible price, both in social and economic terms, that can be avoided, or at least minimized, by advance diagnosis and genetic counseling. Yet conditions that are much rarer and require much more costly intervention often attract more attention from practicing physicians and lay people alike. The clear role of genetics in predisposing significant numbers of individuals to common congenital malformations and chronic adult disorders represents medicine's best opportunity for identifying a subset of the population susceptible to major health problems. Routine consideration of the principles of genetics in evaluating patients and their families can lead to the diagnosis or even the prevention of such diseases through family planning, early intervention, or adoption of appropriate behaviors. In genetics, an ounce of prevention is truly worth a pound of cure.

References

1. Thompson MW, McInnes RR, Willard HF: *Genetics in Medicine*, 5th ed. WB Saunders Co, Philadelphia, 1991

2. Gelehrter TD, Collins FS: *Principles of Medical Genetics*. Williams & Wilkins, Baltimore, 1990

3. *The Metabolic Basis of Inherited Disease*, 7th ed. Scriver CR, Beaudet AL, Sly WS, et al, Eds. McGraw-Hill, New York, 1994

4. Baird PA, Anderson TW, Newcombe HB, et al: Genetic disorders in children and young adults: a population study. *Am J Hum Genet* 42:677, 1988

5. Scriver CR, Neal JL, Saginur R, et al: The frequency of genetic disease and congenital malformation among patients in a pediatric hospital. *Can Med Assoc J* 108:1111, 1973

6. Gardner RJM, Sutherland CR: *Chromosome Abnormalities and Genetic Counseling*. Oxford University Press, New York, 1989

7. White R, Lalouel JM: Chromosome mapping with DNA markers. *Sci Am* 258:40, 1988

8. White R, Lalouel JM: Genetic markers in medicine: DNA sequence variants in the human population reveal genetic basis for metabolic variation. *The Metabolic Basis of Inherited Disease*, 6th ed. Scriver CR, Beaudet AL, Sly WS, et al, Eds. McGraw-Hill, New York, 1989, p 277

9. Harris H: *The Principles of Human Biochemical Genetics*, 3rd ed. Elsevier/North-Holland Press, Amsterdam, 1980

10. Scriver CR, Laberge C, Clow CL, et al: Genetics and medicine: an evolving relationship. *Science* 200:946, 1978

11. Hollstein M, Sidransky D, Vogelstein B, et al: p53 mutations in human cancers. *Science* 253:49, 1991

12. Morell D, Cromartie E, Swift M: Mortality and cancer incidence in 263 patients with ataxia telangiectasia. *J Natl Cancer Inst* 77:89, 1986

13. Swift M, Morell D, Massey RB, et al: Incidence of cancer in 161 families affected by ataxia telangiectasia. *N Engl J Med* 325:1831, 1991

14. Patterson D: The causes of Down syndrome. *Sci Am* 257:52, 1987

15. Hassold T: Chromosome abnormalities in human reproductive wastage. *Trends Genet* 2:105, 1986

16. Epstein CJ: *The Consequences of Chromosome Imbalance: Principles, Mechanisms, and Models*. Cambridge University Press, New York, 1986

17. McKusick VA: *Mendelian Inheritance in Man: Catalogues of Autosomal Dominant, Autosomal Recessive, and X-linked Phenotypes*, 10th ed. Johns Hopkins University Press, Baltimore, 1992

18. Costa T, Scriver CR, Childs B: The effect of Mendelian disease on human health: a measurement. *Am J Med Genet* 21:231, 1985

19. Lyon MF: Sex chromatin and gene action in the mammalian X chromosome. *Am J Hum Genet* 14:135, 1962

20. Wallace DC: Mitochondrial genetics: a paradigm for aging and degenerative diseases? *Science* 256:628, 1992

21. Hall JG: Genomic imprinting: review and relevance to human diseases. *Am J Hum Genet* 46:857, 1990

22. Li E, Beard C, Jaenisch R: Role for DNA methylation in genomic imprinting. *Nature* 366:362, 1993

23. King RA, Rotter JI, Motulsky AG: *The Genetic Basis of Common Disease*. Oxford University Press, New York, 1990

24. Hall JM, Lee MK, Newman B, et al: Linkage of early-onset familial breast cancer to chromosome 17q21. *Science* 250:1684, 1990

25. Froguel P, Vaxillaire M, Sun F, et al: Close linkage of glucokinase locus on chromosome 7p to early-onset non-insulin-dependent diabetes mellitus. *Nature* 356:162, 1992

Acknowledgments

Figure 1 Adapted from *Recombinant DNA*, 2nd ed., by J. D. Watson, J. Witkowski, M. Gilman, et al. Scientific American Books, New York, 1992. © 1992 James D. Watson, Michael Gilman, Jan Witkowski, Mark Zoller. Used by permission.

Figure 2 Reprinted from "Medical Genetics," by R. W. Erbe, in SCIENTIFIC AMERICAN *Medicine*, edited by E. Rubenstein and D. D. Federman, Section 9, Subsection IV. Scientific American, Inc., New York, 1994. All rights reserved. Provided by Mark Kielsma, M.D., Children's Hospital, Buffalo, New York.

Figure 3 Adapted by Talar Agasyan. Reprinted from "Medical Genetics," by R. W. Erbe, in SCIENTIFIC AMERICAN *Medicine*, edited by E. Rubenstein and D. D. Federman, Section 9, Subsection IV. Scientific American, Inc., New York, 1994. All rights reserved.

Figure 4 Dimitry Schidlovsky. Reprinted from "Medical Genetics," by R. W. Erbe, in SCIENTIFIC AMERICAN *Medicine*, edited by E. Rubenstein and D. D. Federman, Section 9, Subsection IV. Scientific American, Inc., New York, 1994. All rights reserved. Adapted from *Recombinant DNA*, 2nd ed, by J. D. Watson, M. Gilman, J. Witkowski, et al. Scientific American Books, New York, 1992. © 1992 James D. Watson, Michael Gilman, Jan Witkowski, Mark Zoller. Used by permission.

Figure 5 Dimitry Schidlovsky.

Figures 6, 7, 8 Talar Agasyan.

Table 1 From *Genetics in Medicine*, 5th ed, by M. W. Thompson, R. R. McInnes, and H. F. Willard. W. B. Saunders Co., Philadelphia, 1991.

CHAPTER 2

Structure, Replication, and Transcription of DNA

David A. Clayton, Ph.D.

T he three central classes of molecules responsible for the integrity and storage of genetic information and its eventual interpretation, or expression, are deoxyribonucleic acid (DNA), ribonucleic acid (RNA), and protein. It has been known for more than a century that DNA exists as a chemically unique macromolecule, and some 50 years ago DNA was identified as the molecule in which organisms store and maintain their genetic information. But DNA alone would not sustain a living cell or the cell's functions; its information must be interpreted to produce other molecules that are needed to maintain life or to generate still other molecules that function in cellular assembly lines to produce the vast complexity of biologic materials found in a typical organism.

The permanent and durable reservoir of genetic information is the DNA molecule, but to be useful, DNA must be copied into another form: RNA. RNA is quite similar in chemical structure to DNA, and the two molecules follow some of the same rules governing chemical life-style and behavior. DNA can be thought of as a book of information and RNA as a discrete photocopy of one or more pages from the book. Some RNA molecules are basic components of the cell's system for synthesizing proteins. Others are information tapes that contain, in a linear fashion, subsets of DNA's chemical information that are needed for the correct ordering of amino acids to build particular protein molecules. In many respects, the utilitarian RNA molecules that serve basic purposes are fairly similar in all cells, tissues, and organisms. It is the RNA information tapes that vary, giving rise to the specialized proteins that are made in different situations and

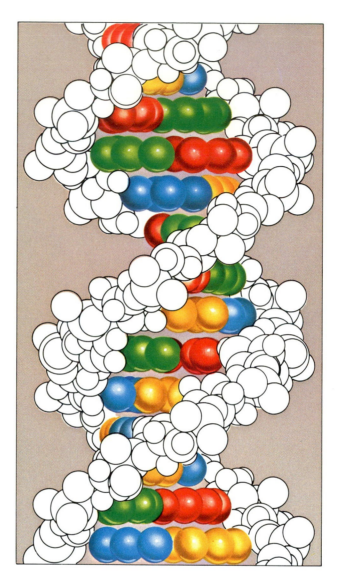

Figure 1 *The DNA molecule consists of an antiparallel double helix made up of nucleotides. The sugar-phosphate backbones of the DNA strands are joined by the pairing of bases.*

that generate the unique characteristics, called phenotypes, associated with different organisms and different parts of any given organism.

Properties, Management, and Propagation of DNA

DNA exists in two cellular locations: in the nucleus, where DNA is in the form of large extended molecules during replication and in a more condensed state at other times in the cell cycle; and in the mitochondrion, in which the organelle genome is a small circular DNA.

Most DNA molecules consist of two polynucleotide chains, or strands, wound around an axis: the well-known double helix [*see Figure 1*]. The backbone of each strand consists of alternating phosphate and sugar links. To each sugar, a flat purine or pyrimidine base is attached [*see Figure 2*]. Each base on one backbone is hydrogen bonded to a base on the other backbone. Each strand of the helix, then, is a sequential arrangement of four kinds of subunits, each composed of a sugar, a phosphate, and one of four bases: the purines adenine and guanine and the pyrimidines thymine and cytosine. The subunits are called deoxyribonucleotides, or often simply nucleotides. DNA sometimes contains bases that are modified; such modifications have been implicated in regulating how the DNA is eventually expressed as protein. For the purposes of this chapter, one can view DNA as being chemically universal, with its uniqueness in each individual instance being based on the particular sequence of the four bases in a linear array. This is best appreciated by realizing that a number of DNA molecules can have the same chemical composition but be crucially different from one another owing to a different ordering of the building blocks within each molecule.

This brings us to a key feature of DNA. Not all base-pair combinations are allowed when two DNA strands are bound together to form the double helix. Adenine (A) pairs (by hydrogen bonding) with thymine (T), and guanosine (G) pairs with cytosine (C) [*see Figure 3*]. Therefore, in a double-stranded DNA molecule, one only needs the information on one

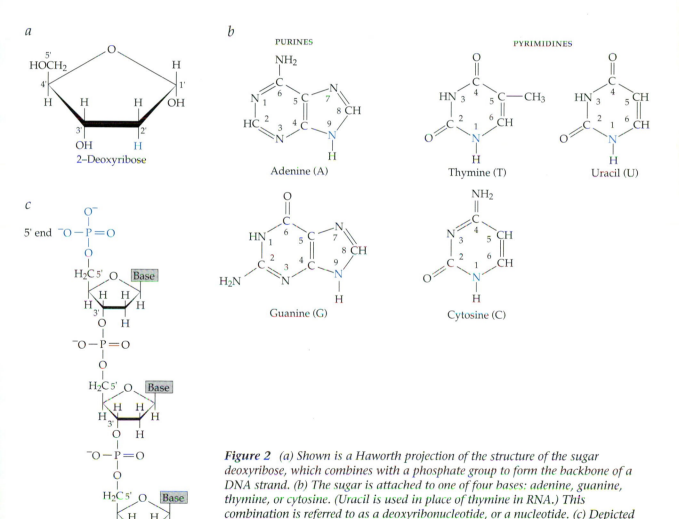

Figure 2 *(a) Shown is a Haworth projection of the structure of the sugar deoxyribose, which combines with a phosphate group to form the backbone of a DNA strand. (b) The sugar is attached to one of four bases: adenine, guanine, thymine, or cytosine. (Uracil is used in place of thymine in RNA.) This combination is referred to as a deoxyribonucleotide, or a nucleotide. (c) Depicted is the chemical structure of a trinucleotide, a single strand of DNA containing only three nucleotides.*

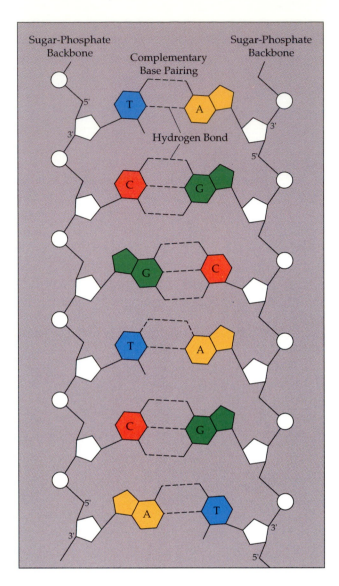

Figure 3 DNA strands are bound to each other by pairing between bases. This process is a selective one: adenine (yellow) bonds only with thymine (blue), and guanine (green) bonds only with cytosine (red).

strand of the helix to predict the exact sequence of subunits on the other, complementary strand. This feature of nucleic-acid pairing is fundamentally important in the expression of genetic information as well. This is because RNA molecules can also base pair with a DNA strand, and they do so by following similar strict base-pairing rules.

Replication

The three most important events in the existence of a DNA molecule are replication, repair, and expression. Replication means simply the duplication of a DNA molecule, which generates two complete and accurate copies of a particular set of genetic information. The process was foreseen in the famous understatement that closed the 1953 paper by Watson and Crick announcing the structure of DNA: "It has not escaped our notice that the specific pairing we have postulated immediately suggests a possible copying mechanism for the genetic material." Given the important insight of complementary base pairing, they recognized that the duplication of a DNA molecule might well proceed by the unraveling of the DNA helix and the subsequent synthesis of new DNA strands, according to the base-pairing rules, to match the two original (parental) strands of the helix. This process characterizes DNA replication for all double-stranded DNAs [*see Figure 4*]. (It is important to note that DNA can also exist in other forms. Some viruses have single-stranded DNA as their genome. Furthermore, DNA is known to exist in both linear and circular forms.)

The general complexity of DNA structural organization can be appreciated by noting the vast differences in DNA content for different organisms [*see Table 1*]. Although replicating a very large genome represents a more formidable task than replicating a very small DNA molecule, the basic principle of strand unwinding and subsequent copying by the appropriate polymer-forming enzyme (called DNA polymerase) is a common feature.

Excellent progress is now being made in understanding the detailed nature of DNA replication in human and other higher cell systems; much of what is known about this process derives, however, from long-term studies with bacterial DNA and with viruses and plasmids that can be propagated in bacteria. The ensemble of protein components, in addition to DNA polymerase, that is required to achieve replication has proved to be much more complex than what one might have anticipated. Such components assist in unwinding the DNA helix and stabilizing it in a conformation that permits the DNA polymerase to track along one of the open strands and build a new strand according to the base-pairing rules. Other proteins are involved in stabilizing the polymerase and helping to bring about the right decisions with regard to synthesizing new DNA. New DNA is made one nucleotide subunit at a time, and the polymerase system is able to select the appropriate building block: a nucleoside triphosphate that will pair correctly with the nucleotide on the strand that is being copied.

DNA Repair

The replication system also contains special components that can correct mistakes, which do occur in the process, albeit at very low frequency. The essential point is that a sophisticated proofreading mechanism exists to ensure that DNA is faithfully replicated. Such a mechanism is crucial for maintaining the integrity of the genetic system as cells divide in a developing organism and for guaranteeing that future generations of a particular species arise on the basis of correct genetic information. The importance of DNA integrity is further underscored by the fact that DNA is the only known macromolecule in living cells for which a system has evolved that is capable of repairing a variety of damage to it after it has been made. In living systems, there are genes encoding proteins that work together as a repair team to maintain the sequence integrity of a DNA molecule. The types of insults that DNA can receive in humans involve free-radical damage, exposure to ultraviolet light, and chemical modifications.

The first step in DNA repair is recognition by a protein molecule that something has gone wrong owing to disruption of a chemical bond in the DNA molecule or a change in its physical and chemical structure. This need not be massive damage. DNA repair systems can even recognize a minor chemical alteration in the base portion of a nucleotide.

Although DNA repair mechanisms are surprisingly complex in terms of the number of different proteins involved, there are essentially only two basic motifs. One type of repair system recognizes damage in a DNA molecule and makes a repair at the specific location either by reversing the event that caused the error or by performing another chemical reaction that restores the original condition. A second type of DNA repair is more drastic. It involves recognition of a damage point, surgical removal of both the site of damage and surrounding DNA sequences, and then rebuilding

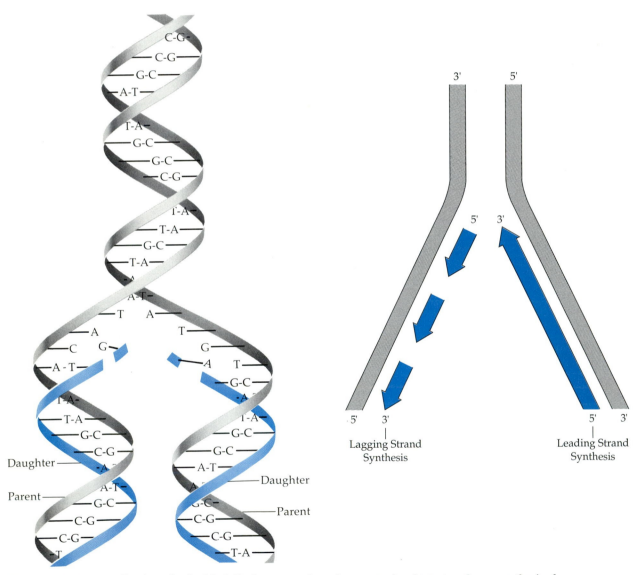

Figure 4 *In DNA replication, the double helix is unwound, and two new daughter strands are synthesized (according to the rules of base pairing) from the two parental strands (left). This process may be represented in the form of a DNA replication fork (right). DNA is always synthesized in the 5'-to-3' direction; thus, synthesis must proceed differently on the two daughter stands. Synthesis on the so-called leading strand is continuous. Synthesis on the so-called lagging strand is not: the new DNA is initially made in the form of short pieces, which are later joined by the enzyme DNA ligase.*

Table 1 DNA Content of Various Cells

Organism	Size of DNA Genome		Maximum Number of Proteins Encoded*	Number of Chromosomes (Haploid)†
	Number of Base Pairs	*Total Length (mm)*		
Prokaryotic				
Escherichia coli (bacterium)	4×10^6	1.36	3.3×10^3	1
Eukaryotic				
Saccharomyces cerevisiae (yeast)	1.35×10^7	4.60	1.125×10^4	17
Drosophila melanogaster (insect)	1.65×10^8	56	1.375×10^5	4
Homo sapiens (human)	2.9×10^9	990	2.42×10^6	23
Zea mays (corn)	5.0×10^9	1710	4.0×10^6	10

*Assuming 1200 base pairs per protein.
†Most insect and human cells are diploid, so they have twice the number of chromosomes shown.

of the DNA molecule in its original configuration. This second type of repair is termed excision repair.

The consequences of severely impaired ability to repair DNA are well documented in at least one human disease, xeroderma pigmentosum. In this disorder there is a defect in the ability to repair DNA damage caused by exposure to ultraviolet light, with the consequent occurrence of skin cancers at very low exposures to natural sunlight. It is currently thought that as many as 10 different gene products can be involved in the pathogenesis of this disease. Although this is a significant number, it is within the realm of current technology to identify the exact molecular defect in a given case, which might then be approachable by gene therapy [*see Chapter 12*].

The capacity to repair a DNA sequence is not perfect, nor is the DNA replication machinery completely accurate in copying DNA. Therefore, mistakes in genetic sequence can be perpetuated. One source of the problem is a very small thermodynamic error rate of the replication enzymes in cells. Depending on the precise location of the genetic damage, the consequences in the somatic cell can be none, minimal, or pathogenic. One such example would be the activation of an oncogene, with a consequent switch to the neoplastic state [*see Chapter 10*]. Of longer-term impact is a change in the germline DNA, which would then be passed on to offspring. Again, depending on the nature of the change in genetic information, the mutation might be of no consequence (as we shall see later, the genetic code itself provides redundancy in this regard), be deleterious, or even improve function. Genetic diversity in the evolution of species derives in part from these small changes in DNA information.

Recombination

DNA can undergo important and elegant exchange events through recombination. Recombination occurs as a normal process in the course of meiosis. It provides a means of shuffling genetic information in ways that can present evolutionary opportunities; it is also the mechanism by which alien DNA elements can become resident in an organism. The basic features of the molecular mechanisms of recombination are complex, and much less is known about the process in mammalian cells than in the classically studied prokaryotic systems. In the latter, it is clear that sequence recognition, usually based on the intrinsic complementary nature of DNA strands, is involved in the process of identifying sequences that can be matched. The matching event must be accompanied by the intervention of specialized enzymes that break the DNA backbone, introduce new pieces of genetic material, and reseal the backbone. Some of these activities are highly specialized for discrete DNA sequences. Others depend on enzymes that are involved in such processes as DNA repair and DNA replication but have the general capacity to recognize DNA and alter its topology in a way that allows a particular reaction to proceed.

Interpreting Genetic Information

A book that is never read has little or no value: DNA's information needs to be read. For that to occur, the DNA molecule (more precisely, the genes it incorporates) is first copied into a more transitory nucleic acid: RNA. The variety of cellular RNA molecules and what they do will be described later, but for now the discussion will focus on the RNA that represents a copy of a particular gene. The details of the fundamental mechanisms by which genes are recognized and properly copied into RNA (for eventual translation into protein) is a topic of intense investigation in the biomedical field [*see Figure* 5].

The first important step in this process is called initiation of transcription. It refers to the act of recognizing a gene and beginning to copy the DNA sequence into the form of an RNA molecule. This is achieved by the combined action of several proteins that interact with the DNA molecule. The first required component is a protein molecule, RNA polymerase, that can synthesize (polymerize) a chain of RNA from nucleoside building blocks much as DNA polymerase does in copying DNA. RNA polymerases can start the synthesis of an RNA chain at any position on a DNA helix in which they are properly situated. It is the physical interaction between a complete RNA polymerase enzyme and DNA that is important and unique for different systems. Only when the polymerase and DNA form a stable complex, dictated by the structures of both the enzyme and DNA, can transcription begin.

The simplest system that can read a gene is one composed of only the gene itself and an RNA polymerase molecule. This pattern occurs in the case of several viruses that infect bacteria. These bacteriophages (or simply phages) contain a special RNA polymerase that, on its own, can recognize a gene in the viral DNA and copy it into a particular form of RNA: messenger RNA (mRNA). The RNA polymerase molecule begins by recognizing a specific sequence of bases (and the consequent structure) in a DNA helix. This so-called promoter sequence encompasses the portions of the DNA molecule that signal the start point of active copying of a gene, thereby promoting this event. These sequences have been studied in detail in many systems; there are features that are held in common as well as features that are unique to particular genes or organisms. The important point is that the viral RNA polymerase, acting alone, is able to recognize a hallmark start signal that is small in size (in this case only about 15 nucleotides). In doing so, the polymerase becomes nestled in the DNA helix and begins to copy one strand of the DNA into an RNA molecule.

Synthesis of nucleic acids is polar in nature: in the language of DNA and RNA structure, everything moves in a 5′ to 3′ direction with respect to the new strand being synthesized [*see Figure 5*]. Note that for a given gene only one strand of the helix is copied; it is termed the coding strand. In almost all cases, then, only one strand of the DNA double helix contains genetic information; the other strand subserves the structural integrity of the molecule and serves as a template for replication and transcription.

Synthesis of the RNA molecule continues across the entire gene until another signal is reached that causes the polymerase to cease functioning

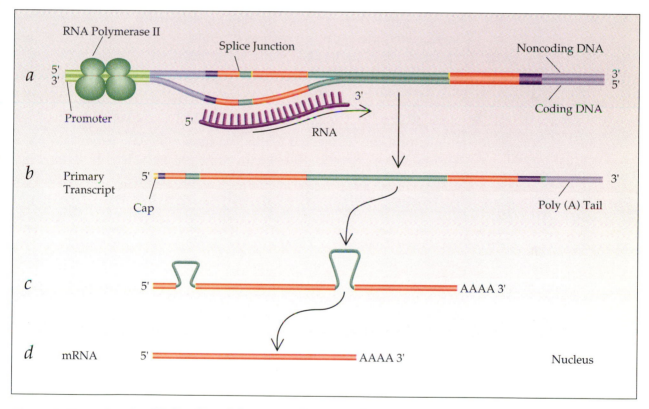

Figure 5 *Shown is a simplified outline of the process of messenger RNA (mRNA) synthesis. (a) The β-globin gene contains three exons (orange) separated by two introns (green), and the boundaries between exons and introns, known as splice junctions, contain specific nucleotide sequences required for proper joining of the exons. The synthesis of RNA from the β-globin gene, as well as from all other genes, proceeds in a 5′-to-3′ direction, whereas the coding strand of the DNA is transcribed in the 3′-to-5′ direction. The enzyme RNA polymerase II (dark green) binds to a promoter region (light green) located 200 to 300 base pairs in the 5′ direction, or upstream, from the point at which RNA synthesis begins. (b) The primary RNA transcript begins with a modified 7-methylguanosine residue, referred to as the cap, and includes a 5′ untranslated region (purple), a coding region of translated exons and introns, and a 3′ untranslated region (purple). Nearly all mRNAs that encode proteins terminate at their 3′ ends with a string of approximately 200 adenosine residues, known as the poly (A) tail, which are added 18 to 20 base pairs downstream from an AAUAAA signal in the 3′ untranslated region. (c) After RNA is synthesized but before it leaves the nucleus, these introns are excised and the exons are spliced together to form mature mRNA. Splicing involves cleavage of the 5′ site of the intron and formation of an intermediate known as a lariat. The 3′ site of the intron is then cleaved, and the two exons to either side of the intron are joined by ligation (d).*

and fall off the DNA molecule. At this point the polymerase can recycle and repeat the act of synthesis or find another gene's promoter and begin transcription of another RNA molecule. Such RNA molecules represent a copy of the DNA genetic information and can now serve the purpose of genetic expression: the synthesis of a protein whose amino acids are in a sequence specified by the sequence of bases in the original DNA molecule.

For a single polymerase protein to perform all the functions required for gene recognition and for copying of genetic information is the exception, not the rule. Even in simple organisms, the process is usually much more complicated and requires additional specialized protein factors that can associate with either the DNA, the polymerase, or both and thereby achieve selective recognition of different genes in the system. As one might anticipate, this has proved to be especially true in mammalian systems. In such systems, there are a large number of proteins, called transcription factors, that in various combinations recognize different types of genes with different efficiencies. Selectivity is achieved by the presence of different combinations of multiple protein factors that recognize elements in the DNA sequence immediately adjacent to the gene. By interacting with DNA and one another, these proteins cause initiation of transcription.

When these processes were first studied, it was assumed that the selective expression of genes in different cells and circumstances would depend on unique proteins that would define the nature of gene expression for a particular class of genes. Although there is some specialization of this type, it has become appreciated that the transcriptional molecular complexes are large, complicated structures. In many cases at least several proteins are involved in addition to RNA polymerase. Selectivity in gene expression is based on the way these proteins interact at a specific gene, and even on the degree to which the DNA is in a physical conformation that makes it accessible to the action of particular proteins. Whereas important transcriptional accessory proteins are held in common for most protein-coding genes, different classes of genes are recognized by different polymerase and accessory protein systems. For example, the RNA molecules that are parts of ribosomes, the organelles on which protein synthesis takes place, are copied from their DNA by one type of polymerase system, whereas the transfer RNAs (tRNAs), which have a different fundamental role in protein synthesis, are transcribed by yet another. A fourth polymerase system is unique to the mitochondrial genome, and there may be specialized cases in which components of one of the four traditional polymerase systems are shared with components from another to transcribe still other types of promoter elements.

Split Genes

In simple organisms, genes usually take the form of a unit stretch of DNA that contains little more than the minimal essential sequence information required to manufacture its protein product. It came as a major surprise when it was discovered in 1977 that the genes in human beings and other metazoans were in fact much larger than they needed to be to encode their protein product. Also, many more and much larger RNA molecules were found in the nucleus of mammalian cells than could be accounted for by the demands of gene expression.

The solution for both of these puzzles lay in the fact that many genes are split. That is, their informational sequences are interrupted by non-coding stretches of DNA—stretches that indeed seem to have no function (this is not always the case, however, and in some special instances there can be genes within genes) [*see Figure 5a*]. Most of the time these interloping sequences (called introns) appear, at first glance, to be an impediment to the flow of transactions involved in expressing genes. They are copied into an RNA form—the primary transcript [*see Figure 5b*]—by the polymerase transcript along with the coding sequences (called exons) and then must be specifically and cleanly removed from the RNA transcript by a precise and complex system that involves multiple components, both proteins and ribonucleoproteins.

Ribonucleoproteins, as the name implies, consist of both RNA and protein moieties. At least several small nuclear ribonucleoproteins (snRNPs) work together, and their combined and concerted action in paring down the primary transcript into a functional coding species— the mature mRNA—is called splicing. There are simple splicing events as well as a more complex series of splicing phenomena. When one looks at the more complicated pattern of splicing, one possible advantage of such complexity is evident. For example, alternative splicing allows the transmission of more than one message from a given genetic locus. That is, a single DNA sequence produces a large RNA molecule. This large preliminary version of the message is recognized by the splicing factors, which then cut and join the sequence at different locations [*see Figures 5c and 5d*]. The cutting and joining events are precise and result in the production of distinctive pieces of information needed to assemble different protein products. The key point is that the splicing machinery recognizes valid coding exon sequences and usually joins all of them together; the introns are thus removed and degraded, and a full-length protein is produced. In some cases, however, the splicing system can purposely skip over selected exons and in this way produce a mature mRNA for a smaller, specialized protein. The end result is increased genetic diversity based on post–RNA synthesis events that generate different end products.

The first molecular components to be identified as critical to the recognition, cutting, and joining of RNA sequences were the ribonucleoproteins. These molecules are typically composed of a small RNA species, usually only several hundred bases (or even less) in length, together with a set of approximately six to 12 protein molecules. The ribonucleoproteins function as a cooperative set of about five individual units, forming a complex called the spliceosome (splicing body). Additional factors required for the operation of the spliceosome include protein molecules that are not intrinsic parts of individual ribonucleoproteins. The spliceosome is a system that has persisted throughout evolution, and it has been conjectured that at one time the splicing body was composed of one large RNA molecule together with a set of proteins. In this model, what remains today in human cells are those portions of the ancestral RNA sequence most active in the process of RNA breakage and rejoining.

Ribozymes

A remarkable finding that followed the discovery of split genes in eukaryotes was that RNA could operate enzymatically on itself, in the absence of any protein. Specialized RNA sequences can fold into structures that function enzymatically and can speed up a reaction associated with RNA breakage and joining by a factor of about 10^{10}. Such RNA enzymes were first discovered as self-splicing and tRNA processing entities in fungal and bacterial systems and have now been termed ribozymes. Ribozymes fulfill other criteria of enzymes as well and must represent an ancient mechanism for manipulating the earliest forms of RNA.

The chemical reaction catalyzed by ribozymes resembles splicing events mediated by ribonucleoproteins, and it has been suggested that ribozymes could be powerful molecular reagents when used therapeutically. A ribozyme and its substrate must meet certain specific sequence requirements if cleavage of the substrate is to occur. Thus, it may be possible to design a specialized ribozyme that could be introduced into human cells to degrade a pathogenic RNA species by enzymatic cleavage. The challenge is to design ribozymes that combine enzymatic specificity and efficiency so that unwanted RNAs can be destroyed while normal cellular RNA species are left unharmed.

Capping and Polyadenylation of RNA

In addition to the exquisite processing events that the initial RNA molecule undergoes, each end of an mRNA molecule must be altered as well [*see Figure 5b*]. At the 5′ end, which was the first to be synthesized and should be thought of as the beginning of the molecule, there is a modification of the base located at the terminus. This modification, which involves the addition of an unusual chemical structure to the 5′-terminal phosphate, is termed capping. Capping of a transcript is in most cases required for it to be used efficiently for translation. Another type of modification occurs at the opposite, or 3′, end of the molecule. This process, termed polyadenylation, involves the addition of adenosine residues so that the RNA has a tail of up to several hundred consecutive adenosines.

The goal, of course, is the formation of a legitimate unit of RNA information that can, in the case of higher cells, exit the nucleus and move to the cytoplasm, which contains the macromolecular machinery necessary to translate the RNA information into a protein product.

Getting the Message Out and Interpreting It

After the RNA copy of the DNA gene has been processed and modified, it is a mature mRNA. It is then ready to leave the nucleus and proceed to the cytoplasm, where it will be translated into a protein molecule.

The RNA molecule represents a copy of the gene and is destined to program the synthesis of a linear, ordered set of amino acids: the primary sequence of the protein product of the gene. There is thus a direct relation among the sets of information in DNA, RNA, and protein, and this relation can be arranged in a colinear fashion (once the extra DNA present in the introns in many eukaryotic genes has been taken into account).

The question then arises: How is the linear information contained in DNA (and mRNA) translated into a linear protein chain? What is the genetic code? The simplest possible information system would be one in which each of the four bases directed the incorporation of one amino acid. A system of this type might work well if there were only four amino acids to be dealt with. A two-base information system raises the number of coding possibilities to 4^2, or 16—still not enough to encode the 20 individual amino acids known to be present in most proteins. And so evolution moved to a three-base minimum system: the triplet genetic code. This system has 4^3, or 64, different possible codons, or triplets, of bases—more than enough to encode 20 amino acids. The system is degenerate in that some amino acids (arginine, leucine, and serine) are encoded by as many as six different triplet combinations. For others (methionine and tryptophan), only one triplet signals the appropriate machinery to insert those amino acids. The rest fall in between [*see Table 2*]. The important thing is that although the genetic code is degenerate, it does not cause errors in protein synthesis, because no single triplet codon specifies more than one amino acid. In addition to specifying the insertion of an amino acid in translation, certain codons, termed stop codons, signal the release of a newly made protein from the translation machinery.

The process of information transfer occurs in a similar way in organisms ranging from bacteria to humans, although complex details of the process vary. In all organisms, however, a good deal of attention is paid to maintaining the integrity of the DNA sequences, the permanent keepers of genetic information. The RNA molecules of various types tend to be used a finite number of times before being degraded by a cell-regulation event. Because of the limited lifespan of RNA molecules and their special functions, there is no apparent need for—nor is there any evidence of the existence of—an RNA repair capacity. Because RNA is made over and over from DNA templates, there is no chance that errors will accumulate in the DNA genetic information store as a result of mutagenic events at the RNA level.

Other safeguards are intrinsically present in the way basic genetic information is expressed. Because many amino acids can be signaled by different, but related, triplets, there can be single-base alterations in particular positions of a codon family (usually the third position) without any change in the amino acid that is encoded. Other changes may be neutral: even if a different amino acid is called for, its physical and chemical properties are similar enough to the original, wild-type amino acid so that the resulting protein may well still be functional.

Finally, although the molecular flow from DNA to RNA to protein is readily conceptualized, the problem of producing a fully functional gene product is made much more complex by the need to fine-tune and polish the primary protein sequence [*see Chapter 3*]. After a protein chain has been synthesized and folded into its final conformation, it may be necessary to modify some of its amino acids. In many cases, such as the phosphorylation of certain amino acid residues, these seemingly minor chemical changes drastically alter the protein's activity. Indeed, the activity of a protein may be largely nullified unless certain modifications occur

Table 2 The Genetic Code: Amino Acids Specified
by mRNA Codons

First Position (5′ End)	Second Position				Third Position (3′ End)
	U	C	A	G	
U	Phe	Ser	Tyr	Cys	U
	Phe	Ser	Tyr	Cys	C
	Leu	Ser	STOP	STOP	A
	Leu	Ser	STOP	Trp	G
C	Leu	Pro	His	Arg	U
	Leu	Pro	His	Arg	C
	Leu	Pro	Gln	Arg	A
	Leu	Pro	Gln	Arg	G
A	Ile	Thr	Asn	Ser	U
	Ile	Thr	Asn	Ser	C
	Ile	Thr	Lys	Arg	A
	Met	Thr	Lys	Arg	G
G	Val	Ala	Asp	Gly	U
	Val	Ala	Asp	Gly	C
	Val	Ala	Glu	Gly	A
	Val	Ala	Glu	Gly	G

Note: Given the position of the bases in a codon, it is possible to find the corresponding amino acid. For example, the codon (5′) AUG (3′) on mRNA specifies methionine, whereas CAU specifies histidine. UAA, UAG, and UGA are termination signals. AUG is part of the initiation signal, and it codes for internal methionines as well.

that enable it to perform its structural or enzymatic function. In other cases, modification can inactivate a protein. But first the protein must be made.

Putting It All Together—from Gene to Protein

The principal initial event in gene expression is the selection of one of four cellular RNA polymerase complexes to copy a particular gene or genes into an RNA chain, which then becomes the working informational macromolecule. The three major transcriptional polymerase systems in the nucleus of human cells are usually referred to as RNA polymerase I, RNA polymerase II, and RNA polymerase III. (There is a fourth RNA polymerase system, which is specific to mitochondrial, rather than nuclear, DNA.) Each of these polymerase systems is complex and is composed of multiple proteins rather than a single, simple polypeptide.

RNA Polymerases

RNA polymerase I is responsible for the production of most ribosomal RNA (rRNA) molecules, which are essential and ancient components of the fundamental unit of translation, the ribosome. RNA polymerase II complexes are responsible for transcribing genes that encode proteins. RNA polymerase III is responsible for the production of one rRNA as well as the other class of important RNA molecules needed for translation, the tRNAs.

There are other small RNA molecules in the cell that are produced by RNA polymerase III, and some of them are important for processing events in the maturation of other RNA molecules. Still other small RNAs are produced by RNA polymerase II, among them RNA components of the small nuclear ribonucleoproteins that function in splicing.

The fourth RNA polymerase system, mitochondrial RNA polymerase, is thought to function only in the mitochondria of eukaryotic cells. It is responsible for the synthesis of all of the mitochondrial gene products—in humans, 37 distinct RNAs and proteins.

In an actively growing cell population, all these polymerase classes are active. RNA polymerase I exemplifies a highly vigorous synthetic system because it must meet the heavy demands for rRNA production to synthesize all the ribosomes in a cell and provide for their continual renewal. The second most abundant RNA class comprises the tRNAs, which accomplish the final step between the recognition of genetic information and the selection of a specific amino acid destined to be part of a long stretch of amino acids in a particular protein. The least abundant RNA class is the mRNA population, which represents whatever protein-encoding genes are being actively copied during a given period. In almost all cases, only a very small fraction of the total number of genes in a cell is being copied, and their mRNAs also tend to be more unstable than other RNA classes.

Transcription

The basic problem of copying the correct DNA strand of a gene can now be addressed. This is, of course, a critical step because in a particular gene, only one strand of the DNA helix contains the appropriate sequence of bases to be copied into an RNA sense strand. The other strand of the DNA helix is complementary to the sense strand, as determined by the DNA base-pairing rules. Its purpose is to maintain the structure and integrity of the duplex DNA and to permit replication and transcription. Usually, copying the wrong strand of the DNA helix would produce an RNA molecule of no value (although there are highly specialized examples where antisense RNA is synthesized that regulates, by base pairing, the availability of complementary sense-strand mRNA). Normally, copying of the wrong strand of DNA does not occur, because there are intrinsic signals in the DNA sequence immediately adjacent to the start point of transcription that are recognized by the polymerase system as an appropriate place to home in on the DNA helix in an orientation that will permit only one possible outcome: the 5'-to-3' biochemical synthesis of the correct strand of RNA. A great deal of effort has been directed toward identifying the essential features of these signal sequences for the polymerase. It is now clear that some signals are routinely found next to the gene; other sequences, some quite distant from the gene, may represent special signposts that are recognized at different points in time and development. The essential concept is that specific regulatory DNA sequences related to the start point of gene transcription are recognized by a complex set of protein molecules that together form what is called a transcriptional initiation complex. When both DNA signals and the proper set of proteins are available, gene expression can ensue.

Once the system is running and a DNA gene is being read, the reaction proceeds until the entire gene sequence is copied into RNA. In fact, transcription usually goes on a little farther. Sometimes this extra transcription contains important information that will be needed later; it almost always includes a short RNA sequence that can be recognized by an enzyme that trims the end of the RNA and further modifies it so that it becomes a mature species (the polyadenylation reaction). At this juncture the other end of the mRNA is also modified by a special enzyme that changes the chemical nature of the 5′ terminal base in the molecule. This capping is necessary to produce a fully functional mRNA. Although the nature of these modifications (as well as some others) is known in detail, a full explanation for why they are required in a mature mRNA molecule is still lacking.

Translation

Two so-called worker RNAs, tRNA and rRNA, operate on the mature mRNA [*see Figure 6*]. Transfer RNAs are intricately folded small RNAs (fewer than 100 bases) that are synthesized and processed in the nucleus. Once they are synthesized, they leave the nucleus and enter the cytoplasm, where all translation takes place. Ribosomal RNAs are transcribed from DNA in a subnuclear organelle called the nucleolus, where they are synthesized in great abundance, usually in the form of large precursor molecules. These molecules are broken down, via a complex pathway, to produce three mature rRNAs (usually termed 28S, 18S, and 5.8S rRNAs on the basis of their size). With the addition of 5S rRNA (made separately), the system thus comprises four different mature rRNA species. These rRNAs are assembled with the ribosomal proteins and move to the cytoplasm as functional ribosomes. Although bacterial ribosomes have been well characterized, they are very complicated structures, usually consisting of 50 or more proteins in addition to the aforementioned RNA molecules. Eukaryotic ribosomes are even more complex, and studying them has been difficult.

Once the requisite parts of the translational machinery are in place in the cytoplasm, namely ribosomes and tRNAs, a gene product can be synthesized. This process of course requires the informational macromolecule, the mRNA from a particular gene. As was explained above, the fundamental unit of genetic language is the triplet codon that specifies a particular amino acid. Each codon is defined as three adjacent bases in the mRNA molecule, and in almost all cases successive codons lie adjacent to one another, with neither intervening spaces nor overlaps. This makes it possible to decipher the genetic message as a linear tape of information. Note again that because the code is degenerate (that is, in most cases a particular amino acid can be specified by more than one triplet sequence), some base changes in genes have no phenotypic effect.

The first step in translation is recognition by the ribosomal system that an mRNA is present. The best evidence suggests that the ribosome (or the largest subunit of the ribosome) recognizes an end of the mRNA molecule: the 5′ end, which was the first part to be transcribed from the gene and which contains the beginning of the genetic message. In some cases, this 5′ end is the very first base of the first informational codon, but in most instances the first codon (called the start codon) is found farther down the molecule, toward the 3′ end. In bacteria, a special recognition sequence is

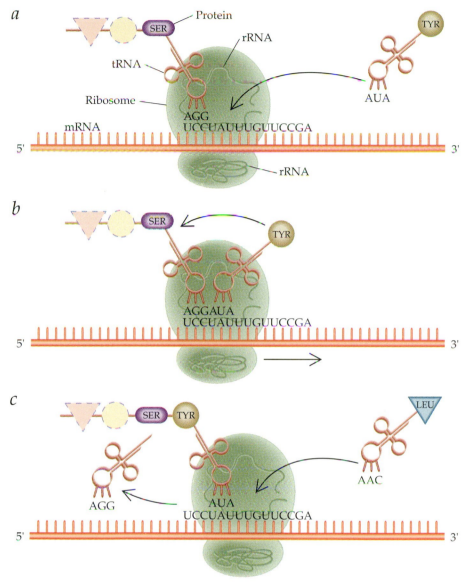

a

Protein

SER

rRNA

tRNA

TYR

Ribosome

AUA

mRNA

AGG
UCCUAUUUGUUCCGA

5'   3'

rRNA

b

SER

TYR

AGGAUA
UCCUAUUUGUUCCGA

5'   3'

c

SER TYR

LEU

AAC

AGG

AUA
UCCUAUUUGUUCCGA

5'   3'

Figure 6 Translation of mRNA into protein requires the presence of two other types of RNA, tRNA and rRNA. tRNAs are the hooks that add amino acids to the growing protein chain; rRNAs are structural components of the ribosome. Each nucleotide triplet, or codon, on the mRNA chain encodes a specific amino acid. Each molecule of tRNA in turn binds only the amino acid corresponding to a particular codon. A tRNA recognizes a codon by means of a complementary nucleotide sequence called an anticodon. Here the addition of one amino acid to a protein chain is shown. (a) An incoming tRNA molecule carrying the amino acid tyrosine binds to the codon exposed at a binding site on the ribosome. (b) The tyrosine forms a peptide bond with serine, the last amino acid on the protein chain. (c) As the ribosome advances one codon, exposing the binding site to the next incoming tRNA, the serine tRNA is released.

present in the mRNA before the first start codon. This recognition element serves as the binding site for the initial attachment of the ribosome. In eukaryotic mRNAs, the 5'-end sequences are variable, and the ribosome system has the capacity to scan the RNA sequence until it recognizes the start codon. In the vast majority of cases this is AUG, which specifies the amino acid methionine. Recognition of the start codon causes the ribosomal machinery to become fully assembled and to lock on to the mRNA, and then to begin its transit for the entire length of the genetic message. Immediately after the AUG start codon is recognized, the appropriate tRNA—one that carries a particular amino acid building block at its 3' end—is recruited [*see Figure 6a*].

The two most important concepts to remember about the tRNA worker molecules are that (1) tRNAs are specifically recognized by enzymes (aminoacyl synthetases) that attach a particular amino acid to the 3' end of the tRNA, and (2) each tRNA incorporates a three-base sequence (the anticodon) that recognizes the mRNA codon by complementary base pairing. (The features of a particular small tRNA sequence that are recognized by the aminoacyl synthetases have yet to be fully elucidated, but in some cases the anticodon is important.) In any case, the enzyme activity that catalyzes the amino acid attachment is very precise, so that a particular tRNA almost always carries, in functional form, its correct amino acid. Such tRNAs carrying amino acids are said to be charged, and they are ready to fulfill their role in protein synthesis.

The next task is for the second codon in the message to be properly translated into its specified amino acid. This is done by the movement of a second tRNA molecule into a second available site on the ribosome [*see Figure 6b*]. Which tRNA is selected depends, again, on the base pairing between codon and anticodon. In all cases, tRNAs that are allowed to associate with ribosome occupancy sites are charged with an amino acid, unless they have done their job and are at the ribosomal exit gate [*see Figure 6c*]. This charging is a two-step process. First, the amino acid is coupled through its carboxyl group to adenosine monophosphate, with adenosine triphosphate (ATP) as the energy source. This intermediate then donates the amino acid to the 3′-acceptor end of the tRNA. This linkage between amino acid and tRNA is higher in free energy than the peptide bond that is subsequently formed between the two amino acids. The excess provides a direct source of energy for peptide bond formation.

The principal feature of translation is the process of bringing in tRNAs that are specified by the codon-anticodon interaction and that have been previously charged with an amino acid. It is a continual process, with the ribosome moving along the mRNA until the new polypeptide chain has been produced. If the gene product is a protein consisting of 100 amino acids, this will require 100 tRNA molecules, each with its correct amino acid attached, and the formation of 99 peptide bonds. The total amount of genetic information required to encode the amino acid sequence of the protein is 300 bases of RNA information, transcribed from and reflecting the information content of the appropriate 300 bases of coding DNA. For many eukaryotic genes, of course, the amount of DNA transcribed is much larger than the mature mRNA, and the transcribed "pre-mRNA" will have been reduced to the correct size and form by splicing. Finally, the stop codon is recognized by a factor that causes the ribosome to be released from the mRNA.

With the end of translation, the desired result—the gene product—is almost in hand. What remains is the folding of the protein into the proper conformation, which is necessary if it is to be biologically active [*see Chapter 3*]. In some cases, correct folding is induced by the amino acid sequence of the protein chain; in other cases the assistance of certain other proteins is required to arrive at a correctly folded final product. As noted above, some proteins undergo postsynthetic modifications that are essential for their biologic activity.

Differences in Organization of Genetic Information

Different biologic systems exhibit different levels of complexity in the organization of their genetic information. In the simplest system, genes would be composed of uninterrupted coding sequences for their initial RNA product, with a minimal amount of additional DNA surrounding the gene so that it could be expressed properly. Prokaryotic cells, viruses, and organellar genomes approach this level of simplicity. One of the more interesting cases is metazoan mitochondrial DNA, in which there are almost no noncoding sequences in the entire genome, apart from the control sequences for DNA replication and the promotion of transcription. In this system, mRNAs are produced that have a start codon right at the 5′ end of the molecule and that terminate in a stop codon followed by only a few additional bases.

In contrast, the gene organization in the nucleus of human cells is much more complicated. Genes can be many times larger than they would have to be to encode their protein product. They are so large because they contain those inserts of noncoding DNA, the introns. Why such a level of complexity should exist in human cells is difficult to answer, but the fact that different gene products can be assembled by alternative modes of piecing together exons—the coding segments—suggests that diversity in function may be the major benefit of having genes in pieces. It seems likely that such flexibility was important early in evolution and that the current complexity in gene expression is a legacy of this process.

General References

Alberts B, Bray D, Lewis J, et al: *Molecular Biology of the Cell,* 2nd ed. Garland Publishing, Inc., New York, 1989

Singer M, Berg P: *Genes & Genomes.* University Science Books, Mill Valley, California, 1991

Stryer L: *Biochemistry,* 3rd ed. W.H. Freeman and Co., New York, 1988

Watson JD, Hopkins NH, Roberts JW, et al: *Molecular Biology of the Gene,* 4th ed. The Benjamin/Cummings Publishing Co., Inc., Menlo Park, California, 1987

Kornberg A, Baker TA: *DNA Replication,* 2nd ed. W. H. Freeman and Co., New York, 1992

Acknowledgments

Quotation on page 30 was reprinted from "Molecular Structure of Nucleic Acids: a Structure for Deoxyribose Nucleic Acid," by J.D. Watson and F.H.C. Crick in *Nature* 171:737, 1953.

Figures 1, 4(left) George Kelvin. From "Medical Genetics," by R. W. Erbe, in SCIENTIFIC AMERICAN *Medicine,* edited by E. Rubenstein and D. D. Federman, Section 9, Subsection IV. Scientific American, Inc., New York, 1994. All rights reserved.

Figure 2 Tom Moore. Adapted from *Molecular Cell Biology,* 2nd ed., by J. Darnell, H. Lodish, and D. Baltimore. Scientific American Books, New York, 1990.

Figure 3 Tom Moore. Adapted from *Recombinant DNA,* 2nd ed., by J. D. Watson, M. Gilman, J. Witkowski, et al. Scientific American Books, New York, 1992. © 1992 James D. Watson, Michael Gilman, Jan Witkowski, Mark Zoller. Used by permission.

Figure 4(right) Talar Agasyan.

Figure 5 Dimitry Schidlovsky. From "Medical Genetics," by R. W. Erbe, in SCIENTIFIC AMERICAN *Medicine,* edited by E. Rubenstein and D. D. Federman, Section 9, Subsection IV. Scientific American, Inc., New York, 1994. All rights reserved.

Figure 6 Dimitry Schidlovsky. Adapted from "The Processing of RNA," by J. E. Darnell, Jr., in *Scientific American* 249(4):90, 1983. © 1983 Scientific American, Inc. All rights reserved.

CHAPTER 3

Elements of Protein Structure

Anne N. Baldwin, Ph.D., Eric M. Shooter, Ph.D.

Proteins are the organic polymers on which all functions of the living organism depend. Some proteins provide the structural framework for the cell and the extracellular support for diverse tissues. Others—the enzymes—make metabolism possible through their role as catalysts. Still other proteins are involved in the regulation of enzyme activity or gene expression, or in the transfer of information from the outside to the inside of the cell.

Each role played by a particular protein is highly specific, and evolution has favored structures that are fine-tuned to perform these roles. Yet an extraordinary unity of design permits a common chemical theme to be used over and over, with variation in detail, to achieve this enormous diversity of function. Indeed, if proteins were not polymers built of shared chemical blocks, it would not be possible for the cell to rely on a simple genetic code to preserve the information for their synthesis, or for a common synthetic apparatus to translate the genetic information into a functional form.

What are some of the essential properties that protein structure must provide?

1. It must provide an extended, diversified surface capable of binding other molecules with high specificity.
2. It must be able to serve as a scaffold to support a variety of chemical functional groups, which can catalyze reactions by serving as electron donors or acceptors or can be chemically modified to provide still more structural diversity.

3. The surface must be able to encode information governing a variety of processes at once, through recognition signals that lead to interactions with other proteins.

4. The three-dimensional structure, or conformation, of each protein molecule must be reproducible. Moreover, the conformation must be stable—and yet not so stable that it cannot be altered or regulated by environmental factors or interaction with other molecules. For instance, the impingement of a single photon on the protein rhodopsin results in a change in the molecule's shape, and this change initiates the process of vision.

5. In some cases, the structure must be able to provide high tensile strength or elasticity. This is achieved by a particular class of proteins that aggregate to form fibers (which withstand longitudinal stress) or are chemically modified to form an elastic mesh.

6. It must be possible to store, in a linear code, all the information needed to achieve the final biologically active three-dimensional structure of the protein.

The Hierarchy of Structural Organization

Nature has solved all these structural problems and more through a hierarchy of structural organization [*see Figure 1*]. At the first level are the 20 different but related amino acids that serve as monomeric building blocks for the formation of a linear polymeric chain. The specific sequence of each protein is its primary structure. As there are 20 possible choices for each position in the sequence, the total number of possible sequences of any given length is very large. Secondary structure consists of a few rather simple patterns of repeating polypeptide structure within a local sequence, notably the α helix, β sheet, and reverse turn. Supersecondary structure refers to a few common motifs of interconnected elements of secondary structure. Tertiary structure describes the arrangement in three-dimensional space of the folded polypeptide chain. For soluble proteins, this arrangement is quite condensed but nonetheless specific. Proteins that fold into a condensed form are known as globular proteins, whereas those whose form is extended and that tend to form insoluble aggregates are called fibrous proteins.

The tertiary structure may consist of more than one folding domain, which may be the true functional building blocks out of which all contemporary proteins have been constructed. Finally, the quaternary structure refers to the arrangement of subunits in an oligomeric protein. A special case of quaternary structure is the extensive aggregation of monomers found in the fibers that form the extracellular matrix of tissues and the cytoskeleton of cells. This polymerization of protein molecules is sometimes referred to as supramolecular structure.

These levels of structural hierarchy, described in greater detail below, have been recognized for many years. Recent work has focused on how the levels are interconnected. The goal, not yet achieved, is to understand how the primary amino acid sequence determines the final folded conformation of the chain and thus specifies the full information content encoded by the surface.

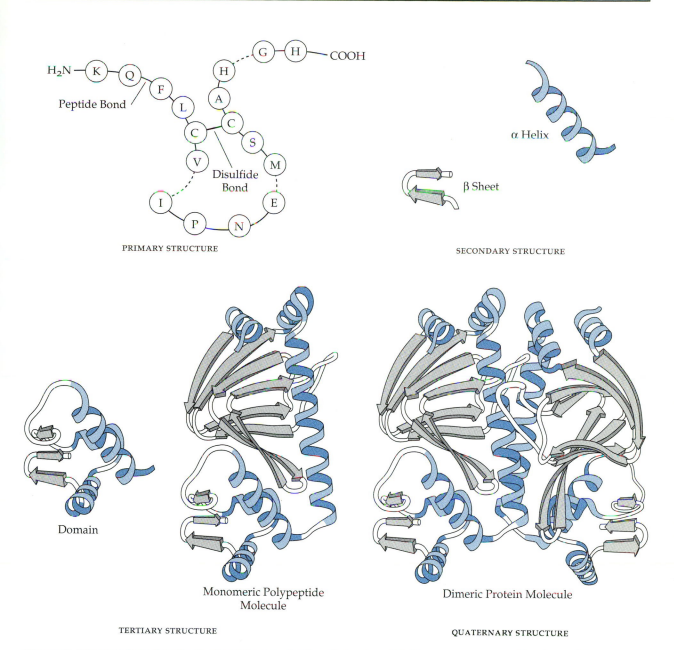

Figure 1 *Illustrated are four levels of protein organizational structure. The linear arrangement of amino acids (indicated by single-letter code) and any intrachain disulfide bonds constitute the primary structure. Folding of parts of a polypeptide chain into regular structures (e.g., α helices and β sheets) generates the secondary structure. Tertiary structure refers to the folding of regions between secondary features to give the overall conformation of the molecule or portions of it (domains) with specific functional properties. Quaternary structure results from association of two or more polypeptide chains into a single polymeric protein molecule.*

This chapter cannot begin to cover all approaches to this problem, or to discuss any of them in depth. The subject is covered in detail in several more thorough reviews.[1-7]

Primary Structure

Every protein consists of an extended chain of amino acids. All amino acids, 20 of which make up proteins in nature, share a structural motif consisting of a carboxyl group and an amino group, both joined to a central carbon atom termed the α (alpha) carbon [*see Figures 2 and 3*]. In the polymeric peptide chain, the carboxyl group of one amino acid is condensed with the amino group of the next amino acid through an amide, or peptide, linkage. The peptide backbone therefore consists of a repeating sequence of atoms: ...-C_α-CO-N-C_α-CO-N-... The amino acids differ from one another in the nature of the side chain, which is also attached to the alpha carbon. All have the L configuration around the α carbon (except in certain peptides, such as the antibiotic gramicidin, that

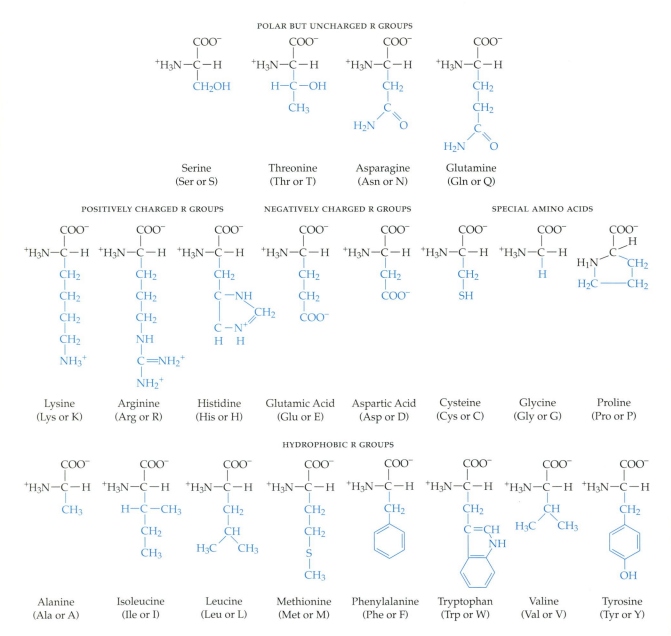

Figure 2 *Shown are the structures of the 20 common amino acids. In each structure, a central carbon atom (the α carbon) is bonded to an amino group (or to an imino group in proline), a carboxyl group, a hydrogen atom, and an R group, or side chain. The R groups are in blue.*

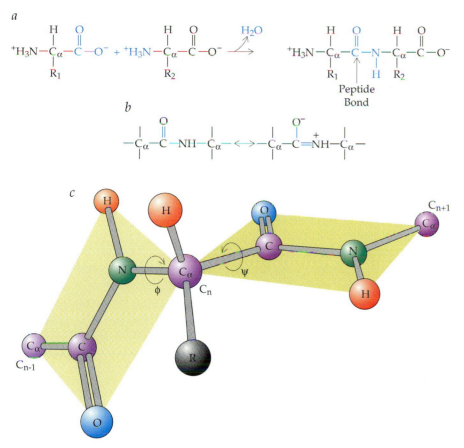

Figure 3 *(a) The peptide bond is formed between the amino group of one amino acid and the carboxyl group of another. This reaction liberates a molecule of water. (b) Because the carboxyl carbon and oxygen atoms are linked by a double bond, the peptide bond between carbon and nitrogen has a partial double-bond character. (c) Rotation is possible about the two covalent single bonds that connect each α carbon to the two adjacent planar peptide units. But some restrictions do apply to the values of ψ and φ. For example, if the pictured adjacent peptide groups were coplanar, then certain oxygen and hydrogen atoms would be separated by less than their van der Waals radii and would repel one another.*

are synthesized in bacteria by a route different from the protein synthetic pathway). The prefix L refers to the fact that L amino acids rotate polarized light in an arbitrarily defined left direction, whereas D amino acids do so in the opposite direction. It is important that all amino acids in proteins have the same chirality, or handedness, in order to form secondary structures, but it is probably chance that they are L rather than D.

It is not known why only 20 of an infinite number of possible amino acid side chains are specified by the genetic code. In any case, this relatively small number allows the sequence of amino acids to be fully specified by a triplet genetic code while providing a reasonably wide range of molecular size, polarity, and specific chemical groups. During earliest evolution, a doublet code, which could specify as many as 16 amino acids, may have been adequate. With the emergence of the peptide-synthesizing apparatus, however, in which amino acids are adapted by specific transfer RNA molecules to translate the nucleotide sequence into a peptide sequence, a triplet code may have become necessary to ensure stability of base pairing.[1]

The peptide bond itself [*see Figure 3a*] provides the backbone for the chain. The planar configuration of this unit results from the partial double-bond character of the bond between the carbonyl (CO) carbon and the nitrogen [*see Figure 3b*]. As a consequence, the peptide group forms a rigid unit. Within the backbone chain, only two bonds permit rotation around them: the bond between the α carbon and the nitrogen and the bond between the α carbon and the carbonyl carbon [*see Figure 3c*]. These two rotations, defined by two dihedral angles ϕ (phi) and ψ (psi), permit a limited range of conformations for the amino acid side chains while maintaining a fairly stable backbone. If there were too much chain flexibility, with too many conformational possibilities, it might never be possible for the protein to fold into a unique tertiary structure. This may be the evolutionary reason for the exclusive presence of α-amino acids, which have their amino group on the carbon immediately adjacent to the carbonyl group, rather than β-amino acids, in which the amino group is two carbon atoms removed. Thus, the electronic properties of the peptide bond permit the translation of information contained in the primary sequence into information contained in a complex but specific three-dimensional array.

The repertoire of 20 amino acids provides a number of functional groups built into different side chains. Acidic and basic side chains can serve as electron donors or acceptors and thus directly increase the rate of an enzymatic reaction through general acid or base catalysis. In addition, amino acids with functional groups can be chemically modified in a variety of ways to serve a wide range of functions. Examples of posttranslational modification include the phosphorylation of tyrosine, serine, and threonine residues; the glycosylation of asparagine, serine, and threonine; the acylation of cysteine residues with long-chain fatty acids; and the addition of a second carboxyl group to glutamic acid, as occurs in the final processing of the prothrombin group of procoagulants (factors II, VII, IX, X) from their precursors.

The primary sequence of a protein may contain structural signals that determine its cellular fate after synthesis, directing it to the secretory pathway or targeting it for compartmentalization in the endoplasmic reticulum, the Golgi apparatus, or mitochondria. There may be signals marking the protein for posttranslational modification, such as phosphorylation, glycosylation, or acylation. Limited proteolytic cleavage at specific sites may be indicated, as in the processing of peptide hormones—for example, the cleavage of proinsulin to form insulin. Other examples include the eventual removal of the signal peptide that is required for transport of secreted proteins across the plasma membrane. Finally, there may be markers that specify the rate of turnover of the protein. In other words, the primary sequence specifies not only the chemical properties of a protein but also a variety of biological properties.

Secondary Structure

Secondary structure is the local, repetitive arrangement of amino acids determined by the repetition of dihedral angles in successive peptide units. The two most common secondary structures are the α helix and the β sheet, first postulated by Pauling and Corey [*see Figure 4*].[8,9] Both are formed by hydrogen bonds between the main-chain N-hydrogen atom of one peptide group and the carbonyl oxygen atom of another. In both structures, the amino acid side chains all point outward. In the case of the α helix [*see Figure 4a*], this hydrogen bond is between two amino acid residues on the same stretch of chain, residue i and residue i+4—the fourth residue away. This structure is very stable, and it is the most common element of secondary structure in globular proteins. The average length is about 11 residues, corresponding to three turns of the helix.

In a β sheet [*see Figure 4b*], the hydrogen bond connects two separate strands and thus remote segments of the same peptide chain. There are two forms of β sheet. In one form, the strands run parallel to each other and are widely separated along the polypeptide chain by either an α helix or some non-α/β structure. In the other, the strands run antiparallel to each other and may be separated by a tight turn or short loop. In both cases, a right-handed twist of each β strand results in a twist or curvature of the sheet.[10] The average length of a single β strand is six residues, about the diameter of an average globular domain (see below). Parallel and antiparallel sheets are equally common and represent about 15 percent of globular structure.[1] Parallel sheets are usually found in the interior of

ALPHA HELIX

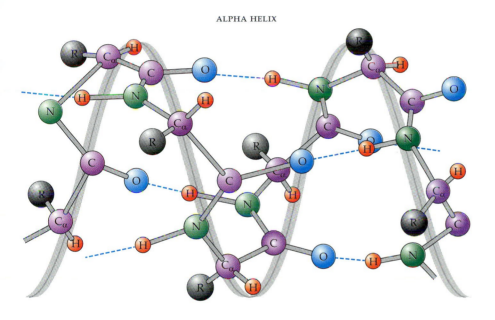

ANTIPARALLEL BETA SHEET

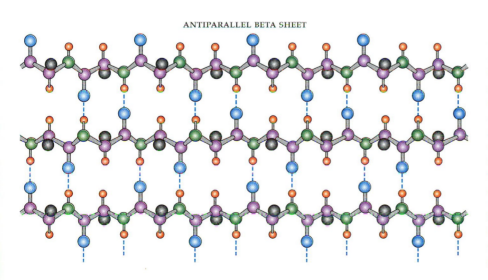

Figure 4 *As the chain of amino acids that makes up a protein is synthesized, regions of it fold spontaneously into α helices (a) and β sheets (b), which constitute the secondary structure; the helices and sheets are assembled in turn to create the tertiary structure. Both the α helix and the β sheet are stabilized by hydrogen bonds (broken colored lines), in which a hydrogen serves as a bridge between oxygen or nitrogen atoms.*

proteins, whereas antiparallel sheets are more often on the surface, with one side facing the interior and the other side the solvent.[6]

Another common feature of proteins is the reverse turn. A turn is composed of four successive residues, the first and the fourth of which are hydrogen-bonded to each other; the second and third are so configured as to reverse the direction of the peptide chain. It is possible to do this in more than one way, depending on the exact orientation of residues in the second and third positions of the turn. The most frequently observed turns are of two types. In type II turns, also known as glycine turns, position 3 must be occupied by glycine because any side chain larger than a hydrogen atom would come too close to the carbonyl oxygen at position 2, causing steric hindrance. In type I turns, or common turns, the carbonyl oxygen is pointed in the opposite direction (relative to the side chain at position 3) and thus does not interfere with the formation of the turn.

Until recently, all segments of the polypeptide chain that were not part of an α helix, a β sheet, or a reverse turn were considered to be nonordered. It is now recognized that even these irregular segments are far from random, although they may be less rigid in conformation than other secondary structures. Often these stretches of chain connect helices or β strands and have the form of loops of variable length. Whereas reverse turns comprise four or five residues, with the backbone groups tightly packed together and the side chains turned out, loops contain from six to 16 residues, with the side chains often packed within the interior of the loop. Loops whose ends are close together in space are referred to as omega loops.[11,12]

Both tight turns and loops are usually located on the surface of proteins. For this reason, in loops at least, the amino acid sequence tends to be less conserved among species than it is for residues in the interior of proteins. Moreover, surface loops may have greater mobility than the more constrained structures in the interior. In immunoglobulins, a cluster of surface loops having highly variable amino acid sequences provides the binding site for a range of different antigens.

CORRELATION OF PRIMARY AND SECONDARY STRUCTURE

Various methods are applied to correlate a primary sequence with secondary structure. Some of these methods are based on the statistical analysis of proteins in the data base of crystal structures.[1] Others are based on the study of synthetic polymers[13] or model peptides[14,15] in which a single position in the chain is filled in turn by each of the 20 amino acids. The tendency of the substituted peptide to form a helical structure in solution is then assessed by some physical measurement, such as a circular dichromism spectrum.

Although each amino acid is sometimes found in any of the secondary structures, depending both on the nearby sequence and to some extent on tertiary interactions,[16] each amino acid has a particular propensity to participate in forming an α helix, a β sheet, or reverse turns. For example, straight-chain aliphatic side chains such as those of alanine and leucine are strong helix promoters, whereas the bulky branched-chain aliphatics, such as valine and isoleucine, fit less easily into an α helix and prefer a β sheet conformation. Short polar residues, such as serine and aspartic acid, are frequently found in reverse turns. The hydroxyl group of serine and the side-chain carboxyl group of aspartate can hydrogen-bond to main-chain carbonyl or amino groups, thus interfering with helix formation.

Glycine is a strong helix breaker for a different reason. Because the α carbon atom is unsubstituted, there is unhindered rotation around the N-C_α and C_α-CO bonds. In thermodynamic terms, the unfolded state has more degrees of freedom or greater entropy, and so a greater price must be paid in free energy to confine a glycine residue to a position within an α helix than to confine another residue. Put more simply, glycine always provides a highly flexible link in the chain. Its lack of "handedness" around the α carbon gives it more conformational freedom. But in other positions, it may be present simply because its small size allows it to fit against bulkier residues in the protein interior, just as it does in the reverse turn.

Proline represents the converse case. Its side chain is locked into a ring structure that includes the α carbon, and so it has fewer conformational possibilities. It is frequently found in turns (but in position 2 rather than the position 3 of glycine), or in a rigid structure known as the proline helix (whose dimensions are different from those of an α helix). Occasionally proline is found within an α helix; in this setting, it causes a bend and destabilizes the structure by breaking hydrogen bonds.

As a result of the rapid progress in cloning new genes and sequencing the DNA, there are many more proteins whose primary sequence is known or has been inferred than there are proteins whose crystal structure has been determined. It has therefore become of great interest to be able to predict secondary, if not tertiary, structure from the sequence. No method is completely effective, because, as mentioned above, any amino acid can be found in any structure; however, several prediction methods have achieved considerable success.

The most widely applied program for predicting secondary structure from a primary sequence is that of Chou and Fasman.[17-19] It begins by searching the sequence for short stretches of helix-forming residues that might nucleate the formation of an α helix. Once a window of five or six residues containing three or more with a high helix-forming propensity has been found, the residues on each side of this nucleus are analyzed and the probable length of helix is determined. This method is from 60 to 70 percent successful in predicting the location of α helices. The longer the segment of predicted helix, the higher the probability that it is correct. A similar approach is taken to identify β strands and reverse turns. This kind of approach does not, however, take into account the fact that an individual amino acid tends to be found at a specific location within a given type of secondary structure.

Supersecondary Structure

It is now recognized that segments of α helix and β strand often combine in specific ways to form recurring structural motifs. One example is the helix-turn-helix motif found in many DNA-binding proteins [*see Figure 5*]. These include the protein that represses expression of genes of bacteriophage λ (the *cro* repressor),[20] a 68 kilodalton (kd) fragment of DNA polymerase I known as Klenow fragment,[21] the restriction endonuclease

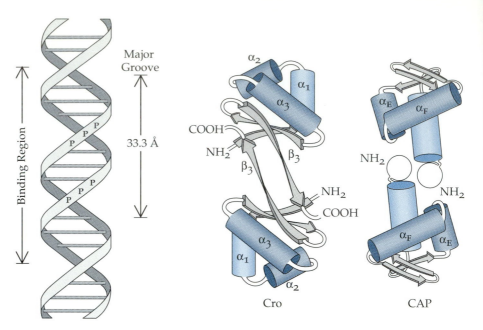

Figure 5 *Shown are the dimeric structures of two DNA-binding proteins with the helix-turn-helix motif in relation to the structure of double-stranded DNA (left). The two proteins are the repressor cro (middle) and the carboxyl-terminal domain of catabolite gene activator protein (CAP) (right). The two α-helices of each helix-turn-helix motif are shaded. In the foreground of each protein, labeled α3 or αF, is the recognition helix, which fits most closely into the major groove of the DNA. Note that the spacing between the two recognition helices of the dimer is very close to the 33.8-Å spacing between the DNA major grooves, but that the orientations of the helices relative to the major groove differ.*

*Eco*RI,[22] and *E. coli*'s catabolite activator protein (CAP)[23]—proteins that are otherwise dissimilar in structure.

The turn in this motif is not a reverse turn but rather a twist, which orients the axis of one helical segment almost perpendicular to the axis of the other. The pair of helices protrudes from the surface of the protein. One of the two helices fits into the DNA major groove at a particular site, the operator region. Specific contacts are made between the amino acid side chains of this helix and the bases within the groove. The other helix makes nonspecific contacts with the phosphodiester backbone of the DNA.[24]

Proteins containing this motif always bind to the DNA as protein dimers. The twofold axis of symmetry of the dimer aligns with the twofold axis of symmetry of the DNA sequence in the operator region, which is at the start of the gene; the helix on one half of the dimer binds to bases in one orientation, and the other half binds to bases with the opposite orientation. A similar two-helix figure is found in calcium-binding proteins, but in these proteins the peptide chain runs in the opposite direction.[25]

In a motif known as the Rossmann fold, three α helices alternate with three parallel β strands [*see Figure 6a*]. In dehydrogenases, two Rossmann folds are combined to form the binding site for the cofactor nicotinamide adenine dinucleotide (NAD).[1,5,26] This has turned out to be a general fold for binding mono- or dinucleotides; it is the most common fold observed in globular proteins.[6]

Another common motif is the four-helix bundle [*see Figure 6b*], in which four helices are connected head to tail, with loops or connecting segments of various lengths. The helices condense so that each lies adjacent to two others that run in the opposite direction; a cross-section of the four helices is roughly a square. One pair of helices is tilted with respect to the other pair, with an angle of about 18 degrees between them. Often the four helices approach one another most closely near one end of the bundle, diverging toward the other end. This divergence creates a natural pocket between the helices. Enzymes take advantage of this pocket to bind a cofactor (such as flavin in the case of cytochrome *c*), or to position catalytic groups. The specific sequence of amino acids within the helix is less important (within packing constraints) than the geometry of the catalytic pocket.

Tertiary Structure

Tertiary structure is the overall spatial arrangement of the polypeptide chain. It is specific and reproducible for each protein. To a first approximation, each molecule of the same sequence has the same spatial conformation. It is not self-evident how a soluble protein achieves its specific fold, but the result is a globular mass in which hydrophobic side chains form the central core, from which water is excluded, and more polar side chains favor the solvent-exposed surface.

The tertiary structure of a protein is defined by the spatial coordinates of the individual atoms. Two methods for determining these coordinates are currently available: x-ray crystallography and nuclear magnetic resonance (NMR). NMR has the advantage of being applicable to protein molecules in solution, but so far it is applicable only for proteins up to about 15 kd in size.[27] Both methods are complex and time-consuming, but

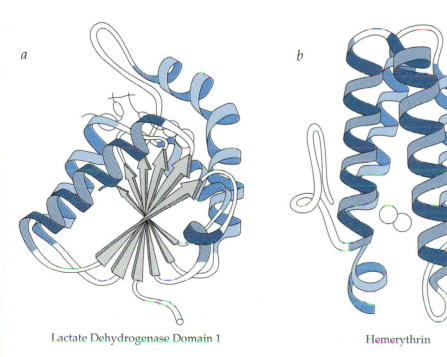

a

b

Lactate Dehydrogenase Domain 1

Hemerythrin

Figure 6 *Schematic drawings of the polypeptide backbones of two proteins illustrate the Rossmann fold (a) and the four-helix bundle (b).*

progress has been made in both fields to speed up the process.[28] A database (the Brookhaven PDB) has been established in which new sets of coordinates are filed and become available by computer access.[29] The list of available structures is updated on a quarterly basis. As of October 1993, approximately 575 structures had been made available, and probably twice that number had been filed but not yet released. Perhaps a third of these represent completely different structures.

Representing a tertiary structure so that it can be readily visualized is a problem. The most accurate method is to build a physical scale model, but this is very laborious. Computer programs have been written to simulate three-dimensional structure, but these are costly to run and have a major disadvantage: it is difficult to see the interior of the structure.

Often one wants to visualize the overall fold of a chain, or the way particular segments of secondary structure relate to each other. The so-called ribbon drawings first introduced by Jane Richardson are particularly valuable for this purpose.[30,31] They allow one to see structural relations among different proteins without getting lost in the complexity of details.

The great challenge in the study of protein structure at present is to predict the fold of a protein segment from its amino acid sequence. It is now evident that a characteristic fold may often be conserved in proteins that show very little overall sequence homology. For example, the myoglobin chain and the two hemoglobin chains (see below) fold into very similar looking structures, even though only 24 out of 141 residues are conserved among the three chains when sperm whale myoglobin is compared with human hemoglobin.[2] Efforts are under way to write computer algorithms to describe these folds for proteins of known structure so that tertiary homologies can be found, but these programs are still at the developmental stage.[32] A promising new method called the profile method has recently been developed.[33,34] Two or more proteins must already be known to be related structurally. Their sequences are aligned, and each residue is assigned a position along the chain. The probability of each of the 20 amino acids occupying that position is calculated, taking into account the rates of mutation of any one amino acid into another. If the crystal structure is known, the calculation can be refined to include information about the secondary structure at each position and whether each residue is found inside or outside the reference protein. This so-called profile can then be aligned with sequences of unknown tertiary structure to see whether they are compatible with the fold of the known structure.

A rapid new method has been developed for comparing the three-dimensional structures of different proteins once the coordinates are known by superimposing one structure on another and analyzing the differences at different resolutions. When the method was used to compare all pairs of structures in the Brookhaven PDB, it revealed a striking similarity in fold between two families of proteins whose relationship had not previously been guessed: the globins, such as hemoglobin, and the DNA-binding portion of certain bacteriophage repressors.[35] This kind of information has been compiled in a new database that groups proteins of known structure into families of common folds.[36]

PROTEIN DOMAINS

In the x-ray structures of globular proteins it is often possible to see regions that are physically somewhat detached from one another, connected only by a single thread of polypeptide. These regions appear to fold independently of one another and are known as folding domains.[37]

Large, complex proteins seem to have evolved through the combining of domains whose size is of the order of 100 amino acid residues. For example, many proteins have a motif that is homologous to the single domain of epidermal growth factor (EGF), a protein that promotes the growth of skin cells and whose three-dimensional structure in solution is known.[38] Blood coagulation factors IX and X incorporate this pattern,[39] as does the low-density lipoprotein (LDL) receptor.[40] Notch, a large membrane-spanning protein required for neuronal differentiation in *Drosophila* (which is believed to interact with surface proteins on other cells to promote cell-to-cell communication), contains 36 consecutive extracellular so-called EGF repeats, each with a unique sequence but with homology to EGF and a conserved pattern of disulfide bonds.[41] The human homologue of the Notch gene, TAN-1, is broken by translocations in some T cell neoplasms, suggesting that the wild-type protein may play a role in normal lymphoid development.[42]

Analysis of the genomic DNA sequence of some of these extracellular and cell-surface proteins has revealed that each repeated motif is encoded by an individual exon, a DNA sequence that is directly translated into a peptide sequence. Exons are set off by intervening sequences, or introns, which are spliced out of the RNA before it is translated and so are not represented in the final protein sequence. The purpose of introns is still unclear, but one consequence may be greater diversity in protein structure [*see Chapter 2*]. It has been postulated that the evolution of complex proteins has occurred by a process termed exon shuffling.[43] Unfortunately, the pattern of introns observed does not always fit this hypothesis neatly. If introns were present at the onset of evolution, it must have been possible to lose them, and also to move them along the genome by "drift." Another school of thought suggests that introns may have been introduced later in the evolution of the protein by viruses or by mobile genetic elements called transposons.[44,45] These hypotheses to account for the origin of introns are not necessarily mutually exclusive.

It has become apparent that the number of unique overall folds that proteins assume is relatively small. It has been estimated that the global number of exons from which all existing protein domains have been derived is somewhere between 1,000 and 7,000.[46] All contemporary proteins have presumably been derived from a small number of original ones, and thus far probably only a small number of the numerous conformational possibilities have been sampled. On the other hand, examples of convergent evolution are known.[47] In some cases, sequence homology between two proteins with related folding patterns is so weak that it is not possible to say whether they shared a common ancestor or evolved independently to a common solution of a functional problem.

Protein domains have been classified into four categories according to their content of secondary structure.[7,48]

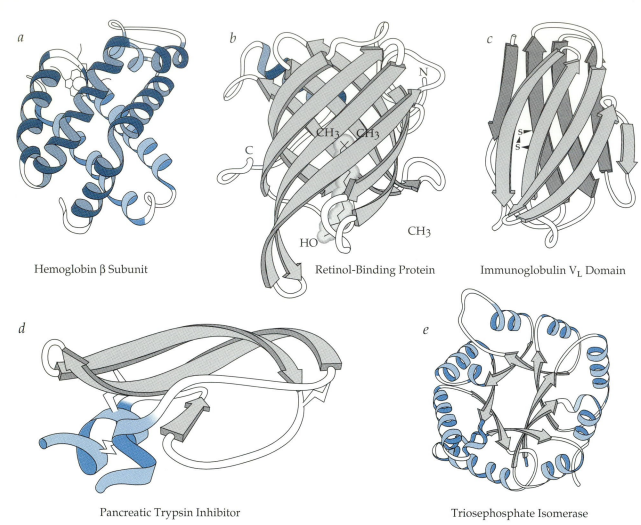

a

Hemoglobin β Subunit

b

N

CH₃   CH₃

C

HO   CH₃

Retinol-Binding Protein

c

S
S

Immunoglobulin V_L Domain

d

Pancreatic Trypsin Inhibitor

e

Triosephosphate Isomerase

Figure 7 *The four categories into which protein domains are classified are all-α domains (a), all-β domains (b), including Greek-key barrels (c), α + β domains (d), and α/β domains (e).*

1. All-α domains contain only the α helix [*see Figure 7a*]. They include the single domains of cytochrome *c*, parvalbumin, myoglobin, and hemerythrin, and the four subunits of hemoglobin. Helices have the general shape of cylinders, and pack together around a central core, with one face of each helix in the interior of the protein, and one face exposed to solvent. The arrangement can usually be described by a polyhedron in which the helices are aligned along the ribs of the figure.[7,49]

2. All-β domains, made up almost exclusively of β sheets, are of two different types. In proteins such as chymotrypsin or retinol-binding protein, β strands are connected by tight turns so that each strand alternates in direction with its immediate neighbors and moreover follows the frequently observed rule that near-neighbors in a primary sequence tend to be found spatially close in the tertiary fold. The result is a two-sheet or β-barrel structure [*see Figure 7b*]. Other all-β domains, known as Greek-key β barrels and represented by superoxide dis-

mutase and the immunoglobulins, do not follow this spatial rule [*see Figure 7c*]. It has been postulated that they arose by the collapse of an extended single β strand folded back on itself.[25]

3. Domains termed α + β have both the α helix and the β sheet, with the two types of secondary structure segregated along the chain. Examples are carbonic anhydrase, cytochrome b_5, ribonuclease, and bovine pancreatic trypsin inhibitor [*see Figure 7d*].

4. In α/β domains, α helices and β strands alternate along the chain. An example would be the Rossmann fold described above. In addition, there is a family of proteins known as α/β barrel proteins, of which the first example was triosephosphate isomerase, an enzyme involved in the metabolism of glucose. Some 17 proteins with this structure are now known. They include functionally diverse enzymes such as pyruvate kinase, enolase, and tryptophan synthetase *a*. The common structural feature is a circular barrel with parallel β strands running through the center and α helices on the outside [*see Figure 7e*]. It is suggested that all members have evolved from a common ancestor.[50]

Domains seem to have functional as well as structural significance. In enzymes, the active site is commonly partitioned between domains: one domain may bind a specific cofactor and an adjacent domain the substrate. Enzymes that function with a metal cofactor, such as the zinc-requiring enzyme carboxypeptidase,[51] display such architecture. This observation supports the idea that proteins have been built up on a modular basis.

TOPOLOGY OF THE PROTEIN SURFACE

The surface of a globular protein plays a critical role in its activity because it is the surface that interacts with other molecules, whether small substrates or other proteins. These interactions are always very specific: the protein surface has been selected to fit its binding partners. An enzyme not only brings reactive substrates into close proximity but also often discriminates among closely related substances. In addition, reactive side chains, such as acids or bases, are positioned on the surface in a precise geometry with respect to substrates, enabling them to facilitate electron transfers or in some cases to accept a reactive group as an intermediate.

In addition to enzyme substrates, a great variety of other small molecules bind to specific proteins. Some are regulators of enzyme activity. Others are extracellular ligands that, by binding to a cell-surface receptor, set off a cascade of reactions within the cell, eventually triggering a transcriptional change in the nucleus that leads to a new pattern of protein expression. Receptors such as those that bind adrenergic mediators typify this group of proteins.

In the case of enzymes, the substrate-binding sites are generally found in a pocket or cleft of the surface. The surface involution not only permits more extensive contacts between the protein surface and the substrates but also provides a local environment from which solvent can readily be excluded. Moreover, within a pocket a relatively small movement of amino acid side chains can have a large effect on the reactants. Such motion can result in an induced fit that favors the geometry of the transition state.

Quaternary Structure

Enzymes are frequently made up of subunits each of which is an individual polypeptide chain. The quaternary structure is defined by the arrangement of these monomeric subunits in the oligomeric complex. The subunits often can assume different conformations depending on their mode of association with one another; the reactivity of the complex therefore depends on the subunits' interactions. The equilibrium between the different states can be shifted by the binding of small molecules to one or more of the subunits. Small changes in the structure of one subunit are thus transmitted to the other subunits in the oligomeric complex and thereby amplified, often with dramatic changes in function. A comparison of the properties of myoglobin, an all α-helical protein, with hemoglobin, a protein comprising four myoglobinlike subunits, illustrates this point.

The folding of the eight α-helical regions in myoglobin creates a hydrophobic pocket for the almost flat heme group. A ferrous (Fe^{2+}) ion is held in the center of the heme group, but just outside the plane of the heme, by its coordination to the four pyrrole rings in heme and to a histidine residue sticking out from one of the α helices, the F helix.[52] The structure of the deoxy- form of myoglobin is relatively constrained. When an oxygen molecule binds to the ferrous ion on the side of the heme opposite the histidine residue, the electronic state of the iron changes and it moves into the plane of the heme group. This movement, which is less than 1Å, is transmitted through the histidine to the F helix. The subsequent movement of this helix disrupts hydrogen bonds and other interactions in various parts of the molecule, and the structure becomes less constrained. The chain of events is reversed when the oxygen molecule leaves myoglobin.

In hemoglobin, the four myoglobinlike subunits occupy the four corners of a tetrahedron and are held together by many interactions between residues on opposite surfaces of the subunits. Hemoglobin exists in two widely different quaternary packing arrangements, the deoxy- and oxy-forms. In the absence of oxygen, the ferrous ion in each of the four separate heme groups lies (as in myoglobin) out of the plane of the group. The structure of each deoxyhemoglobin chain is (as in myoglobin) quite constrained, and the affinity for O_2 is low. As a consequence, it is rather difficult for the first oxygen molecule to enter one of the heme pockets. The entry and binding of this first oxygen molecule, however, has the same effect as the binding of oxygen to myoglobin: the ferrous ion moves, taking with it the F helix, and the structure is loosened.

These structural changes in a single protomer have additional effects in the tetrameric hemoglobin molecule. Here the interaction among subunits strongly favors a state in which all subunits are in either the deoxy- or the oxy- form. An equilibrium exists between the deoxy- form of the tetramer and the oxy- form. In the absence of O_2, the equilibrium strongly favors the deoxy- form. On the other hand, bound O_2 stabilizes the oxy-form of each monomer, and so the binding of even one O_2 pulls the equilibrium between the tetrameric forms toward the oxy- form. Because the oxy- form has a higher affinity for oxygen, the second oxygen molecule can bind more easily to its heme group than the first one could.

The sigmoid shape of the oxygen-binding curve of hemoglobin reflects these "cooperative" interactions.

The binding of a small organic ion, 2,3-diphosphoglycerate, to deoxy-hemoglobin provides additional stability to this form and ensures that its oxygen-binding curve is in the appropriate range of oxygen tension to allow hemoglobin to bind oxygen in the lungs and release it in the tissues.[53]

A change in conformation that leads to a shift in equilibrium between two oligomeric forms, thus amplifying the change, is known as an allosteric transition. It is usually initiated by the binding of a small effector molecule, such as oxygen or diphosphoglycerate in the case of hemoglobin.

It has become apparent that many complex biochemical reactions are carried out by oligomeric protein complexes. For example, the replication of DNA requires a large number of different enzymatic functions. Some seven different proteins that take part in this process have been identi-fied,[54,55] and at least 20 proteins are isolated as a complex; clearly, they are in tight association in the cell. Similarly, signal-transduction pathways may involve large complexes of proteins. For example, the interleukin-2 receptor in activated T cells seems to be an oligomeric protein with a number of different polypeptide chains whose particular functions are as yet unknown. In fact, the distinction between an oligomeric protein and an organelle becomes blurred as soon as one permits the association of other chemical components, such as lipid or nucleic acid. For example, the various proteins associated with ribosomes are organized in a spatially defined and specific way, and this is undoubtedly true for membrane-as-sociated complexes as well, in spite of the relative fluidity of the lipid bilayer. Much future work will undoubtedly focus on understanding these complex structural relations.

Forces Stabilizing the Tertiary Fold

All globular domains have in common the property of being tightly packed. Evidently the conformational structure of the folded polypeptide is stabilized by the exclusion of water from the surface of hydrophobic side chains. Nonpolar chains therefore tend to fold into the core of a globular protein, with the charged (and uncharged but polar) residues on the outside, in contact with the aqueous solvent. This so-called hydropho-bic interaction is the most important factor in holding a protein in its native conformation.[56]

Amino acid residues have been ranked according to their hydrophobic tendency. A thermodynamic scale can be obtained by measuring the partition of a particular amino acid between water and some organic solvent chosen to mimic the interior of the protein. Alternatively, a scale can be constructed based on knowledge of the crystallographic data base. The hydrophobicity scale of Kyte and Doolittle[57] is frequently used to analyze protein sequences of unknown three-dimensional structure. For example, a sequence of 19 to 22 residues of high hydrophobicity indicates the presence of a membrane-spanning segment of polypeptide.

Occasionally, a charged residue is found in the interior of a protein. It is nearly always paired, however, with another residue of opposite charge to form a so-called ion pair or salt bridge. These structures stabilize the conformation through electrostatic attraction. Statistically, the contribution of ion pairs to conformational stability is small, but in individual cases an ion pair may make an important contribution to stability.[58]

Residues such as serine, threonine, asparagine, and glutamine are polar although they carry no net charge. These residues are able to participate in hydrogen bonds. In serine, for example, the oxygen of the hydroxyl group has a partial negative charge and the hydrogen has a partial positive charge. This hydrogen can form a bridge with another oxygen, such as a main-chain carbonyl oxygen, which also has a partial negative charge. Simultaneously, a hydrogen from an amide or amino group can share the extra pair of electrons on the oxygen atom, thus forming a second hydrogen bond. An analysis of structures in the database[59] revealed that most hydrogen bonds that can be formed are in fact present. Each one contributes only a little energy of stabilization to the protein, because for each intraprotein hydrogen bond formed, a hydrogen bond with water is broken. There are so many hydrogen bonds, however, that the cumulative effect can be large.

Disulfide bonds (between the sulfur atoms of two cysteine residues) play an obvious role in stabilizing the structure of some proteins. They are particularly prevalent in small extracellular proteins, such as peptide hormones, and in the extracellular domains of membrane-bound proteins. In one experiment, extra disulfide bonds have been introduced into T4 lysozyme, whose crystal structure is known, at positions where little or no strain should result from the disulfide bridge.[60] A comparison of the stability of these mutant proteins with the wild-type protein shows that each disulfide bond can contribute as much as 20 kcal of stability to the protein.[60] A more usual figure, however, is 3 to 5 kcal.

Packing arrangements are critically important because solvent is almost entirely excluded from the interior of a globular protein. How the packing of side chains contributes to the folded structure is under active investigation from both a theoretical and an experimental point of view.[61,62]

The difference in free energy between the folded and unfolded forms of a protein is very small compared with the total energy of the molecule.[63] For this reason, changes in conformation can occur without much energy cost or gain, and these changes are readily reversible. This quasi-stability of protein conformation gives rise to a structure that is in constant fluctuation. In some cases, movement akin to Brownian motion plays an essential role in the function of the protein. For example, movement of the hemoglobin chain enables oxygen to gain access to the heme group, which is otherwise buried in the hydrophobic interior of the protein.[64] In a sense, the hemoglobin molecule breathes.

Some enzymes show larger conformational changes. Kinases, for example, bind their substrates, ATP and a phosphate acceptor, to two separate domains linked by a hinge region. When the substrates bind, these domains rotate with respect to each other, bringing the substrates closer together within the cleft between the two domains. In the case of phosphoglycerate kinase, this rotation amounts to 7.7°.[65] This mechanical action involving the whole protein is made possible by the relative rigidity of α helices. Proteins containing only β sheet are more flexible and tend to convert binding energy into mechanical action that affects more local regions of the polypeptide chain. The secondary structure of a particular protein must have been selected to meet the mechanical needs of its catalytic function. It has been postulated that mechanical action is a fundamental cause of the catalytic rate enhancement achieved by enzymes and may be a reason for the large size of most enzymes.[66]

Amphiphilic Sequences

The pattern of hydrophobic and hydrophilic residues along a particular stretch of sequence is often a valuable clue to both the secondary structure and its tertiary interactions. For example, a β strand that has a strictly alternating pattern of hydrophobic and hydrophilic residues is likely to be found on the surface of a protein, with the hydrophobic side chains oriented toward the interior. A sequence in which the polar side chains face in one direction and the nonpolar ones in another is called amphiphilic.

Helices as well as β strands are often amphiphilic. An α helix can be analyzed by means of a so-called helical wheel [*see Figure 8a*]. In many proteins, clustered hydrophobic residues on one side of such a wheel indicate a surface that interacts with another helix or that faces the protein core or the lipid components of a membrane.[67]

A classic example is the leucine zipper structure[68] [*see Figure 8b*] found in such proteins as the nuclear oncoproteins Jun and Fos, which combine to form a heterodimer pair. Leucine, with its long aliphatic side chain, is an essential component of a stretch of helix on the surface of each protein. The leucine residues are distributed along the chain so that their side chains extend out from the same side of the helix. The hydrophobic side chains on one protein pack against hydrophobic side chains on the surface of the other protein. It has been shown that the helices of Fos and Jun are aligned in a parallel orientation to form a coiled coil.[69] An adjacent domain of each protein binds to a regulatory sequence of DNA.

The Process of Protein Folding

The mechanism by which a nascent protein chain folds into the proper conformation is not completely understood at this time, but it is clear that the factors controlling the process must be closely related to those that determine the final structure.

From the now classic work of Anfinsen,[70,71] it has been known for some time that the primary sequence of amino acids contains sufficient information to direct the folding process to the biologically active conformation, at least for small, globular, single-domain proteins that are not covalently modified after folding. When RNase A was denatured and reduced in urea and later refolded under oxidizing conditions, protein with the activity of the native enzyme was recovered. This result was later confirmed with chemically synthesized ribonuclease.[72,73] The folding and unfolding transitions were identical, showing that the pathway of folding was fully reversible. The active, folded protein therefore represented an equilibrium state that had the lowest free energy attainable under the conditions tested.

Reversibility has held true for all unprocessed single-domain proteins studied to date. The transition between unfolded and folded states is cooperative. Usually only two states have been seen, but in a few cases an intermediate can be detected: the so-called molten globule state, which is discussed below.[74] More complex transitions are expected for multidomain proteins. (A domain is defined here as a contiguous stretch of amino acid residues that folds into a compact structure and that can be physically distinguished from other regions of the protein by visual inspection of the x-ray structure.)

The test of reversibility does not work for proteins that are modified after folding. Many of the peptide hormones are synthesized as extended polypeptide chains that are later cleaved proteolytically to form the mature protein. Preproinsulin folds reversibly, but the shorter mature protein, which consists of two separate polypeptide chains joined by disulfide bonds, does not.[75] Proteases such as subtilisin and α-lytic protease are also synthesized as inactive precursors, which cannot degrade them-

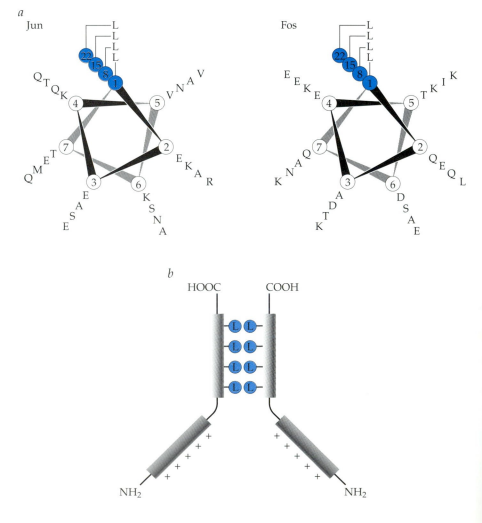

Figure 8 (a) Shown are the helical wheel regions of the nuclear oncoproteins Jun and Fos. Because there are about 3.5 amino acids per helical turn, each seventh amino acid is in register; the residues labeled 1, 8, 15, and 22 are all leucines. These hydrophobic leucines are on one face of the helix and charged amino acids on the other, endowing the helix with an amphiphilic character. The two helices interact with each other to form a so-called leucine zipper (b). Leucine residues 1, 8, 15, and 22 occupy position d as described in the text; residue 5 occupies position a. In a dimeric coiled coil, leucine is favored at position d and branched-chain amino acids (e.g., the valines in Jun) at position a.

selves or prematurely degrade other proteins. It has been shown that the propeptide sequence of each one plays a role in the correct folding of the active protein.[76,77] Propeptide added back to the mature protein permits reversible folding.

As pointed out above, for a small single-domain protein in dilute solution, folding occurs spontaneously and is under thermodynamic control. It is not certain, however, whether the spontaneously folded structure always represents the global free-energy minimum. (Most attempts to calculate protein structure by energy minimization have failed for technical reasons.[78]) It is possible to imagine that a particular structure, such as one containing a polypeptide knot, might be more stable than the observed structure but is almost impossible to achieve because of the high energy of activation of the folding process. This is equivalent to saying that there is a kinetic barrier. In the case of α-lytic protease, the propeptide accelerates the rate-limiting step in the folding of the mature protein by a factor of 10^7. Without this propeptide, the correctly folded form of the mature protein is not kinetically accessible, even though it is thermodynamically stable.[77]

For a protein to sample all the conformations possible as a result of the allowed rotations in each amino acid residue along the chain would require an almost infinite amount of time.[79] Yet a protein folds within seconds. There must, then, be folding intermediates.

Models of Protein Folding

Currently, two models for the mechanism by which a protein folds explain different sets of observations. These models are not necessarily incompatible, but they have not yet been brought together in a unified theory.

The first of these is the so-called framework model.[80] It is based on the idea that short regions of polypeptide with a propensity to form secondary structure fluctuate rapidly between structured and unstructured forms. When two elements of α helix or β sheet interact through favorable tertiary contacts, they stabilize each other. For example, in native bovine pancreatic trypsin inhibitor, there are three disulfide bonds. One of these, linking Cys 31 with Cys 50, joins a segment of α helix with a segment of β strand. Two synthetic peptides representing the separate sequences of the two segments show no evidence of secondary structure by circular dichroism. However, if they are joined by oxidation of the cysteines to form a heterodimer, α-helical structure can be detected.[81] This finding supports the notion that elements of secondary structure can stabilize each other.

The second model is based on the observed properties of the molten globule intermediates that are found at equilibrium in a few special cases of protein unfolding/folding reactions. These intermediates are compact as judged by hydrodynamic measurements, but the side chains have considerable mobility.[82-87] Appreciable secondary structure already appears to be present. It is not yet clear exactly what this structure is, however, or whether—as suggested in the model—all proteins go through a similar state in the process of folding.

From Sequence to Folding

New insight into how amino acid sequence determines the final fold of a protein comes from the recent synthesis of novel polypeptide chains. To test the ability to predict the tertiary fold from sequence, several groups have now synthesized polypeptide chains predicted to form four-helix bundles, starting in each case with a sequence that lacks homology to any known proteins.[88,89] Each helix in the bundle was designed to be amphiphilic so that the helices would interact with each other. Indeed, they do appear to fold as predicted.

Protein Folding in the Cell

The preceding paragraphs have outlined what is known about how protein molecules fold into an active conformation in dilute solution in vitro. Within the living cell, however, there are additional constraints on the process. To start with, the space is very limited and highly compartmentalized; the aqueous phase is far from dilute! Second, the precise timing of any step in the folding process is critical. Unfolded proteins have a great tendency to aggregate, especially in concentrated solution. The nascent peptide chain must therefore be kept in an unfolded state so that it will not misfold or aggregate before its synthesis is complete and before correct folding to the active conformation can occur. In some cases, folding must be further delayed until the protein has been transported into the proper organelle, a process that may involve threading it through a membrane.

It is now known that folding is mediated by a series of proteins called chaperones.[90,91] These are highly conserved proteins found universally, in both eukaryotic and prokaryotic cells. Some were first identified as proteins that are induced to high levels when cells are exposed to high temperature, but these so-called heat-shock proteins are now known to be expressed constitutively as well and to be essential for growth at any temperature. Homologous proteins in *E. coli*, first identified as cellular proteins required for replication of bacteriophage λ, have been called chaperonins.

There are two broad classes of these proteins, the Hsp70 class and the Hsp60 class. The Hsp70 proteins (DnaK and DnaJ in *E. coli*) are monomeric or dimeric proteins that bind to the newly synthesized, unfolded peptide chains to prevent misfolding or aggregation. In eukaryotes, Hsp70 is also needed to keep proteins competent for import into such organelles as mitochondria. In contrast, Hsp60 (GroEl in *E. coli*) is an oligomeric protein built from two rings, each formed by seven monomers. Hsp60 seems to stabilize partially folded proteins in a more compact state that may be akin to the molten-globule state discussed above.

Recently, a chaperone-mediated folding pathway has been reconstituted in vitro with chaperonins purified from *E. coli*.[92,93] In this system, the denatured protein binds first to DnaK in an extended conformation. When a second chaperone, DnaJ, is added, the folding peptide assumes a more compact configuration. It is transferred from the DnaK/DnaJ complex to one involving GroEl and a second protein, GroES. The transfer is accompanied by the hydrolysis of ATP and requires an additional protein factor, GrpE. Further condensation of the folding peptide presumably takes place on the surface of the GroEl/ES complex. ATP is required again for the release of the fully folded peptide.

GroEl can carry out more than one cycle in the refolding of the model protein rhodenase, and thus behaves like a catalyst. The fact that this pathway parallels the in vitro refolding pathway in the absence of chaperone factors suggests that it may truly reflect the in vivo process.

Supramolecular Structure: Fibrous Proteins

Beyond the level of quaternary structure as it applies to soluble proteins is the polymerization of protein monomers to form insoluble aggregates. Polymeric fibrous proteins are the building blocks for the cytoskeleton, which gives the cell its shape and organizes many of its components. Outside the cell, the fibrous proteins form the extracellular matrix, which is responsible for tissue organization. In this context, a "monomer" may be a single polypeptide chain, but it is more often itself an oligomeric protein, referred to as a protomer.

Polymerization of monomers is a process more akin to crystallization than to the folding of globular protein chains. It begins with a slow association of a few monomers (nucleation), which is followed by the spontaneous rapid addition of more monomeric units. For this kind of polymerization to occur, there must be surface regions on each monomer that are mutually complementary. The nucleation step occurs only at a critical protein concentration.[94-96] Actin[94] and tubulin[97-99] are examples of globular proteins that self-aggregate in this way. Sickle cell hemoglobin is another well-studied example.[100]

Other classes of fibrous proteins have very special primary sequences that promote intertwining of two or more peptide chains to increase the tensile strength of individual fibrils. These sequences are repetitive, and the monomers that result are highly extended. In collagen, the most abundant protein in vertebrates and the major component of connective tissue, three strands intertwine to form a triple helix. In myosin and tropomyosin, two parallel α helices intertwine to form a coiled coil structure. Three-stranded coiled coils also exist: fibrinogen[101] and laminin[102] are heterotrimers containing three-stranded coiled coils, and the gp17 tail fiber of bacteriophage T7 is a homotrimer.[103] A four-stranded coiled coil has been found in fibrous proteins secreted by insects.[104] These proteins usually have globular domains at the ends of the helices and polymerize into large, insoluble aggregates. Posttranslational modification and cross-linking between monomers are common.

Each of these systems is very complex. The regulation of the polymerization is only poorly understood at this time. In most cases determination of a precise three-dimensional structure has been elusive because of the insolubility of the fibers and the difficulty of obtaining crystals. However, the cloning of genes has provided information on the variations of sequence tolerated by each system and on the function of different domains.

Proteins representative of the three classes of structure will be described only very briefly here.

Actin and Tubulin

Actin and tubulin are globular proteins that polymerize to form fibers involved in cellular structure and movement. Actin is a major constituent of muscle fibers; tubulin is the major component of microtubules, which form the spindle body that directs the movement of chromosomes during mitosis; both actin and tubulin are found in the cytoskeleton of cells (along with the so-called intermediate filaments and various other proteins). Actin and tubulin also play similar molecular roles: each provides a supporting structure against which an energy-producing molecular motor moves. In the case of actin, the motor is myosin; in the case of tubulin, the motor is either dynein or kinesin.

The polymerization of both actin and tubulin is a reversible process. This is important physiologically, because it enables the cell to reorganize its cytoskeleton almost instantaneously in response to changes in the cell cycle.

Each monomer of actin or tubulin is asymmetric, and so the fibers they form have polarity. Movement occurs in one direction only. Myosin moves toward the (+) end of fibrous actin; dynein moves toward the (–) end of microtubules and kinesin toward the (+) end.

Monomeric actin has been crystallized as a complex with ATP and bovine pancreatic DNase I,[105] and the structure has been determined to 2.8 Å resolution. The actin monomer has two domains, with ATP and Ca^{2+} binding in a cleft between them. The atomic structure of ADP-actin determined from this complex was used to construct a model of filamentous actin that explains earlier 10 Å-resolution x-ray data obtained from fibers oriented in a capillary tube.[106] It shows a two-stranded helix stabilized by extensive hydrophobic interactions between each monomer and those above and below it on the same strand and by a loop that intercalates with residues of the opposing strand, forming a dense hydrophobic plug. Residues known to be involved in binding to myosin form a patch on the outside of the helical filament.

An open-ended F-actin filament contains thousands of actin protomers. This is a direct consequence of the fact that nucleation has a much less favorable equilibrium than does fiber elongation. To a first approximation, actin follows the theory of polymer self-assembly based on an equilibrium between the pool of monomers and the growing chains.[94] Likewise, tubulin assembles by self-polymerization of α,β dimers (two almost identical monomers) into threadlike protofilaments, which in turn associate to form hollow microtubules. The dynamic properties of these polymers cannot, however, be fully described by simple equilibria.

The rate of polymerization in each case is enhanced by the binding of other proteins, but none of these is required for polymerization to occur. Gelsolin speeds the nucleation step in actin polymerization.[107] Microtubule-associated proteins MAP1, MAP2, and tau probably enhance tubulin polymerization by stabilizing structures already formed.[99] They also affect the form of the aggregate. Tubulin can aggregate into a variety of structures. MAPs, as well as polycations and such basic proteins as histones, favor a ring-shaped structure in vitro. The role of these various forms of tubulin is not understood at this time.

The polymerization process involves the hydrolysis of a nucleotide triphosphate that accompanies the addition of each monomeric unit to the growing chain. The actin monomer binds ATP, which is hydrolysed on polymerization; hydrolysis of tightly bound guanosine triphosphate (GTP) accompanies the addition of each tubulin monomer to the growing microtubule. Somewhat surprisingly, however, in both actin and tubulin the hydrolysis of the triphosphate is not tightly coupled to the addition of monomer but lags behind it.[108] Indeed, under special conditions globular actin, or G actin, can assemble into filaments in the total absence of nucleotide; clearly, the energy for polymerization is not derived from the hydrolysis.

Both of these polymerizations have been studied extensively in vitro in an effort to understand the role of the nucleotide. For both actin and tubulin, when the nucleotide bound to monomer is in the diphosphate form, the critical concentration for polymerization is much higher than when the bound nucleotide is in the triphosphate form. This implies a difference in conformation of the protein monomer that affects the nucleation step. As a consequence, monomers added nearly always have nucleotide bound as triphosphate. Only subsequently does the nucleotide undergo hydrolysis and the protein monomer change its conformation.

In the presence of nucleotide, both actin and tubulin monomers exchange with polymer at steady state in a process referred to as treadmilling.[109,110] The kinetics of this process have been hard to explain. Recently developed techniques have now made it possible to trace the polymerization and depolymerization of individual filaments by direct visualization,[111,112] and this has led to a model for the monomer exchange. Individual nucleated tubulin filaments can be seen to alternate between periods of growth and rapid breakdown. It is thought that the last monomer added, with its bound nucleotide still in the triphosphate form, forms a cap. When occasionally the GTP diffuses off, the structure behind it is destabilized. A phase transition occurs, accompanied by rapid depolymerization, until the chain is once again capped. This abrupt transition is known as catastrophe, and its reversal has been termed rescue.[113]

The random alternation between elongation and rapid shortening gives rise to dynamic instability, a process believed to be biologically important in the rapid assembly and disassembly of microtubules during mitosis and meiosis.[113,114] It has been postulated that the shifts between polymer and monomer states of the mitotic spindle provide the free energy required to move chromosomes during mitosis,[115,116] but other proteins are likely to be needed as well.

Collagen

Collagen performs a function entirely different from that of tubulin or actin. Its primary role is to provide strong but elastic structure. Actually, collagen is a family of closely related proteins, of which 14 types have thus far been distinguished.[117] All of them are extracellular proteins, built to last. Polymerization into fibrils, which occurs only after carefully regulated secretion of the protomer, is irreversible, because the fibrils are insoluble.

All collagens share a common, unique element of structure: the triple helix, in which three separate polypeptide chains are tightly interwound. The collagen protomer is actually a polypeptide trimer. Formation of the triple helix depends on very stringent sequence constraints. When the three strands intertwine, the side chain of every third residue of each chain is oriented toward the interior of the compound helix. This is sterically possible only if glycine occupies that position. Therefore, every third residue of each chain must be glycine, and the glycine residues on the three strands must be staggered along the triple helix. Mutation of even a single glycine can prevent folding and cause the procollagen to remain in a gelatinlike conformation. Along with any normal but unpolymerized chains, it is then degraded in a process referred to as procollagen suicide. Such dominant negative mutations can cause severe, even lethal, disorders, such as so-called brittle bone disease, or osteogenesis imperfecta.[118]

Proline and hydroxyproline (which is formed by posttranslational modification of proline) account for a large percent of the other two residues in collagen's reiterated sequence, Gly-X-Y. They add rigidity to the structure and extend the pitch of the triple helix (since steric hindrance would prevent closer packing). The synthetic polymer poly-L-proline forms a single helix in solution that has dimensions very similar to those of the individual collagen strands. With glycine at every third position, however, such a single-stranded helix would not be stable. There are no hydrogen bonds within the so-called proline helix; the helical structure is the result of steric repulsion between the pyrrolidone rings and the relatively low entropy of the unfolded state. In the collagen triple helix, hydrogen bonds likewise form not between amide groups on the same chain (as in an α helix) but rather between chains, thereby stabilizing the triple-helical structure. The hydroxy groups of 4-hydroxyproline further stabilize the triple helix in some way not yet understood. Without them, helix formation does not occur at physiologic temperatures.

The three strands of a collagen helix do not need to be identical in sequence; indeed, in several of the common types of collagen, two gene products are combined. For example, type I collagen, found in skin, tendon, bone, and cornea, contains two strands of one kind ($\alpha 1$) and one strand ($\alpha 2$) having a different sequence. A collagen type is fully described by its Roman numeral along with the stoichiometry of the different chains, indicated by a subscript. The composition of type I collagen is given by the formula $[\alpha 1(I)]_2 \alpha 2$; type II collagen, found in cartilage and some other tissues and comprising three identical chains, is described as $[\alpha 1(II)]_3$. The different types of collagen structure and their distribution have been reviewed elsewhere.[119,120]

The different collagen chains vary in length as well as in sequence. In the most abundant fibrillar collagens, each of the three intertwined polypeptide chains is approximately 1,000 residues long; in other collagen, such as type IV collagen, the helix is shorter and is sometimes interrupted by short nonhelical stretches. (Type IV collagen, found in basement membranes, forms a flexible mesh rather than fibrils.) Within a single triple helix, however, the three chains must match in length in order to be in correct register.

The highly repetitive sequence makes registration a problem for spontaneous helix formation. The cell has solved this problem by the addition of propeptide sequences at each end of the triple-helix domain. At the C-terminal end these propeptides bind together to form a trimeric globular domain that is stabilized by interchain disulfide bonds. Posttranslational modification occurs after the globular domains have come together but before the triple helix has formed. Hydroxylation of proline and lysine is catalyzed by specific oxidases that contain iron and require ascorbic acid.[2] Glycosylation, whose function is still unknown, also occurs. Once these modifications have been made, helix formation occurs spontaneously, beginning at the C-terminal end. The rate-limiting step for this propagation is the *cis-trans* isomerization of prolines, which is probably catalyzed by a specific prolyl isomerase.[121] This isomerization is necessary because proline exists as a mixture of two stereoisomers, and only the *trans* form fits in the triple helix of collagen.

After secretion of the collagen protomer from the cell, the prosequences are trimmed off by specific proteases. Cleavage of the N- and C-terminal propeptides decreases the solubility of the protein 2,000-fold.[118] Outside the cell, collagen protomers are incorporated into fibrils, and then into thicker fibers much as rope is made from smaller strands. As in the case of actin and tubulin, the polymerization is a nucleated process, with a lag phase followed by rapid growth. A critical concentration of monomer is required. Although fibrils formed in vivo may contain different types of collagen and other proteins of the extracellular matrix, purified collagen forms fibrils in vitro: the information for correct polymerization must be contained in the monomeric structure.

Cross-linking connects the fibrils formed in vivo. Hydroxylysine (formed, as noted above, by posttranslational modification before formation of the helix) is further oxidized to an aldehyde by an extracellular enzyme and cross-links the strands through an aldol condensation. Additional cross-linking is achieved by disulfide bridges between cysteine residues, which continue to be added as the animal ages. Mature collagen is much less flexible than the immature tropocollagen, which still lacks these modifications. Cross-linking between strands of different triple helices not only strengthens the aggregate but also reinforces each monomer by making the individual polypeptide chains topologically inseparable. The triple helices of adjacent protomers align in a staggered way, which is regulated by repetitive units. In interstitial collagens, each repetitive unit is 234 residues long.

The gene structure of collagens is under active investigation.[119-122] Types I, II, III, V, and XI, which are all fibril forming collagens, are encoded by multi-exon genes that seem to have evolved by repeated duplication of a protogene, 54 nucleotides long, that specifies an 18-residue polypeptide: six repeats of the pattern Gly-X-Y. The length of this exon may have been highly conserved so that the triple-helical protomers could align themselves in a correctly staggered way to form fibrils and higher orders of structure. The gene of type IV collagen, which forms not fibrils but rather a flexible three-dimensional network in basement membranes, has a different structure. The exons vary much more in size than do those of the fibrillar collagens, and some of the codons for the Gly in the repeat are split by introns.[122] The significance of the latter observation is not known. The genes for the short-chain collagens, $\alpha 1$(VIII) and $\alpha 1$(X), have large exons encoding the entire triple helical and C-terminal nonhelical domains.[122]

Myosin and Tropomyosin

The third type of structure found in fibrous proteins is the coiled coil, exemplified by the two-stranded tail of myosin and by tropomyosin. It is a motif found in conjunction with globular domains in a wide variety of such multidomain, multifunctional proteins as fibronectin, laminin, integrin, and fibrinogen. The function of the coiled coil is both to connect different polypeptide chains and to form extended, relatively rigid structures that often aggregate in turn to form fibers. The emphasis on each of these two functions covers a full spectrum, from the short leucine zippers of globular proteins to the long coiled coil of myosin fibers. The coil stabilizes the α helices, which in isolation would be only marginally stable in solution. The stability of the structure also varies in proportion to the length of the coil: apparently, each molecular species has evolved to optimize the stability of strand interaction for a particular role.

Myosin is the motor that drives muscle contraction and various other molecular and cellular movements. It contains three gene products: a heavy chain and two different light chains that assemble into a hexameric protein incorporating two copies of each polypeptide. In an electron micrograph one sees two adjacent globular "heads" at one end of a single long, rodlike tail. Each head turns out to be a globular domain at the N-terminal end of the heavy chain and to be associated with one of the two light chains. The remainder of each heavy chain forms an α helix. The helical tails of the two heavy chains, aligned in a parallel orientation, twist around each other to form the coiled coil. In muscle fibers these tails associate further, both longitudinally and laterally, to form myosin fibrils. In the fibril the protomers are aligned in a staggered manner so that the heads can bind to specific sites at regular intervals along an actin fiber. Movement of the myosin fiber relative to the actin fiber is achieved by a conformational change in the myosin head (or in the hinge region between the head and the tail), accompanied by the hydrolysis of ATP (which is distinct from the hydrolysis accompanying actin polymerization). The release of the head from the actin-binding site and its reattachment at a new site farther along the fiber permit this motion to be repeated, so that incremental movements are combined.[123]

The α-helical coiled coil was first recognized in two other fibrous proteins: tropomyosin and α-keratin. Tropomyosin is a regulatory protein of the muscle system. It binds to actin, fitting longitudinally into the groove of the actin helix, and also to troponin, a calcium-binding protein involved in the regulation of muscle contraction. This complex is the so-called thin filament of muscle. Tropomyosin resembles the tail of the myosin molecule, and because it is a simpler molecule and was the first of these proteins to be crystallized, it has been studied extensively. The resolution of the x-ray structure is limited by the high water content of the crystals, but has been refined by modeling to 15 Å.[124]

It had been noted by Francis Crick as long ago as 1953 that the sequence of tropomyosin, and also that of keratin, was based on a periodicity of both hydrophobic and charged amino acids, a heptad repeat.[125] He predicted that two helices would form a coiled coil with a so-called knobs-in-holes packing of the hydrophobic residues on one side of each helix. This packing stabilizes the dimeric structure—and also the helical structure of each chain—by excluding solvent, just as hydrophobic interactions stabilize the folded structure of a globular protein.

The residues in the heptad repeat are traditionally labeled alphabetically, *a* through *g*. Residues *a* and *d* are the two hydrophobic residues that align on the same face of the helix—often leucine and alanine. Residues *e* and *g*, on either side of the hydrophobic interface, tend to be acidic and basic, respectively. When two helices are aligned in parallel and in register, with one rotated with respect to the other, residue *a* faces residue *d* on the opposing helix. The *a-d* pairs in both orientations provide hydrophobic contacts at each complete turn of the helices. The external, oppositely charged residues *e* and *g* further stabilize the interaction by forming a salt bridge on each side, and they may be important for determining the register of the chain.

The precise packing of the hydrophobic side chains determines the strandedness of a coiled coil.[126] Isoleucine, with a branched side chain, and leucine promote different packing conformations. Isoleucine at the *a* position coupled with leucine at the *d* position favors dimer formation, as in leucine zippers; reversal of this pattern favors formation of a tetrameric coiled coil, and isoleucine at both positions favors trimer formation.

For two parallel helices to interact over a long stretch of sequence, each helical axis must be slightly curved. Curvature within a single helix results from the fact that hydrogen bonds are not uniform in length but are shorter on the side of the hydrophobic residues. This kind of curvature is commonly seen in the helices of globular proteins.[127] When two parallel helices are brought together by a hydrophobic interface, curvature results in supercoiling. For optimal knobs-in-holes packing, two parallel helices should have exactly 3.5 residues per turn, so that residue *a* and *d* on each helix are vertically aligned. In fact, this conformation is achieved in some proteins by a left-handed supercoil superimposed on the right-handed helices.

The degree of supercoiling varies from one protein to another. The pitch of the coiled coil therefore varies in a sequence-dependent way. In the case of tropomyosin, the average number of residues per turn of α helix is 3.63 to 3.64, slightly more than the average in helices of globular proteins. The helices cross each other at an angle of about 28°.[128] The average pitch of the supercoil is 14 nm (140 Å), which allows each half turn of the tropomyosin supercoil to bind to a single actin monomer.[129] Clearly, the exact dimensions of the coiled coil are critical for the specific interactions of tropomyosin with the actin helix. Undoubtedly, the same principle applies to other fibrous protein systems.

Tropomyosin polymerizes in a longitudinal sense. At each end of the coiled coil, molecules overlap by eight or nine residues. These joints are probably nonhelical.[125]

Similar short nonhelical regions are also seen at the ends of intermediate filaments, another set of coiled-coil proteins. In the case of lamin, a nuclear protein that polymerizes to create a structural net on the inside of the nuclear membrane, these nonhelical ends contain sites for the control of polymerization. Lamin forms a scaffold thought to be involved in the organization of chromatin. At the onset of mitosis, this scaffold depolymerizes rapidly. The reaction occurs when the lamin polymer is phosphorylated at specific serine and threonine residues close to the ends of the helical coiled coil.[130] This phosphorylation step illustrates how the basic chemical and physical properties of a monomeric protein can be altered to change its structural role within the cell.

Relation of Structure and Function

Information about the structure of proteins is accumulating at an increasing rate. Improvements in x-ray–diffraction and NMR technologies have speeded up the process of structure analysis. Site-directed mutagenesis has made it possible to study the effects of specific sequence changes on the properties of a protein. The rules of protein folding are beginning to emerge, and methods for predicting structure are improving steadily.

We have said very little, except in the case of hemoglobin, about the importance of conformational change in the functioning of proteins. This is likely to be an area of intense study in the future, for instance in connection with the cascades of phosphorylations and dephosphorylations through which information is transferred from one part of the cell to another. Still under active investigation is the exact mechanism by which a signal is transferred via a receptor across a cell membrane. In some cases, this clearly involves oligomerization of the receptor; in other cases, that is not yet clear. In any case, a conformational change on the cytoplasmic side must enable the receptor to interact with other proteins. Conformational changes also provide critical switches in subsequent steps of the signal-transduction cascade and in the regulation of transcription. In these areas and many more, the details of dynamic protein structure will be of great interest.

References

1. Schultz GE, Schirmer RH: *Principles of Protein Structure*. Springer-Verlag, New York, 1979, p 8

2. Stryer L: *Biochemistry*, 3rd ed. WH Freeman and Co, New York, 1988

3. Creighton TE: *Proteins: Structures and Molecular Properties*, 2nd ed. WH Freeman and Co, New York, 1993

4. Richardson JS: The anatomy and taxonomy of protein structure. *Adv Prot Chem* 34:167, 1981

5. Rossmann MG, Argos P: Protein folding. *Annu Rev Biochem* 50:497, 1981

6. Richardson JS, Richardson DC: Principles and patterns of protein conformation. *Prediction of Protein Structure and the Principles of Protein Conformation*. Fasman GD, Ed. Plenum Press, New York, 1989

7. Chothia C, Finkelstein AV: The classification and origins of protein folding patterns. *Annu Rev Biochem* 59:1007, 1990

8. Pauling L, Corey RB, Branson HR: The structure of proteins: two hydrogen-bonded helical configurations of the polypeptide chain. *Proc Natl Acad Sci USA* 37:205, 1951

9. Pauling L, Corey RB: Configurations of polypeptide chains with favored orientations around single bonds: two new pleated sheets. *Proc Natl Acad Sci USA* 37:729, 1951

10. Chothia C: Conformation of twisted β-sheets in proteins. *J Mol Biol* 75:295, 1973

11. Leszczynski J, Rose GD: Lopps in flobular proteins: a novel category of secondary structure. *Science* 234:849, 1986

12. Fetrow J, Rose GD: Loops in globular proteins. *Protein Folding*. Gierasch LM, King J, Eds. American Association for the Advancement of Science, Washington, DC, 1990, p 18

13. Sueki S, Lee S, Powers SP, et al: Helix-coil stability constants for the naturally occurring amino acids in water: 22. Histidine parameters from random poly(hydroxybutyl)glutamine-co-L-histidine. *Macromolecules* 17:148, 1984

14. Marqusee S, Baldwin RL: α-Helix formation by short peptides in water. *Protein Folding*. Gierasch LM, King J, Eds, Amererican Association for the Advancement of Science, Washington, DC, 1990

15. O'Neil KT, DeGrado WF: A thermodynamic scale for the helix-forming tendencies of the commonly occurring amino acids. *Science* 250:646, 1990

16. Wilson IA, Haft DH, Getzoff ED, et al: Identical short peptide sequences in unrelated proteins can have different conformations: a testing ground for theories of immune recognition. *Proc Natl Acad Sci USA* 82:5255, 1985

17. Chou PY, Fasman GD: Conformational parameters for amino acids in helical, β-sheet, and random coil regions calculated from proteins. *Biochemistry* 13:211, 1974

18. Chou PY, Fasman GD: Prediction of protein conformation. *Biochemistry* 13:222, 1974

19. Chou PY, Fasman GD: Prediction of β-turns. *Biophys J* 26:367, 1979

20. Andersson WF, Ohlendorf DH, Takeda Y, et al: Structure of the *cro* repressor from bacteriophage λ and its interaction with DNA. *Nature* 290:754, 1981

21. Freemont PS, Friedman JM, Beese LS, et al: Co-crystal structure of an editing complex of Klenow fragment with DNA. *Proc Natl Acad Sci USA* 85:8924, 1988

22. Frederick CA, Grable J, Melia M, et al: Kinked DNA in crystalline complex with EcoRI. *Nature* 309:327, 1984

23. McKay DB, Steitz TA: Structure of catabolite gene activator protein at 2.9 A resolution suggests binding to left-handed B-DNA. *Nature* 290:744, 1981

24. Brennan RG, Matthews BW: Structural basis of DNA-protein recognition. *Trends Biochem Sci* 14:286, 1989

25. Richardson JS, Richardson DC: The origami of proteins. *Protein Folding*. Gierasch LM, King J, Eds. American Association for the Advancement of Science, Washington, DC, 1990

26. Rao ST, Rossmann MG: Comparison of super-secondary structures in proteins. *J Mol Biol* 76:241, 1973

27. Wuthrich K: Protein structure determination in solution by NMR spectroscopy. *J Biol Chem* 265:22059, 1990

28. Eisenberg D, Hill CP: Protein crystallography: more surprises ahead. *Trends Biochem Sci* 14:260, 1989

29. Bernstein FC, Koetzle TF, Williams GJB, et al: The protein data bank: a computer-based archival file for macromolecular structures. *J Mol Biol* 112:535, 1977

30. Richardson JS: Describing patterns of protein tertiary structure. *Methods Enzymol* 115:341, 1985

31. Richardson JS: Schematic drawings of protein structure. *Methods Enzymol* 115:359, 1985

32. Thornton JM, Gardner SP: Protein motifs and data-base searching. *Trends Biochem Sci* 14:300, 1989

33. Luthy R, McLachlan AD, Eisenberg D: Secondary structure-based profiles: use of structure-conserving scoring tables in searching protein sequence databases for structural similarities. *Proteins* 10:229, 1991

34. Luthy R, Bowie JU, Eisenberg D: Assessment of protein models with three-dimensional profiles. *Nature* 356:83, 1992

35. Holm L, Ouzounis C, Sander C, et al: A database of protein structure families with common folding motifs. *Protein Sci* 1:1691, 1992

36. Subbiah S, Laurents DV, Levitt M: Structural similarity of DNA-binding domains of bacteriophage repressors and the globin core. *Current Biology* 3:141, 1993

37. Janin J, Chothia C: Domains in proteins: definitions, location and structural principles. *Methods Enzymol* 115:420, 1985

38. Montelione GT, Wuthrich K, Nice EC, et al: Solution structure of murine epidermal growth factor: determination of the polypeptide backbone chain-fold by nuclear magnetic resonance and distance geometry. *Proc Natl Acad Sci USA* 84:5226, 1987

39. Leytus SP, Foster DC, Jurachi K, et al: Gene for human factor X: a blood coagulation factor whose gene organization is essentially identical with that of factor IX and protein C. *Biochemistry* 25:5098, 1986

40. Yamamoto T, Davis CG, Brown MS, et al: The human LDL receptor: a cysteine-rich protein with multiple Alu sequences in its mRNA. *Cell* 39:27, 1984

41. Wharton KA, Johansen KM, Xu T, et al: Nucleotide sequence from the neurogenic locus notch implies a gene product that shares homology with proteins containing EGF-like repeats. *Cell* 43:567, 1985

42. Ellisen LW, Bird J, West DC, et al: TAN-1, the human homolog of the Drosophila notch gene, is broken by chromosomal translocations in T lymphoblastic neoplasms. *Cell* 66:649, 1991

43. Gilbert W: Why genes in pieces? *Nature* 271:501, 1978

44. Dujon B: Group I introns as mobile genetic elements: facts and mechanistic speculations—a review. *Gene* 82:91, 1989

45. Lambowitz AM, Perlman PS: Involvement of aminoacyl-tRNA synthetases and other proteins in group I and group II intron splicing. *Trends Biochem Sci* 15:440, 1990

46. Dorit RL, Schoenback L, Gilbert W: How big is the universe of exons? *Science* 250:1377, 1990

47. Sawyer L, Shotton DM, Campbell JW, et al: The atomic structure of crystalline porcine elastase at 2.5 A resolution: comparison with the structure of a-chymotrypsin. *J Mol Biol* 118:137, 1978

48. Levitt M, Chothia C: Structural patterns in globular proteins. *Nature* 261:552, 1976

49. Finkelstein AV, Ptitsyn O: Why do globular proteins fit the limited set of folding patterns? *Prog Biophys Mol Biol* 50:171, 1987

50. Farber GK, Petsko GA: The evolution of α/β barrel enzymes. *Trends Biochem Sci* 15:228, 1990

51. Quiocho FA, Lipscomb WN: Carboxypeptidase A: a protein and an enzyme. *Adv Protein Chem* 25:1, 1971

52. Perutz MF: Stereochemical mechanism of oxygen transport by haemoglobin. *Proc R Soc Lond* 208:135, 1980

53. Benesch R, Benesch RE: Intracellular organic phosphates as regulators of oxygen release by haemoglobin. *Nature* 221:618, 1969

54. Kornberg A: *1982 Supplement to DNA Replication.* Freeman, San Francisco, 1982, p S101

55. McHenry CS: DNA polymerase III holoenzyme of E. coli. *Annu Rev Biochem* 57:519, 1988

56. Kauzman W: Some factors in the interpretation of protein denaturation. *Adv Protein Chem* 14:1, 1959

57. Kyte J, Doolittle RF: A simple method of displaying the hydropathic character of a protein. *J Mol Biol* 157:105, 1982

58. Burley SK, Petsko GA: Weakly polar interations in proteins. *Adv Protein Chem* 39:125, 1988

59. Baker EN, Hubbard RE: Hydrogen bonding in globular proteins. *Prog Biophys Mol Biol* 44:97, 1984

60. Matsumura M, Signor G, Matthews BW: Substantial increase of protein stability by multiple disulphide bonds. *Nature* 342:291, 1989

61. Ponder JW, Richards FM: Tertiary templates for proteins: use of packing criteria in the enumeration of allowed sequences for different structural classes. *J Mol Biol* 193:775, 1987

62. Lim WA, Sauer RT: Alternative packing arrangements in the hydrophobic core of λ repressor. *Nature* 339:31, 1989

63. Baldwin RL, Eisenberg D: Protein stability. *Protein Engineering.* Oxender DL, Fox CF, Eds. Alan R Liss Inc, New York, 1987, p 127

64. Case DA, Karplus M: Dynamics of ligand binding to heme proteins. *J Mol Biol* 132:343, 1979

65. Harlos K, Vas M, Blake EEF: Crystal structure of the binary complex of pig muscle phosphoglycerate kinase and its substrate 3-phospho-D-glycerate. *Proteins* 12:133, 1992

66. Williams RJ: Are enzymes mechanical devices? *Trends Biochem Sci* 18:115, 1993

67. Segrest JP, De Loof H, Dohlman JG, et al: Amphipathic helix motif: classes and properties. *Proteins* 8:103, 1990

68. Landschulz WH, Johnson PF, McKnight SL: The leucine zipper: a hypothetical structure common to a new class of DNA binding proteins. *Science* 240:1759, 1988

69. O'Shea EK, Rutkowski R, Kim PS: Evidence that the leucine zipper is a coiled coil. *Science* 243:538, 1989

70. Anfinsen CB, Scheraga HH: Experimental and theoretical aspects of protein folding. *Adv Protein Chem* 29:205, 1975

71. Anfinsen CB, Haber E, Sela M, et al: The kinetics of formation of native ribonuclease during oxidation of the reduced polypeptide chain. *Proc Natl Acad Sci USA* 47:1309, 1961

72. Gutte B, Merrifield RB: The total synthesis of an enzyme with ribonuclease A activity. *J Am Chem Soc* 91:501, 1969

73. Hirschmann R, Nutt RF, Veber DF, et al: Studies on the total synthesis of an enzyme V. The preparation of enzymically active material. *J Am Chem Soc* 91:507, 1969

74. Kuwajima K: The molten globule state as a clue for understanding the folding and cooperativity of globular-protein structure. *Proteins* 6:87, 1989

75. Givol D, DeLorenzo F, Goldberger RF, et al: Disulfide interchange and the three-dimensional structure of proteins. *Proc Natl Acad Sci USA* 53:676, 1965

76. Zhu XL, Ohta Y, Jordan F, et al: Pro-sequence of subtilisin can guide the refolding of denatured subtilisin in an intermolecular process. *Nature* 334:483, 1989

77. Baker D, Sohl JL, Agard DA: A protein-folding reaction under kinetic control. *Nature* 356:263, 1992

78. Creighton TE: Up the kinetic pathway. *Nature* 356:194, 1992

79. Levinthal C: Are there pathways for protein folding? *J Chim Phys* 65:44, 1968

80. Kim PS, Baldwin RL: Specific intermediates in the folding reactions of small proteins and the mechanism of protein folding. *Annu Rev Biochem* 51:459, 1982

81. Oas TG, Kim PS: A peptide model of a protein folding intermediate. *Nature* 336:42, 1988

82. Ptitsyn OB: Protein folding: hypotheses and experiments. *J Protein Chem* 6:273, 1987

83. Shortle D, Meeker AK: Mutant forms of staphylococcal nuclease with altered patterns of guanidine hydrochorchloride and urea denaturation. *Proteins* 1:81, 1986

84. Shortle D, Meeker AK: Residual structure in large fragments of staphylococcal nuclease: effects of amino acid substitutions. *Biochemistry* 28:936, 1989

85. Goto Y, Fink AL: Conformational states of β-lactamase: molten globule states at acidic and alkaline pH with high salt. *Biochemistry* 28:945, 1989

86. Kuwajima K, Hiraoka Y, Ikeguchi M, et al: Comparison of the transient folding intermediates of lysozyme and α-lactalbumin. *Biochemistry* 24:874, 1985

87. Craig S, Hollecker M, Creighton TE, et al: Single amino acid mutations block a late step in the folding of β-lactamase from Staphylococcus aureus. *J Mol Biol* 185:681, 1985

88. Hecht MH, Richardson JS, Richardson DC, et al: De novo design, expression, and characterization of Felix: a four-helix bundle protein of native-like sequence. *Science* 249:884, 1990

89. Hill CP, Anderson DH, Wesson L, et al: Crystal structure of α_1: implications for protein design. *Science* 249:543, 1990

90. Gething MJ, Sambrook J: Protein folding in the cell. *Nature* 355:33, 1992

91. Ang D, Liberek K, Skowyra D, et al: Biological role and regulation of the universally conserved heat shock proteins. *J Biol Chem* 266:24233, 1991

92. Langer T, Lu C, Echols H, et al: Successive action of DnaK, DnaJ, and GroEl along the pathway of chaperone-mediated protein folding. *Nature* 356:683, 1992

93. Pain R: Further up the kinetic pathway. *Nature* 356:664, 1992

94. Oosawa F, Kasai M: A theory of linear and helical aggregation of macromolecules. *J Mol Biol* 4:10, 1962

95. Oosawa F, Asakura S: *Thermodynamics of the Polymerization of Protein.* Academic Press, New York, 1975

96. Frieden C: The regulation of protein polymerization. *Trends Biochem Sci* 14:283, 1989

97. Timasheff SN, Grisham LM: In vitro assembly of cytoplasmic microtubules. *Annu Rev Biochem* 49:565, 1980

98. Purich DL, Kristofferson D: Microtubule assembly: a review of progress, principles, and perspectives. *Adv Protein Chem* 36:133, 1984

99. Olmsted JB: Microtubule-associated proteins. *Annu Rev Cell Biol* 2:421, 1986

100. Noguchi CT, Schechter AN: Sickle hemoglobin polymerization in solution and in cells. *Annu Rev Biophys Biophys Chem* 14:239, 1985

101. Doolittle RF, Goldbaum DM, Doolittle LR: Designation of sequences involved in the coiled-coil interdomainal connections in fibrinogen: construction of an atomic scale model. *J Mol Biol* 120:311, 1978

102. Sasaki M, Kato S, Kohno K, et al: Sequence of the cDNA encoding the laminin B1 chain reveals a multidomain protein containing cysteine-rich repeats. *Proc Natl Acad Sci USA* 84:935, 1987

103. Steven AC, Trus BL, Maizel JV, et al: Molecular substructure of a viral receptor-recognition protein: the gp17 tail-fiber of bacteriophage T7. *J Mol Biol* 200:351, 1988

104. Atkins EDT: A four-stranded coiled coil model for some insect fibrous proteins. *J Mol Biol* 24:139, 1967

105. Kabsch W, Mannherz HG, Suck D, et al: Atomic structure of the actin:DNase I complex. *Nature* 347:37, 1990

106. Holmes KC, Popp D, Gebhard W, et al: Atomic model of the actin filament. *Nature* 347:44, 1990

107. Yin HL, Hartwig JH, Murayama K, et al: Ca^{++} control of actin filament length: effects of macrophage gelsolin on actin polymerization. *J Biol Chem* 256:9693, 1981

108. Carlier MF: Role of nucleotide hydrolysis in the polymerization of actin and tubulin. *Cell Biophys* 12:105, 1988

109. Wanger M, Keiser T, Neuhaus JM, et al: The actin treadmill. *Can J Biochem Cell Biol* 63:414, 1985

110. Margolis RL, Wilson L: Opposite end assembly and disassembly of microtubules at steady state in vitro. *Cell* 13:1, 1978

111. Horio T, Hotani H: Visualization of the dynamic instability of individual microtubules by dark field microscopy. *Nature* 321:605, 1986

112. Walker RA, O'Brien ET, Pryer NK, et al: Dynamic instability of individual microtubules analysed by video light microscopy: rate constants and transition frequencies. *J Cell Biol* 107:1437, 1988

113. Mitchison T, Kirschner M: Dynamic instability of microtubule growth. *Nature* 312:237, 1984

114. Mitchison TJ, Kirschner MW: Some thoughts on the partitioning of tubulin between monomer and polymer under conditions of dynamic instability. *Cell Biophys* 11:35, 1987

115. Inoue S, Sato H: Cell motility by labile association of molecules: the nature of mitotic spindle fibers and their role in chromosome movement. *J Gen Physiol* 50(suppl):259, 1967

116. Salmon ED: Spindle microtubules: thermodynamics of in vivo assembly and role in chromosome movement. *Ann NY Acad Sci* 253:383, 1975

117. Shaw LM, Olsen BJ: FACIT collagens: diverse molecular bridges in extracellular matrices. *Trends Biochem Sci* 16:191, 1991

118. Prockop DJ: Mutations that alter the primary structure of Type I collagen: the perils of a system for generating large structures by the principle of nucleated growth. *J Biol Chem* 265:15349, 1990

119. Burgeson RE: New collagens, new concepts. *Annu Rev Cell Biol* 4:551, 1988

120. Vuorio E, de Crombrugghe B: The family of collagen genes. *Annu Rev Biochem* 59:837, 1990

121. Kivirikko KI, Myllyla R: Post-translational processing of procollagens. *Ann NY Acad Sci* 460:187, 1985

122. Yamaguchi N, Mayne R, Ninomiya Y: the α1(VIII) collagen gene is homologous to the α1(X) collagen gene and contains a large exon encoding the entire triple helical and carboxyl-terminal non-triple helical domains of the α1(VIII) polypeptide. *J Biol Chem* 266:4508, 1991

123. Warrick HM, Spudich JA: Myosin structure and function in cell motility. *Annu Rev Cell Biol* 3:379, 1987

124. Phillips GN Jr, Fillers JP, Cohen C: Tropomyosin crystal structure and muscle regulation. *J Mol Biol* 192:111, 1986

125. Crick FHC: The packing of α-helices: simple coiled coils. *Acta Crystallogr* 6:689, 1953

126. Harbury PB, Zhang T, Kim PS, et al: A switch between two-, three-, and four-stranded coiled coils in GCN4 leucine zipper mutants. *Science* 262:1401, 1993

127. Barlow DJ, Thornton JM: Helix geometry in proteins. *J Mol Biol* 201:601, 1988

128. Cohen C, Parry DA: α-Helical coiled coils and bundles: how to design an α-helical protein. *Proteins* 7:1, 1990

129. McLachlan AD, Stewart M: The 14-fold periodicity in α-tropomyosin and the interaction with actin. *J Mol Biol* 103:271, 1976

130. Peter M, Heitlinger E, Haner M, et al: Disassembly of in vitro formed lamin head-to-tail polymers by CDC^2 kinase. *EMBO J* 10:1535, 1991

Acknowledgments

Figure 1   Dimitry Schidlovsky. Adapted from *Immunology*, by J. Kuby. W. H. Freeman and Co., New York, 1992.

Figures 2 and 3   Tom Moore. Adapted from *Molecular Cell Biology*, 2nd ed., by J. Darnell, H. Lodish, and D. Baltimore. Scientific American Books, New York, 1990.

Figure 4   Tom Moore. Adapted from "Proteins," by R. F. Doolittle, in *Scientific American* 253(4):98, 1985. © 1985 Scientific American, Inc. All rights reserved.

Figures 5, 6, 7a, and 7c   Dimitry Schidlovsky. Adapted from *Proteins: Structures and Molecular Properties*, 2nd ed., by T. E. Creighton. W. H. Freeman and Co., New York, 1993.

Figures 7b and 7e   Dimitry Schidlovsky. Adapted from *Introduction to Protein Structure*, by C. Branden and J. Tooze. Garland Publishing, Inc., New York, 1991.

Figure 7d   Dimitry Schidlovsky. Adapted from "The Anatomy and Taxonomy of Protein Structure," by J. S. Richardson, in *Advances in Protein Chemistry* 34:167, 1981.

Figure 8a   Tom Moore. Adapted from "The Leucine Zipper: A Hypothetical Structure Common to a New Class of DNA Binding Proteins," by W. H. Landschulz, P. F. Johnson, and S. L. McKnight, in *Science* 240:1759, 1988.

Figure 8b   Tom Moore. Adapted from *Recombinant DNA*, 2nd ed., by J. D. Watson, J. Witkowski, M. Gilman, et al. Scientific American Books, New York, 1992. © 1992 James D. Watson, Jan Witkowski, Michael Gilman, Mark Zoller. Used with permission.

CHAPTER 4

The Genetic Basis of Antibody Diversity

Philip Leder, M.D.

The powerful biologic strategy that generates the diversity of immunoglobulins (and T cell receptors) is unquestionably one of the most remarkable genetic mechanisms that has yet been identified. Imagine the basic paradox that confronted immunologists in the early 1970s in having to account in genetic terms for the fact that each vertebrate animal has the capacity to synthesize tens or hundreds of millions of different antibody molecules. Given the assumption—commonly held at the time—that genes consisted of a linear array of nucleotide sequences, read off one by one, to construct such a repertoire would require all or virtually all of the genome.

The answer to the paradox emerged over the course of the next decade. In essence, it is that the genes ultimately specifying the structure of each antibody are not present as such in germ cells or in the cells of the early embryo. Rather than harboring a set of complete and active antibody genes, these cells contain bits and pieces of the genes: a kit of components. The components are shuffled in the B cells of the immune system as those cells develop and mature. The shuffling can lead to a different result in each of millions of lines of cells. Individual mutations amplify the diversity. The result is that in the mature descendants of each cell line, a unique gene is assembled to express its information in the form of a unique antibody. This is the immune system's means of dealing with a virtually unlimited array of antigens. This explanation, which has been unraveled in terms of the immunoglobulin molecules, is largely valid for the T cell receptor as well.

The Structure of Antibodies

Antibodies, like other proteins, are made up of the subunits called amino acids. There are 20 kinds of amino acid, which can be linked together in any combination to form a protein chain. The amino acid composition of a chain and the sequence in which the amino acids are arrayed along the chain determine how the chain folds in three dimensions and perhaps combines with other chains. Substituting one amino acid for another or altering the sequence changes the protein's properties.

The amino acid composition and sequence of a protein chain are prescribed by a gene, which is a segment of another kind of chain: a molecule of the nucleic acid DNA. The subunits of DNA are four nucleotides, each incorporating one of four bases: adenine (A), guanine (G), thymine (T), or cytosine (C). The nucleotides are assembled to form a strand of DNA, and the sequence of their bases along the strand defines the information carried by the gene. The information is deciphered by means of the genetic code, whose code words (codons) are triplets of bases, such as CTG or AGC. In general, each codon specifies an amino acid, and a long series of codons supplies instructions for assembling an entire protein chain consisting of hundreds of amino acids. The information in DNA, however, is not translated directly into a protein. First it is transcribed into a single strand of the similar nucleic acid RNA; this molecule (messenger RNA) is translated into protein.

Immunoglobulins, the antibody molecules, have structural features that reflect their function. An antibody molecule is made up of two kinds of related protein chains, designated light and heavy [see Figure 1]. When the amino acid sequences of light chains from various antibodies were compared, the chains were found to have a peculiar property. The sequences of chains from different antibodies are different from one another, but the differences are confined to the first half of each chain. The remainder of the chain has essentially the same sequence in all antibodies of a given type.

The presence of both variation and constancy in a single protein turned out to have great functional significance. Indeed, an antibody is a bifunctional molecule. Each chain has a variable region (about half of a light chain and a quarter of a heavy chain) and a constant region. It is the variable regions of the chains that fold up in space to form an antibody-antigen combining site [see Figure 2]. Changing the amino acid sequence in the variable region changes the combining site's chemical structure and thereby changes the affinity of the antibody for an antigen.

The constant region of an antibody molecule of a particular type serves the same function in every molecule of that type. For example, there are two types of light chain in most vertebrate animals, kappa and lambda. The constant region of each kappa or lambda light chain is identical to the constant region of other chains of the same type.

In addition, each antibody molecule has one of five types of heavy chain: mu, delta, gamma, epsilon, or alpha. The heavy-chain type defines the class of the immunoglobulin as IgM, IgD, IgG, IgE, or IgA [see Table 1]. In secreted antibodies of the IgM type, for example, all the heavy chains have the same mu constant-region sequence and all the light chains have the same kappa or lambda constant-region sequence. Their variable re-

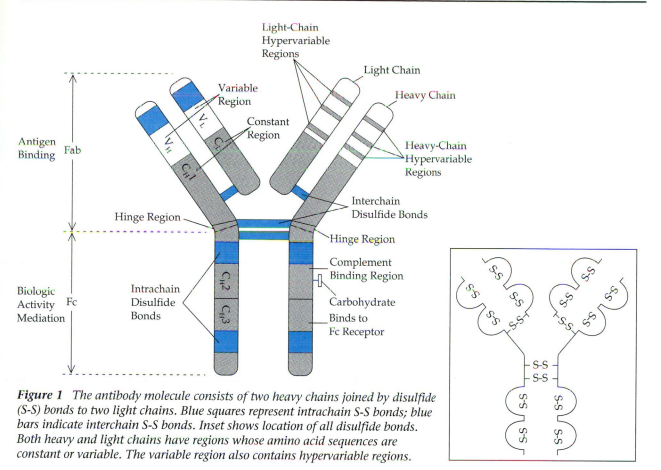

Figure 1 *The antibody molecule consists of two heavy chains joined by disulfide (S-S) bonds to two light chains. Blue squares represent intrachain S-S bonds; blue bars indicate interchain S-S bonds. Inset shows location of all disulfide bonds. Both heavy and light chains have regions whose amino acid sequences are constant or variable. The variable region also contains hypervariable regions.*

gions, on the other hand, differ from one antibody to the next, reflecting their different antigenic specificities.

The constant region of the heavy chains determines the effector function of an antibody. Consider an antibody whose variable region is specific for an antigen found on ragweed pollen. If the heavy chain is of the delta type, the IgD antibody remains associated with the surface of the cell that makes it. If the gamma heavy chain is present, the resulting IgG antibody is likely to circulate in the blood. With an epsilon chain, IgE may bind to the surface of a cell that releases histamine, giving rise to the symptoms of hay fever or asthma, when the antibody interacts with the ragweed antigen. All the antibodies are specific for the same antigen—the ragweed antigen. The same effector functions are found in antibodies directed against other antigens: the effector function is independent of the variable region.

The Genetics of Diversity

It was the structural features of antibodies that offered the first clues to the genetic source of their diversity.

The Dreyer-Bennett Hypothesis

William J. Dreyer and J. Claude Bennett, working at the California Institute of Technology in the mid-1960s, recognized that a million different

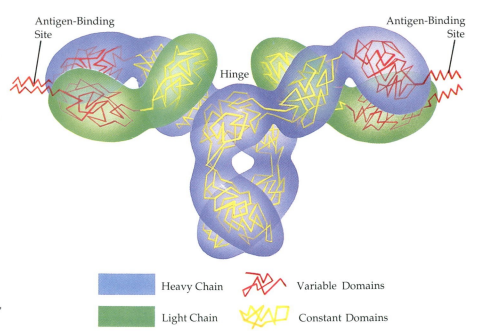

Figure 2 An antibody molecule is a Y-shaped protein made up of four polypeptide chains (top). Two heavy chains (blue) extend from the stem of the Y into the arms; two light chains (green) are confined to the arms. Each polypeptide has both constant regions (white and yellow) and variable regions (red). All antibodies of a given type have the same constant regions, but the variable regions differ from one clone of B cells to another. At the end of each arm, the heavy- and light-chain variable regions fold to create an antigen-binding site. The schematic model shows the domain structure of an antibody molecule (bottom); the domains share a characteristic folding pattern, which is also seen in T cell receptor proteins and proteins of the major histocompatibility complex.

Antigen-Binding Site   Antigen-Binding Site

Hinge

Heavy Chain   Variable Domains

Light Chain   Constant Domains

antibodies could be generated by combining 1,000 different light chains with 1,000 different heavy chains.[1] How, they wondered, might the genetic information for this diversity of proteins be organized? Above all, what organization could account for the strange variable-and-constant structure of each chain?

Consider just the problem of one type of light chain. There might conceivably be 1,000 genes, each gene specifying one of 1,000 light chains. In that case, however, some mechanism must have operated in the course of evolution to preserve unchanged the sequence of the constant-region half of each of the 1,000 genes while the other half of each gene (the half encoding the variable region) was allowed to mutate wildly. Such a mechanism seemed unlikely because there is no obvious biologic reason

Table 1   Properties of Antibodies

Property	IgG	IgM	IgA	IgE	IgD
Heavy chains (subgroups)	Gamma ($\gamma 1$, $\gamma 2$, $\gamma 3$, $\gamma 4$)	Mu	Alpha ($\alpha 1$, $\alpha 2$)	Epsilon	Delta
Light chains	Kappa or lambda	Kappa or lambda	Kappa or lambda	Kappa or lambda	Kappa or lambda
Molecular formula	$\gamma_2\,\kappa_2$ or $\gamma_2\,\lambda_2$	$(\mu_2\,\kappa_2)_5$ or $(\mu_2\,\lambda_2)_5$	$(\alpha_2\,\kappa_2)_n$ or $(\alpha_2\,\lambda_2)_n$ (n = 1, 2, or 3)	$\varepsilon_2\,\kappa_2$ or $\varepsilon_2\,\lambda_2$	$\delta_2\,\kappa_2$ or $\delta_2\,\lambda_2$
Structure	Monomer	Pentamer	Monomer, dimer, or trimer	Monomer	Monomer
Concentration in serum (mg/dl)	1,250	120	280	0.3–30.0	0.002–0.200
Half-life in serum (days)	23	5	6	3	2.5
Localization	Serum, amniotic fluid	Serum	Serum, secretions, colostrum, saliva, tears, GI tract	Serum	Serum
Function	Secondary response	Primary response	Protects mucous membranes	Protects against para-sites (?)	?

for any given constant-region amino acid sequence to have been conserved. Comparisons of immunoglobulins in different individuals and species indicate that there is little evolutionary pressure to maintain absolute identity among constant-region sequences; a change of a few amino acids in the constant region seems to have no ill effect.

This reasoning led the investigators to a hypothesis. Instead of assuming that the genetic information for an antibody light chain is specified by a continuous array of codons, they suggested that the light chain is encoded in two discontinuous stretches of DNA, one for the variable region and the other for the constant region. They proposed further that there are several hundred or several thousand separately encoded variable-region genes in the DNA of germ cells—but only one constant-region gene.

By postulating a single constant-region gene, the Dreyer-Bennett proposal showed how essentially the same sequence might be conserved to appear in every constant region of a given type in a given species. If there is only one constant-region gene, any mutation in it must immediately alter the amino acid sequence of every light chain. Also implicit in the proposal was the notion that the information in the separate genetic elements must somehow come together to form a contiguous and coherent genetic message and then a single protein chain.

This proposal initially attracted considerable criticism. It called for split genes and for mechanisms to join them, both of which were then quite without precedent. Yet the idea proved to be essentially correct.

Early Experiments

Initial studies using hybridization kinetic analysis undertook to test the hypothesis. The strategy was to detect and isolate the initial product of an antibody gene: its messenger RNA. A strand of DNA artificially copied from that messenger (by means of the enzyme reverse transcriptase) would serve as a probe with which to detect the antibody genes in embryonic cells and estimate how many such genes are present. This would test the central prediction of the Dreyer-Bennett hypothesis: that there is only one constant-region gene, or at most a few, as opposed to the many genes required by the more straightforward genetic models.

The technique of hybridization kinetics is based on the fact that two stretches of nucleic acid with complementary nucleotide sequences hybridize, or bind to each other. If one of the sequences has been labeled with atoms of a radioactive isotope, the hybrid molecules can be identified by their radioactivity. The speed with which a radioactive DNA probe finds and hybridizes with any complementary DNA molecules (the hybridization kinetics) is an indirect but effective measure of the number of such complementary molecules in the preparation.

Measurement of the rate at which the probe (DNA copied from the RNA specifying the constant region of the mouse light chain) hybridized with DNA representing the entire genome of the mouse embryo yielded results indicating clearly that there are very few copies of the light-chain constant-region gene, perhaps no more than two in each cell.[2,3] Similar results were soon obtained in a number of other laboratories. Clearly the Dreyer-Bennett hypothesis had to be taken seriously.

If there are only a few copies of the constant-region gene and many separately encoded variable-region genes, some mechanism must operate to bring the information together in a coherent sequence. The most economical way would be at the level of the gene, that is, to join two sequences of DNA that are separate in an embryonic cell to form a single active sequence in the nucleus of a mature, antibody-producing lymphocyte. Such a rearrangement of DNA in the course of the differentiation and development of somatic, or body, cells is termed somatic recombination.

Further Advances

The mid-1970s was a period of extraordinary developments in molecular genetics. A major advance in 1973 was the first successful application of new recombinant DNA techniques to insert foreign DNA into a bacterium or a bacterial virus and thereby clone a single gene in quantity [see Chapter 5]. It was immediately clear to investigators working with more cumbersome genetic techniques that gene cloning would make it possible to isolate antibody genes and determine their structure in a direct way. One group decided to adapt the bacteriophage (bacterial virus) called phage λ (lambda) for this purpose. Introducing a series of crippling mutations to ensure the safety of the material, the workers were soon able to report the first successful cloning in a bacteriophage of a mammalian gene: a mouse gene for globin, the protein of the hemoglobin molecule.

A group in Switzerland exploited the cloning strategy to isolate the mouse genes for the lambda light chain in both embryonic and antibody-producing cells.[4] The results showed that the constant-region gene and the variable-region gene are indeed encoded far apart in the DNA of cells that do not synthesize antibodies. In an appropriate antibody-producing plasmacytoma, the two genes are much closer together. The rearrangement does not, however, bring the variable-region and the constant-region genes together to form a continuous sequence. Instead, the variable-region gene (V) is still about 1,500 nucleotides away from the constant-region gene (C); between them, and abutting the V gene, is a segment called the J (for joining) sequence.

Another cloning effort was directed toward the kappa light-chain genes of the mouse [see Figure 3].[5,6] The investigators undertook to examine this system because more than 95 percent of mouse antibodies incorporate the kappa chain, making it the major source of mouse light-chain diversity. The experimenters cloned both the embryonic and the active forms of the kappa variable-region and constant-region genes. Then, by means of a rapid DNA-sequencing technique, they determined the nucleotide sequences of the genes.

A large number of V genes were identified in the embryonic DNA. They seem to fall into families, with each family being made up of genes whose nucleotide sequences are closely retained. This study and a similar one indicate that as many as several hundred variable-region genes may be present in mouse-embryo DNA. Each of the V genes, whether kappa or lambda, retains certain structural features that appear to be of considerable significance. For example, each gene is divided into two discrete coding sequences separated by a short intervening sequence. The first coding sequence specifies a hydrophobic leader, 17 to 20 amino acids long, that is thought to be important for the transport of the antibody molecules through the cell membrane. The leader is a part of the original protein product of the active light-chain gene but is cleaved away as the nascent antibody passes through the membrane.

The other coding region of the V gene specifies most of the variable region, but not all of it. The nonleader part of the V gene encodes only 95 of the 108 amino acids of the kappa chain's variable region. As earlier findings had suggested was the case in the lambda system, in the kappa DNA the remaining portion of the variable region is encoded by a sequence well downstream from the V gene, near the single constant-region gene, exactly at the site to which the V gene is joined to make an active immunoglobulin gene. This short sequence, the J sequence, is repeated with slight but significant variations five times at intervals of about 300 nucleotides. (Further studies of the mouse lambda system showed a somewhat different arrangement. Instead of one constant-region gene, there are four C genes, each with its own J gene. In the human lambda system, there are six C genes.)

Kappa Light Chain

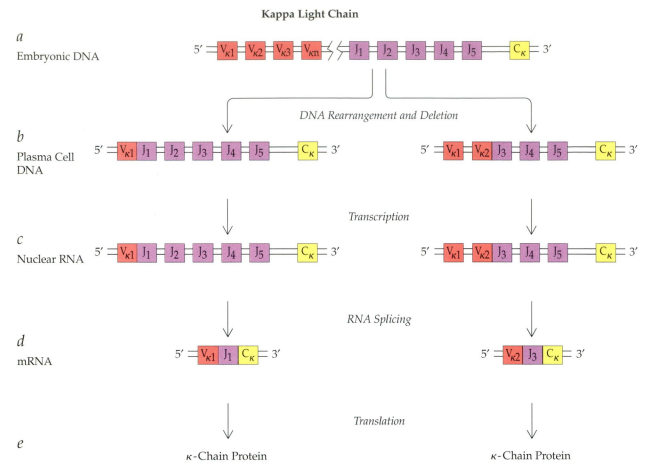

Figure 3   *Rearrangement of embryonic DNA during B cell differentiation gives rise to a variety of plasma cell lines that encode different kappa light chains. The variable region of the chain is encoded by V and J sequences, the constant region by a C gene. The embryonic DNA contains more than 200 V (variable) genes, each one separated by a short intervening sequence from a leader sequence (the leaders are not shown). The V segments are separated by a long noncoding stretch of DNA from five J (for joining) sequences. The Js are separated by an intervening sequence from a single C (constant) gene (a). In the pathway on the left, differentiation of the embryonic cell to a plasma cell results in deletion of the intervening V genes, so that $V_{\kappa1}$ is joined with the J_1 gene (b). The linked $V_{\kappa1}J_1$ segment codes for one of more than 1,500 possible kappa light-chain variable regions. The plasma cell DNA us transcribed into nuclear RNA (c). Splicing of the nuclear RNA produces messenger RNA with the $V_{\kappa1}$, J_1, and C genes linked together (d), ready for translation to a kappa light-chain protein (e). The alternative pathway at right (b to e) shows another of the many possible pathways leading to a different kappa light chain with a different specificity of the variable region.*

Now the potential of the kappa system to develop diversity begins to become clear.[7] The joining of one of several hundred V genes—say 150 to be conservative—to one of five J genes can generate 150×5, or 750, different active genes for a light-chain variable region. Evidence from a number of laboratories indicates that this is exactly the way the sequences are shuffled. One of the V genes is joined to one of the J sequences; the extra Vs and Js and the long noncoding spacer between them are deleted. The finished active gene is encoded in three separate sequences: a leader gene, a V/J gene, and a C gene. The sequences are assembled by RNA splicing to form a coherent light-chain messenger RNA.

The 750-fold diversity is multiplied by another source of variation. Careful comparisons of the amino acid sequences of light chains revealed a particularly high degree of diversity in a region close to the site of V/J joining. The amino acids around position 96 form one of the three regions of the light chains that had earlier been designated as hypervariable. The light chains fold up in such a way that the hypervariable regions form the antibody-antigen combining site.

At least some part of the variation in this region can now be explained by the fact that the V/J recombination site is not precisely defined. A V gene and a J gene can apparently be joined at different crossover points. As a result, the codon for amino acid 96 (the nominal V/J junction) and the codons adjacent to it can change depending on what part of the sequence is supplied by the embryonic V region and what part by the J region. If one makes the assumption that alternative joining sites can increase the diversity tenfold, the total number of potential V/J combinations becomes $150 \times 5 \times 10$, or 7,500.

Signal Sequences

Certain features of the sequences of the light-chain genes have been conserved and seem likely to be of functional significance. In particular, a pattern of signal-like sequences is found on the 3', or downstream, side of the V genes and on the 5', or upstream, side of the J genes [*see Figure 4*]. Each such sequence has a stretch of about nine nucleotides (a nonamer) of which a large proportion are either A or T.[7,8] The nonamer is followed, at an interval of either about 12 base pairs (one turn of the DNA helix) or about 23 base pairs (two turns), by a seven-nucleotide sequence, or heptamer: CACTGTG or GTGACAC. The nonamer and the heptamer can be visualized as forming a stem structure in which the sequences would be complementary according to the rules of base pairing (A with T and G with C), bringing the V and J genes together at the base of the stem. It is then easy to see how the genes might be joined by some kind of DNA-recombination system, with the signal sequences being deleted.

The flexibility of the recombinational system, although powerful in its ability to generate diversity, does have its price. V and J genes are occasionally brought together aberrantly, yielding an inactive gene. This may in part explain the phenomenon called allelic exclusion. Each somatic cell has two sets of chromosomes, with one member of each chromosome pair supplied by the mother and the other by the father. The corresponding copies of a given gene on the two chromosomes are called alleles. In an antibody-producing cell it is usually the case that only the antibody genes on one copy of the chromosomes carrying such genes undergo somatic recombination and are finally translated into protein; the alleles on the other chromosome are ordinarily excluded from the rearrangement process and are not expressed. Occasionally, however, an antibody-producing cell has two sets of rearranged antibody genes. Apparently, in such cases, the genes on one chromosome were recombined aberrantly, forming an inactive antibody gene, and the active gene was thereby generated in a second try, with the so-called spare chromosome serving as the backup.

It is also possible that the lambda light-chain genes serve as a fail-safe system for misjoined kappa genes. Studies show that there is a clear order

a

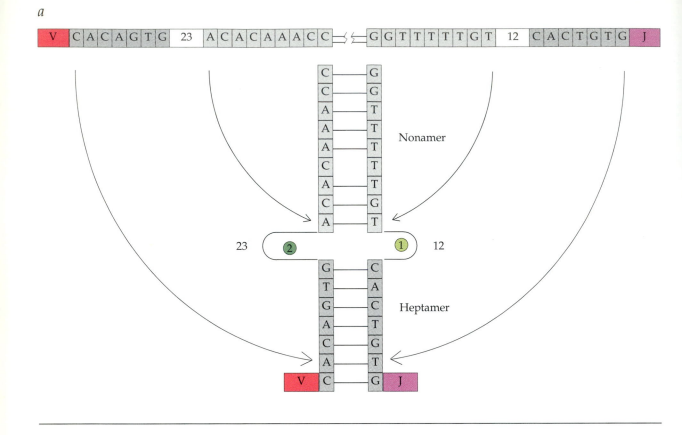

b

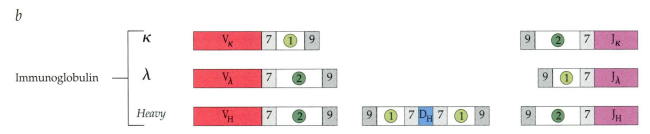

Figure 4 *Recombination signals in embryonic DNA serve to ensure that the correct gene segments are joined during the formation of specific antibody light and heavy chains. For the light chains, the V and J segments are brought together (a). For the heavy chain, a similar mechanism operates, but it includes signals for the additional sequence designated D (for diversity). The recombination signals consist of a conserved heptamer and nonamer separated by either 12 base pairs (one turn of the DNA helix) or 23 base pairs (two turns). Typical recombination signals observed for the kappa and lambda light chains and the heavy chain are shown (b).*

of events in the formation of a light-chain gene. First the kappa genes rearrange. If they fail to form an active gene, the lambda system begins to rearrange.

These findings led to the intriguing proposal that the appearance of a functional antibody in a cell acts as a signal precluding further V/J joining.[9] In the absence of the signal, the cell keeps trying. In humans, with six lambda J/C sequences on each chromosome 22, there are in effect 12 lambda genes per cell. Together with the two kappa genes (one on each chromosome 2), that would mean the cell has 14 opportunities to form an active light-chain gene.

The Heavy Chain

In the heavy chain, the formation of the variable region is governed by the same principles that apply in the light chain, but the potential for diversity is even greater: an extra piece of genetic information multiplies the combinatorial possibilities [*see Figure 5*]. When investigators cloned the active heavy-chain variable-region DNA of an antibody-producing cell and determined its structure, they found that a sequence of at least 13 nucleotides exactly at the V/J junction could not be accounted for by either the V or the J genes in the embryonic DNA.[10-12] They reasoned that this segment must be supplied by a stretch of embryonic DNA they called the D (for diversity) gene. They noted that the D segment's location in the active gene corresponds to the major portion of the third hypervariable region of the heavy chain.

Also noted in the embryonic heavy-chain DNA were the nonamer-heptamer sequences that seem to serve in light-chain DNA as signals for V/J joining. The arrangement of those signals in light-chain DNA had indicated that the spacing between the nonamer and the heptamer had to be different on the V side and the J side of the stem structure (about 12 nucleotides on one side and 23 on the other) for recombination to take place. In the heavy chain, however, the V and the J signals were both found to have spacers about 23 nucleotides long. It was therefore predicted that when the D genes were identified in embryonic DNA, they would be found to be flanked by recombination signals having the 12-nucleotide spacing. In this way, the joining of V to D and of D to J would conform to the 12/23 rule.

The D segments presented a problem in cloning. Their coding sequences were too short for them to serve as a hybridization probe for detecting their embryonic counterparts. This problem was solved by taking advan-

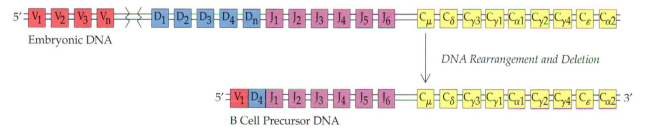

Figure 5 *The active heavy-chain gene is assembled from four sets of sequences in the embryonic DNA: V, D, J, and C. There are several hundred V sequences, 10 to 20 D sequences, and six J sequences. Somatic recombination brings together one of the several hundred V sequences, a D sequence, and a J sequence to code for the variable region of the chain. As in the case of the light-chain gene, the constant (C) region DNA is downstream, separated by a noncoding sequence. In the heavy chain, however, there are nine C sequences, each one coding for a different constant region. In the pathway shown, when the embryonic cell differentiates into a B cell precursor, various V and D genes are deleted, so that V_1, D_4 and J_1 are joined to form one of the many possible heavy-chain genes. Rearrangement that leads to the joining of particular V, D, and J segments occurs in response to an antigenic challenge and is directed by specific recombination signals [see Figure 4]. Final assembly of coding sequences is accomplished by RNA processing [see Figure 8].*

tage of an aberrant intermediate product of V/D/J recombination: a human D segment that had somehow been joined incorrectly to a J gene. The D gene had been processed by the recombinatory enzymes on only one side (the side next to the J gene), and so its opposite flank carried with it a large segment of embryonic DNA. The aberrant segment made an excellent probe for cloning embryonic D sequences.

When the structure of the DNA in these clones was determined, the D sequences were found to be surrounded by recombination signals with 12-nucleotide spacers, fulfilling the predictions of the 12/23 rule. Then, with the cloned D segment as a probe, the human genome was searched for sequences with which it would hybridize. The search detected a large D-gene family consisting of at least five closely related sequences. There are indications that this is only one of several such families of D genes.

The formation of the active gene for the heavy-chain variable region can generate an extraordinarily large number of genetic possibilities. One group has estimated that there are as many as 80 embryonic heavy-chain V genes in man. The group found six active J genes within 8,000 nucleotides of the human mu C gene. Although one cannot confidently extrapolate the number of human D genes from what is now known, it can be assumed that the D families have about 50 members. Somatic recombination, then, could generate approximately $80 \times 6 \times 50$, or 24,000, genetic combinations. Another factor of about 100 (a very rough estimate) is contributed by recombinatorial flexibility: alternative codons at the two crossover points of V/D and D/J recombination. The total then comes to about 2.4 million possible different heavy chains.

In addition to the sources of diversity referred to above, there is yet another mechanism that operates especially at the level of heavy-chain gene assembly. It involves the insertion of an apparently random sequence of bases at the junction between the joined V/D and D/J segments. These additions are called N regions because they consist of added nucleotides that are not complementary to those present in the genome. Rather they are added in a nontemplated manner, by a special enzyme (terminal deoxynucleotidyl transferase) present in early lymphoid cells. The addition of these N sequences carries all the advantages (in terms of generating additional diversity) and limitations (in terms of generating out-of-frame translations) of the flexible joining mechanism in light-chain gene assembly.

Taken together with the 7,500 combinatorial possibilities available to the human kappa light chain (150 for the complement of V genes, five for the J genes, and 10 for recombinational flexibility), the 2.4 million heavy chains yield a total of some 18 billion (2.4 million multiplied by 7,500) possible antibodies. They can be generated from perhaps 300 separate genetic segments in the embryonic DNA.

Somatic Mutation

The enormous diversity generated by means of recombination may be supplemented by yet another mechanism: solitary somatic mutation, which introduces sporadic single-nucleotide changes throughout the variable-region DNA in the course of somatic development. Immunoglobulin genes are highly unstable in antibody-producing cells. When clones of mature lymphocytes were propagated and successive generations were screened for new antigen-binding specificity, it was found that the immunoglobulin genes underwent mutation at the remarkable rate of once per 10,000 cells per generation. Other experiments have isolated active genes whose variable-region DNA differs by one nucleotide or two from the embryonic DNA sequences that were its source.

These findings support a suggestion made about 25 years ago that some proportion of antibody diversity is the result of single-nucleotide mutation in the variable-region DNA of developing lymphocytes. Two groups have found evidence to suggest that the mutations accumulate as the lymphocyte passes through progressive stages in its development.

The gene shuffling that can generate billions of variable-region genes is matched by two additional processes that explain how a single variable region can be joined successively to a series of heavy-chain constant regions. A precursor of the antibody-producing cells, the pre-B cell, makes a mu heavy-chain constant region linked to a specific variable region (a product of V/D/J recombination). This heavy chain at first remains inside the pre-B cell. Then, after the onset of light-chain and delta heavy-chain synthesis, both the mu and the delta heavy chains combine with the light chains to form complete IgM and IgD molecules. The next stage in development is distinguished by the concurrent appearance of both IgM and IgD on the cell surface. Both antibodies have the same variable regions and so both are directed against the same antigen.

Clonal Selection

The subsequent steps in lymphocyte development are apparently antigen-driven [*see Figure 6*]. The primary event of the immune process is called clonal selection.[13] An antigen binds to a receptor—the best-fitting antigen-combining site among millions or billions of surface immunoglobulins. By this interaction, the cell displaying the selected immunoglobulin is driven further along its developmental path. It proliferates to form a clone of antibody-producing B cells.

In the course of B-cell maturation, the IgM and IgD disappear from the cell surface and either IgM, IgG, IgE, or IgA is instead secreted by the cell. Each of those classes of immunoglobulins has a different heavy-chain constant region, but antibodies of any class that are synthesized in a given cell have the same variable regions, namely, the ones that were assembled in the precursor and that formed the combining site selected by the antigen. Because each heavy chain gives the antibody a different effector function, the same combining site can take part in different immune reactions. The process by which the same variable region appears in association with different heavy-chain constant regions is called heavy-chain class switching. The lymphocyte depends on two mechanisms to carry out class switching. One mechanism is based on differential RNA transcription and splicing, the other on a version of DNA recombination.

How is it that IgM can appear successively in two forms, one bound to the lymphocyte membrane and the other secreted? Structural studies detected differences between the membrane-bound mu chain and the secreted one. More detailed studies showed that the membrane-bound form ends in a short sequence of hydrophobic amino acids, which evi-

Figure 6 Differentiation of antibody-producing cells is traced, beginning with the pre-B cell. At each stage, the major genetic events are listed (left), along with the pertinent gene-shuffling mechanisms (right). The heavy chain is manufactured first, then the light chain (kappa or lambda). IgM and IgD are displayed on the cell surface. When a specific antigen is recognized and bound by a surface antibody, the cell is driven further in development: it proliferates to form a clone of mature B cells, which are specialized to synthesize large amounts of protein. Now the expression and the arrangement of the heavy-chain constant-region gene may change, so that different types of antibody are produced. In most cases, the variable regions remain the same and the antibody continues to be directed against the same antigen, but point mutations can accumulate to change the variable regions in the course of maturation.

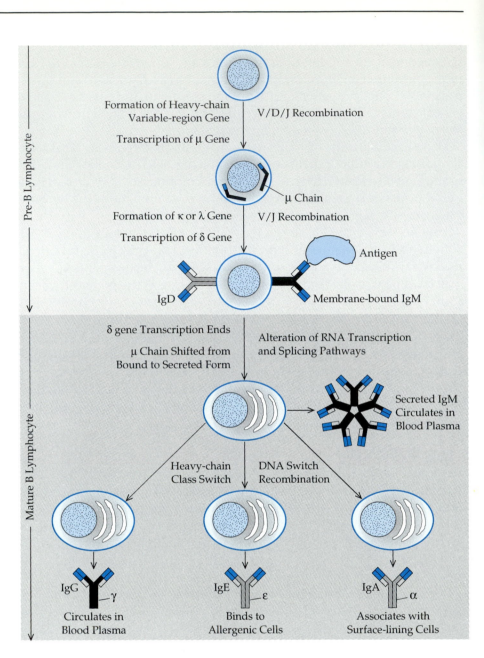

dently anchor the antibody in the cell's membrane through their affinity for the hydrophobic lipids of the membrane.[14-17] The secreted mu chain lacks the hydrophobic sequence. Further work showed that two forms of messenger RNA are synthesized from the mu gene. In one form, the message stops just short of two small coding segments that specify the anchor sequence; in the other form, the segments coding for the anchor sequence are included.

Mechanisms of Shuffling

Each heavy-chain constant region is encoded in from three to six separate coding domains separated by short intervening sequences of non-informational DNA. As is the case with most other split genes, the primary transcript of the heavy-chain genes includes both the coding sequences and the intervening sequences. RNA processing thereupon splices the coding sequences to one another, eliminating the noninformational segments. The primary transcript of the mu gene sometimes includes the coding sequence for the hydrophobic anchor; if it is present, the enzymes that process the RNA splice it to the end of the main mu messenger so as to exclude a so-called stop codon that would otherwise halt translation at the end of the main message. If the primary RNA transcript lacks the anchor sequence, no splicing takes place; the stop codon preceding the anchor sequence is recognized and the secretable form of the mu chain is synthesized. Later evidence indicates that many of the other heavy chains, and perhaps all of them, have a similar arrangement that allows them either to be anchored to the membrane or to be secreted.

The simultaneous appearance of mu and delta chains is likely to be caused by similar splicing alternatives [*see Figure 7*]. Transcription proceeds through the variable-region DNA and then through the several domains of the mu gene. A certain fraction of the primary transcripts end in a way that yields mu chains, as described above. Another fraction of the transcripts continue for a few thousand nucleotides and therefore include not only the V/D/J and mu sequences but also the delta sequence. Among the many options for splicing such transcripts, one is to splice the V/D/J DNA directly to the beginning of the delta-gene transcript. In this way, two messenger RNAs are formed simultaneously; one specifies the mu heavy chain and one the delta chain, but both encode the same variable region. Translation of the two RNAs into protein leads to the simultaneous display on the cell surface of IgM and IgD that have the same antigen specificity.

A second mechanism that shuffles heavy-chain genes depends on the rearrangement of DNA sequences to accomplish the remaining steps of the heavy-chain class switch [*see Figure 8*].[18-20] In contrast to the rather precise nature of the V/J and V/J/D joining events, the recombination process that leads to the expression of a particular heavy-chain class has a much greater degree of freedom.

Consider the switch from the mu chain to the alpha chain (from IgM to IgA). The active heavy-chain gene is arranged so that the variable-region coding sequence is a long way (about 8,000 nucleotides) from the first constant-region sequence (which is the first mu sequence). Ordinarily, this noncoding spacer region is excised from the primary RNA transcript for the mu chain. Although the spacer region has no known coding function, it does have a stretch of about 2,000 nucleotides that includes series of repeated nucleotides of various sizes.

This 2,000-nucleotide segment with the repeated blocks is similar in sequence to a stretch of DNA far downstream, adjacent to the alpha gene. Switching from IgM to IgA must involve recombination of these distant similar sequences; they apparently serve as switch signals to join the V/D/J sequence to the alpha coding sequence, deleting mu and the other constant-region genes. Since there are no coding sequences within the switch regions, the exact crossover points in the recombination event can apparently vary widely within the region. Other workers have found analogous switch regions adjacent to the gamma genes and have suggested that these regions constitute a signal for the switch from mu to gamma.

HEAVY-CHAIN GENE EXPRESSION

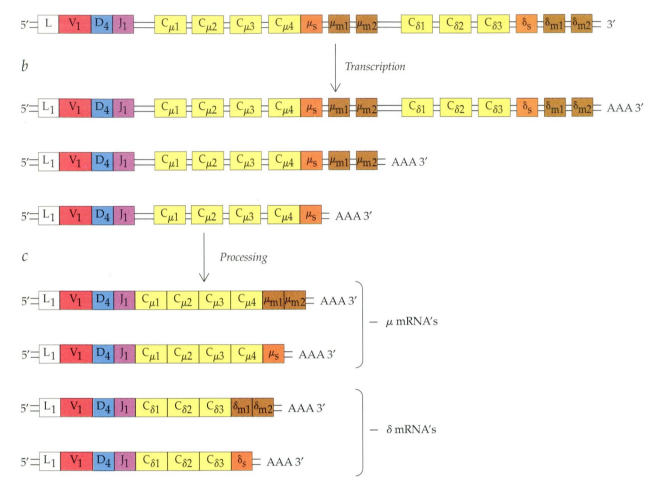

Figure 7 *RNA transcription and processing account for the appearance of membrane-bound and secreted forms of IgM and IgD and for the simultaneous appearance of both types of heavy chain. The DNA of B cells that express both IgM and IgD heavy chains contains rearranged C_μ and C_δ genes (a). Several nuclear RNA transcripts are produced from this DNA (b): some transcripts contain both C_μ and C_δ segments; others contain only the C_μ or C_δ segments; and still others either carry or lack the segment that encodes the hydrophobic tail that anchors the antibody in the cell's membrane (μ_m or δ_m). Splicing events remove intervening, noncoding RNA and generate IgM and IgD mRNAs that code for either the membrane-bound ($C_{\mu m}$, $C_{\delta m}$) or the secreted ($C_{\mu s}$, $C_{\delta s}$) forms of the IgM or IgD heavy chains (c).*

SCID Mice and Recombination-Activating Genes

It stands to reason that the mechanisms for generating diversity in the immune system depend on a variety of enzymes and associated proteins. Note that the immune system includes not only the antibodies of the humoral branch but also the T cell receptors of the cellular branch, the diversity of which is comparable to that of antibodies and is generated by very similar mechanisms. Moreover, it is likely that elements of the immunoglobulin-gene recombinatorial system are borrowed from recombinatorial mechanisms that operate outside the immune system.

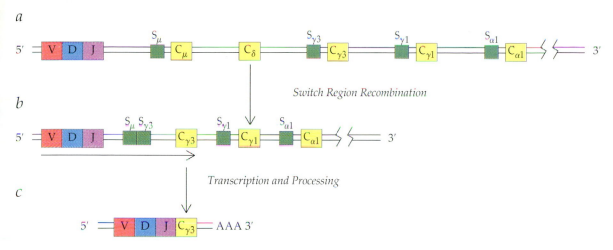

Figure 8 *The heavy-chain class switch is accomplished by DNA recombination. In this hypothetical model of heavy-chain class switching to $C_{\alpha}3$, the heavy-chain constant regions (yellow) and the switch regions (light green) are indicated (a). The switch region is a stretch of DNA that directs the deletion events. In this model, recombination of switch regions S_{μ} and $S_{\alpha}3$ and deletion of the intervening DNA occur first to produce a DNA sequence in which the gene for $C_{\alpha}3$ has been brought into close proximity to the VDJ segment (b). Further processing and transcription of this DNA yields the mRNA encoding IgG3 (c).*

The discovery of several genes and the creation of mutant strains of mice have borne out this expectation. In particular, the discovery of the SCID (severe combined immunodeficiency) mutation in certain mice and the discovery of two genes that are essential for generating diversity in antibody (and T cell receptor) molecules are notably instructive.

One finding was that the genetically defective mice are unable to assemble an adequate number of normal genes for antigen receptors.[21,22] This finding led to the hypothesis that the SCID mutation impairs the V/D/J recombination event. Further work in several laboratories bore out the hypothesis.[23-25] It turns out that because of the mutation, the mice form coding joints (i.e., joints between the coding sequences rather than between the noncoding signal sequences) at a rate some 100 times lower than that at which they form signal joints. D and J remain separate instead of joining in the earliest stages of the development of pre-B and pre-T cells. The result is a severe deficiency in the assembly of antigen-receptor genes.

Recent work has established that two recombination-activating genes, RAG-1 and RAG-2, are required for V/D/J recombination to take place.[26,27] Indeed, in the hematopoietic system, the two genes are found only in cells that carry out V/D/J recombination. Their function is to make the proteins required for the assembly of the genes encoding the proteins that, in mature B and T cells, recognize antigens and mount an appropriate immune response.

The role of the recombination-activating genes has been further clarified by the so-called knockout mice developed by two groups.[28,29] The technique is to disrupt, or knock out, a particular gene and see what the effect is, thereby ascertaining indirectly the function of the gene. It is a technique that works especially well in studying the immune system because mice with an immune system impaired by a knockout can nonetheless live if they are protected from infection.

In 1992 two groups reported that they had knocked out RAG-1 and RAG-2 in mice. They found that disrupting either gene made the mice severely immunodeficient—the equivalent of SCID mice—because most of their lymphocytes were immature and so could not function properly in mounting an immune response.

Medical Applications

The role of antibodies as practical reagents in the diagnosis of disease is well established, especially in the case of monoclonal antibodies. The application of these reagents as potential therapeutic agents has not developed as quickly, primarily because of the obvious limitations of administering murine or other nonhuman antibodies to an immunocompetent patient. Several approaches relying on recombinant DNA technology are being taken in efforts to solve this problem [*see Chapter 11*].

For example, it is possible to use only the smallest portion of a murine monoclonal antibody gene (the complementarity-determining regions, concerned with antigen binding) to convey the antibody's specificity into the framework of otherwise human heavy- and light-chain genes. Thus one can produce so-called humanized antibodies in which the major portion of the antibody molecule corresponds to the human sequence. Other techniques—which involve cycling human antibody genes through a bacteriophage, allowing the selection of useful heavy- and light-chain combinations—may make it possible to produce human monoclonal antibodies without taking the classical rodent monoclonal approach.

Such reagents may be useful in the treatment of viral as well as bacterial infections and in targeting cancer cells with appropriate toxins fused to immunoglobulin molecules. Indeed, the ability to target cells reliably with cell-specific antibodies of high affinity has implications that include the development of diagnostic imaging procedures as well as therapies for a variety of inflammatory, allergic, and—possibly—autoimmune diseases.

References

1. Dreyer WJ, Bennett JC: The molecular basis of antibody formation: a paradox. *Proc Natl Acad Sci USA* 54:864, 1965

2. Faust CH, Diggelmann H, Mach B: Estimation of the number of genes coding for the constant part of the mouse immunoglobulin kappa light chain. *Proc Natl Acad Sci USA* 71:2491, 1974

3. Leder P, Honjo T, Packman S, et al: The organization and diversity of immunoglobulin genes. *Proc Natl Acad Sci USA* 71:5109, 1974

4. Brack C, Tonegawa S: Variable and constant parts of the immunoglobulin light chain gene of a mouse myeloma cell are 1250 nontranslated bases apart. *Proc Natl Acad Sci USA* 74:5652, 1977

5. Seidman JG, Leder A, Edgell MH, et al: Multiple related immunoglobulin variable-region genes identified by cloning and sequence analysis. *Proc Natl Acad Sci USA* 75:3881, 1978

6. Seidman JG, Leder P: The arrangement and re-arrangement of antibody genes. *Nature* 276:790, 1978

7. Max EE, Seidman JG, Leder P: Sequences of five potential recombination sites encoded close to an immunoglobulin kappa constant region gene. *Proc Natl Acad Sci USA* 76:3450, 1979

8. Sakano H, Huppi K, Heinrich G, et al: Sequences at the somatic recombination sites of immunoglobulin light-chain genes. *Nature* 280:288, 1979

9. Alt FW, Enea V, Bothwell AL, et al: Activity of multiple light chain genes in murine myeloma cells producing a single functional light chain. *Cell* 21:1, 1980

10. Davis MM, Calame K, Early PW, et al: An immunoglobulin heavy-chain gene is formed by at least two recombinational events. *Nature* 283:733, 1980

11. Maki R, Traunecker A, Sakano H, et al: Exon shuffling generates an immunoglobulin heavy chain gene. *Proc Natl Acad Sci USA* 77:2138, 1980

12. Kataoka T, Kawakami T, Takahashi N, et al: Rearrangement of immunoglobulin gamma 1-chain gene and mechanism for heavy-chain class switch. *Proc Natl Acad Sci USA* 77:919, 1980

13. Burnet FM: *The Clonal Selection Theory of Acquired Immunity.* Cambridge University Press, London, 1959

14. Early P, Rogers J, Davis M, et al: Two mRNAs can be produced from a single immunoglobulin mu gene by alternative RNA processing pathways. *Cell* 20:313, 1980

15. Alt F, Bothwell ALM, Knapp M, et al: Synthesis of secreted and membrane-bound immunoglobulin mu heavy chains is directed by mRNAs that differ at their 3′ ends. *Cell* 20:293, 1980

16. Rogers J, Early P, Carter C, et al: Two mRNAs with different 3′ ends encode membrane-bound and secreted forms of immunoglobulin-bound and secreted forms of immunoglobulin mu chain. *Cell* 20:303, 1980

17. Singer PA, Singer HH, Williamson AR: Different species of messenger RNA encode receptor and secretory IgM mu chains differing at their carboxy termini. *Nature* 285:294, 1980

18. Davis MM, Kim SK, Hood LE: DNA sequences mediating class switching in alpha-immunoglobulins. *Science* 209:1360, 1980

19. Dunnick W, Rabbitts TH, Milstein C: An immunoglobulin deletion mutant with implications for the heavy-chain switch and RNA splicing. *Nature* 286:669, 1980

20. Takahashi N, Kataoka T, Honjo T: Nucleotide sequences of class-switch recombination region of the mouse immunoglobulin gamma 2b-chain gene. *Gene* 11:117, 1980

21. Hirayoshi K, Nishikawa SI, Kina T, et al: Immunoglobulin heavy chain gene diversification in the long-term bone marrow culture of normal mice and mice with severe combined immunodeficiency. *Eur J Immunol* 17:1051, 1987

22. Witte PL, Burrows PD, Kincade PW, et al: Characterization of B lymphocyte lineage progenitor cells from mice with severe combined immune deficiency disease (SCID) made possible by long term culture. *J Immunol* 138:2698, 1987

23. Kim M-G, Schuler W, Bosma MJ, et al: Abnormal recombination of IgH D and J gene segments in transformed pre-B cells of SCID mice. *J Immunol* 141:1341, 1988

24. Malynn BA, Blackwell TK, Fulop GM, et al: The SCID defect affects the final step of the immunoglobulin VDJ recombinase mechanism. *Cell* 54:453, 1988

25. Okazaki K, Nishikawa S-I, Sakano H: Aberrant immunoglobulin gene rearrangement in SCID mouse bone marrow cells. *J Immunol* 141:1348, 1988

26. Schatz DG, Oettinger MA, Baltimore D: The V(D)J recombination activating gene, RAG-1. *Cell* 59:1035, 1989

27. Oettinger MA, Schatz DG, Gorka C, et al: RAG-1 and RAG-2, adjacent genes that synergistically activate V(D)J recombination. *Science* 248:1517, 1990

28. Mombaerts P, Iacomini J, Johnson RS, et al: RAG-1 deficient mice have no mature B and T lymphocytes. *Cell* 68:869, 1992

29. Shinkai Y, Koyasu S, Nakayama K, et al: Restoration of T cell development in RAG-2-deficient mice by functional TCR transgenes. *Science* 259:822, 1993

General Reference

Max E: Immunoglobulins: molecular genetics. *Fundamental Immunology*, 2nd ed. Paul WE, Ed. Raven Press, New York, 1989, p 235

Acknowledgments

This article has been adapted from "The Genetics of Antibody Diversity," by Philip Leder, in *Scientific American* 246(5):102, 1982. © 1982 Scientific American, Inc. All rights reserved.

Figures 1 through 5, 7, 8   From "Antigens, Antibodies, and T cell Receptors," by C. Terhorst and J. David, in SCIENTIFIC AMERICAN *Medicine*, edited by E. Rubenstein and D. D. Federman, Section 6, Subsection II. Scientific American, Inc., New York, 1994. All rights reserved.

Figure 1   George Kelvin.

Figure 2   Dana Burns. Data from "The Molecules of the Immune System," by S. Tonegawa, in *Scientific American* 253(4):122, 1985. © 1985 Scientific American, Inc. All rights reserved. Computer graphic model and photograph by A. J. Olson, Ph.D. © 1985 Research Institute of Scripps Clinic. Used by permission.

Figure 3   Wendy Wolf and Talar Agasyan.

Figure 4   Dana Burns and Wendy Wolf.

Figure 5   Wendy Wolf and Talar Agasyan. Data from "The Molecular Genetics of the T Cell Antigen Receptor and T Cell Antigen Recognition," by M. Kronenberg, G. Siu, L. E. Hood, et al, in *Annual Review of Immunology* 4:529, 1986.

Figure 6   Tom Moore. Adapted from "The Genetics of Antibody Diversity," by Philip Leder, in *Scientific American* 246(5):102, 1982. © 1982 Scientific American, Inc. All rights reserved.

Figures 7, 8   Wendy Wolf and Talar Agasyan.

CHAPTER 5

Gene Cloning

John L. R. Rubenstein, M.D., Ph.D.

Recombinant DNA technology—and with it the ability to isolate genes, to sequence and alter them, to learn how they function, to express them as proteins that can be characterized and then perhaps modified and produced in large amounts—has revolutionized biology and promises to have a similarly profound effect on medical practice. "The central experimental maneuver in these manipulations is the cloning of genes," as Robert A. Weinberg has put it, "and it is cloning, more than any other single factor, that has changed the face of biology."

To clone is to multiply asexually—more specifically, to grow a colony of bacteria from a single bacterial cell. Gene (or molecular) cloning is essentially the process of amplifying a particular gene selectively by incorporating it into a bacterial cell and cloning the bacterium. Sometimes, the gene thus cloned is a known one and the objective is to characterize it or synthesize its protein product; at other times, the objective is to identify a hitherto unknown disease gene. To understand the achievements and the promise of molecular medicine, one needs to have some feel for the techniques of gene cloning.

A Little History

In the early 1970s, several groups at Stanford University and the University of California at San Francisco first reported successful recombinant DNA experiments and the cloning of DNA in bacteria. Their achievement was made possible by the convergence of several conceptual and technological advances. The advances that contributed most directly to the advent of cloning included the identification, by the 1960s, of small circular DNAs called plasmids, which carry genes for bacterial resistance to antibiotics. Throughout the 1960s, the physical chemistry of DNA was being elucidated, and important advances in understanding the energetics and kinetics of DNA base-pairing were being worked out by several groups. Important advances in polymer biophysics led to the development of physicochemical methods for purifying supercoiled plasmid DNA. A critical step was the discovery and characterization of restriction endonucleases in the late 1960s by Hamilton Smith, Werner Arber, and Daniel Nathans. These bacterial enzymes (the best known is *Eco*RI, named for *Escherichia coli*, its source) cut DNA at specific sites within specific nucleotide sequences. In 1967, several groups purified DNA ligase, an enzyme capable of covalently joining pieces of DNA. Then, improved ways of getting naked DNA into *E. coli* were developed.

Each of these discoveries contributed to a series of clever experiments designed by several groups in the early 1970s. (Actually, the original theoretical prescription for gene cloning was written in 1969 by a graduate student at Stanford named Peter Lobban; his experimental studies with Dale Kaiser were not published until after other workers had built on his insight to carry out the first gene-cloning experiments.) In 1972, Paul Berg's group successfully inserted genes from bacteriophage λ (lambda) and *E. coli* into the SV40 virus genome. Janet Mertz and Ron Davis then demonstrated that DNA digested by *Eco*RI had cohesive ("sticky") ends, which could readily be joined with DNA ligase [*see Figure 1*]. Stanley Cohen and Herbert Boyer put all these elements together by joining pieces of two plasmids, one encoding resistance to tetracycline and the other resistance to kanamycin. They thus created a chimeric, or recombinant, DNA mole-

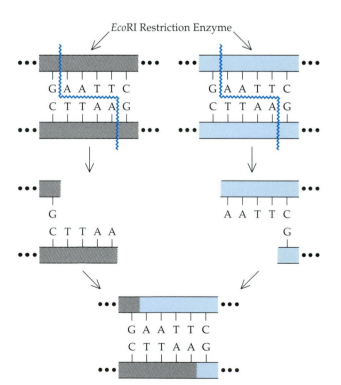

EcoRI Restriction Enzyme

Figure 1 *The* EcoRI *restriction enzyme makes staggered but symmetric cuts in the DNA, leaving four-base tails on the end of each fragment. These fragments tend to adhere to complementary single-stranded tails, regardless of the source of the DNA, and are therefore called sticky ends.*

cule. They introduced it into *E. coli*, where the genes encoding resistance were expressed: the bacteria were now resistant to both tetracycline and kanamycin. The door was thus opened to the era of genetic engineering.

Elements of Gene Cloning

The cloning of genetic material begins with the insertion of the DNA one seeks to clone into a cloning vector and the propagation of this chimeric DNA molecule in a host organism. The process leads to the amplification of specific DNA fragments more than 10^{10}-fold, making possible the isolation and chemical characterization of specific DNA sequences. Moreover, because cloning permits the production of milligram quantities of a given piece of DNA, a broad range of in vitro manipulations of gene structure—or genetic engineering—becomes possible.

Cloning Vectors

A cloning vector is a DNA molecule that has three major characteristics. First, it is capable of replicating independently of the host chromosome in at least one organism; second, organisms containing the vector can be grown preferentially because the vector confers on the organism some readily identifiable physical or chemical properties, or both; third, additional DNA can be inserted into the vector. Cloning vectors fall into two general classes: plasmid vectors and phage vectors [*see Figure 2*].

PLASMID VECTORS

Plasmids are small extrachromosomal circles of double-stranded DNA that replicate independently in bacteria. Often they encode proteins that confer resistance to antibiotics. A typical plasmid vector is a naturally occurring or redesigned plasmid incorporating a replicon that encodes an origin of DNA replication, a gene encoding an enzyme that inactivates an antibiotic, and a cloning site. One of the earliest vectors was pBR322.[1,2] Most plasmid cloning vectors are designed to replicate in *E. coli* [*see Figure 3*]. All the enzymes required for the replication of the plasmid DNA are produced by the host bacterium, although the plasmid's replicon helps regulate the initiation of replication.

The replicon is a region of about 1,000 base pairs encoding the site at which DNA replication is initiated as well as a set of regulatory elements involved in controlling how many copies of the plasmid are made within any given bacterium[3]; mutations in specific parts of the replicon can increase this plasmid copy number. For instance, the pBR322 plasmid, which has a pMB1 replicon, has a copy number of from 15 to 20 plasmids per cell—a low copy number; pBluescript SK(–), with a mutated form of the same replicon, has a copy number of from 500 to 700 plasmids per cell—a high copy number. For most purposes, high–copy number plasmids are preferable because of the increased amplification of the cloning vector.

The next essential element for plasmid cloning vectors is a selectable marker. Most plasmid vectors encode a gene that confers on bacteria resistance to an antibiotic (or two or even more such genes).[3] A variety of such genes are available off the shelf. Their expression enables the host bacterium to grow in media containing particular antibiotics and thus to

a

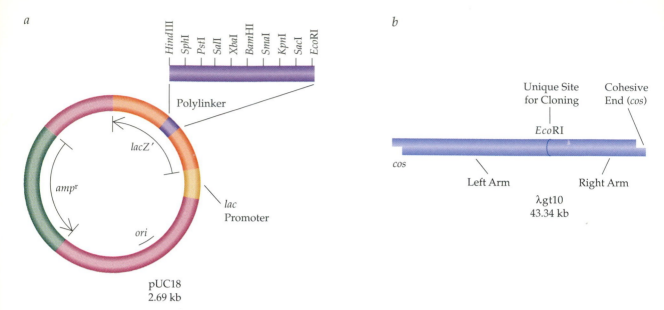

b

Figure 2 *Shown are typical cloning vectors. (a) This is a typical plasmid vector used for propagating cloned DNA fragments. Important features of plasmid vectors include an origin of replication (ori) that permits the efficient replication of plasmids to hundreds of copies per cell, a drug-resistance gene (amp^r for ampicillin resistance) to allow selection of cell clones carrying the plasmid, and restriction enzyme cleavage sites for the insertion of foreign DNA fragments. Modern vectors often carry an array of restriction sites in a polylinker. In plasmids of the popular pUC family, the polylinker is situated within a fragment of the E. coli lacZ gene (lacZ'), which encodes β-galactosidase. The polylinker does not disrupt the lacZ reading frame, and in an appropriate E. coli host expression of this lacZ fragment leads to synthesis of active β-galactosidase enzyme. When these E. coli are grown on an agar plate containing a colorless compound called X-gal, cleavage of the X-gal by the enzyme produces an insoluble blue product, so that E. coli colonies with plasmids that do not have an insert of foreign DNA in their polylinker are blue. However, insertion of a foreign fragment into the polylinker usually shifts or terminates the lacZ reading frame in the plasmid, β-galactosidase is not produced, and the resulting plasmid yields colorless colonies that are easily distinguished on the agar plates. (b) The phage λ vector λgt10 is commonly used for cDNA cloning. Phage structural genes are clustered on the left and right arms of the phage genome. Sequences in the middle are dispensable for purposes of phage replication. In lambda-based cloning vectors, these dispensable sequences are removed and replaced with restriction enzyme sites for cloning of complementary DNA. In addition to the phage structural genes that permit replication, λ vectors also retain the single-stranded cohesive ends (cos) that are required for phage DNA packaging.*

be selected from bacteria that do not harbor the plasmid. For example, pBR322 encodes both the ampicillin-resistance gene (*amp^r*) and the tetracycline-resistance gene (*tet^r*); bacteria harboring native pBR322 are able to grow in a medium containing both ampicillin and tetracycline. Cloning vectors must also contain at least one cloning site, where the foreign DNA is inserted. A cloning site is a specific DNA sequence that is recognized and cut by a restriction endonuclease. The endonuclease is an enzyme that binds to DNA at a recognition sequence and hydrolyzes the phosphodiester bonds on both strands of the DNA.[3-8] There are three classes of restriction enzymes, one of which (class II) is preferred for recombinant DNA work. Class II restriction enzymes recognize a sequence of from four to eight nucleotides. Such restriction sites usually have twofold symmetry. That is, the recognition sequence on one strand of the DNA is the mirror image of the sequence on the complementary strand: in other words, restriction sites are palindromes. Another important feature of these enzymes is that many of them do not cut the DNA in the middle of the restriction site; this feature produces DNA molecules with overhanging ends.

The restriction enzyme *Eco*RI, isolated from *E. coli*, cleaves DNA wherever it sees the sequence 5'-GAATTC-3'. The plasmid pBR322 has only one *Eco*RI site. It is in the promoter region of the tetracyline-resistance gene, tet^r, so that when pBR322 is cut by *Eco*RI, the circular plasmid is converted to a linear structure and tet^r is disabled (but amp^r remains intact).

The *Eco*RI endonuclease scans the pBR322 molecule until it finds the GAATTC sequence, where it severs the phosphodiester bond between the

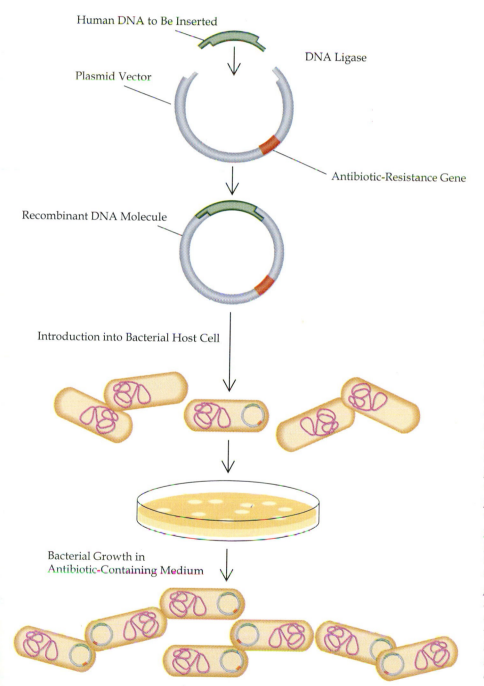

Figure 3 *An* Escherichia coli *plasmid that contains a single recognition site for the restriction enzyme* EcoRI *as well as a bacterial gene that confers antibiotic resistance can be used as a vector for a human gene. After* EcoRI *cuts the plasmid, the fragments from the plasmid vector and its insert can be covalently joined by the action of the enzyme DNA ligase. The plasmid can, in turn, replicate within a bacterial host to produce many copies of the fragment of DNA, and the bacteria themselves reproduce. Growth of the bacteria on plates containing antibiotics selects for those cells that contain copies of the plasmid with its human insert. The human gene can then be recovered when the plasmid is cut by a restriction enzyme.*

deoxyguanosine and the deoxyadenosine (G/AATTC) on both strands of the DNA, creating a four–base pair (AATT) single-stranded overhang. The phosphate group that originally bridged the deoxyguanosine and the deoxyadenosine remains attached to the deoxyadenosine.

As noted earlier, the *Eco*RI site is a palindrome, so that the overhanging single-stranded ends are complementary to each other and can hybridize, or anneal to each other, by base-pairing. Such complementary single-stranded ends of DNA molecules are commonly referred to as sticky ends. Although they can anneal to each other, short overhangs (fewer than 15 base pairs), cannot hybridize stably at physiologic temperatures; stable joining requires the formation of a phosphodiester bond between the ends of the DNA molecules. The enzymes called DNA ligases perform exactly this type of reaction, and so a DNA ligase must be supplied to covalently join pieces of DNA.

With its two sticky ends, the *Eco*RI-cleaved, linear pBR322 molecule could close on itself and thus revert to its circular form. Since the objective is to make the plasmid a vector—a carrier for another piece of DNA that one seeks to clone—the plasmid DNA is treated with a phosphatase to remove its terminal phosphate groups. Elimination of these phosphates prevents the linear vector from cyclizing in the absence of another piece of DNA.

Now the DNA to be cloned can be inserted into the vector. This DNA fragment, having been cleaved from its source by *Eco*RI, has *Eco*RI sticky ends, and they retain their terminal phosphate groups. The fragment to be inserted anneals to the vector, and DNA ligase catalyzes the covalent joining of the vector DNA to the new piece of DNA. In this manner, the new DNA is inserted into the *Eco*RI site of pBR322. This is perhaps the most critical step in all types of gene cloning; it is a general method for inserting genes into cloning vectors as well as assembling a number of pieces of DNA to create new genes.

Imagine that the new piece of DNA is a 1,000 bp DNA fragment encoding the insulin gene. Mixed with the vector DNA, annealed and ligated with it, the insulin gene becomes a passenger on the vector molecule, ready for the next step in its cloning.

Now the vector, carrying its inserted insulin gene, is introduced into bacteria. This process, termed DNA transformation, can be accomplished by several techniques, of which the most efficient is electroporation[9]: the chimeric DNA is mixed with bacteria in a cuvette, and an electrical potential is created across the walls of the container. Through a mechanism that is not fully understood, the DNA enters the bacteria. The bacteria are then grown in the presence of ampicillin. Those that harbor the recombinant pBR322 plasmid (and thus the *amp*[r] gene) will proliferate, whereas any bacteria that were not transformed with the recombinant plasmid will die. The bacteria can be cultured in liquid medium or on ampicillin-containing agar plates; the latter make it possible to isolate individual colonies, or clones, of bacteria that contain the cloning vector.

These clones can be characterized in several ways. First, given that the insertion of the insulin gene into the *Eco*RI site of the pBR322 vector disabled the *tet*[r] gene, bacteria harboring the plasmid should be resistant to ampicillin but sensitive to tetracycline. This provides a simple assay for identifying ampicillin-resistant bacterial clones that contain vectors carrying the insulin gene. For a more definitive test, individual bacterial clones can be cultured and their DNA isolated and examined. There are a variety of ways to separate the vector DNA from bacterial chromosomal DNA. Once the plasmid DNA has been purified, its structure can be analyzed to verify that the insulin gene was indeed ligated into the pBR322 *Eco*RI site. This can be done by digesting the DNA with *Eco*RI and then electrophoresing the products of the reaction through an agarose gel. If the pBR322 is carrying the insert, *Eco*RI will cut the two *Eco*RI sites that mark the junctions between the insert and the vector, converting the circular molecule into two linear fragments. The pBR322 fragment is 4,322 bp in length, and the fragment encoding the insulin gene is 1,000 bp long. Larger pieces of DNA migrate through the agarose matrix more slowly than smaller pieces of DNA. The DNA is then visualized by staining the gel with ethidium bromide, which becomes highly fluorescent when it is intercalated into DNA. Thus, electrophoresis resolves the two products of the latest *Eco*RI reaction and verifies whether the pBR322 cloning vector has incorporated the insulin gene.

PHAGE VECTORS

Almost all phage vectors [*see Figure 2*] are based on bacteriophage λ, a bacterial virus that infects *E. coli*. Phage vectors were developed because their several potential advantages over plasmid vectors were recognized. For one thing, phages introduce their genes into bacteria with notable efficiency. (After all, that is their way of life.) Second, because many phage species have large genomes, they can be exploited to clone larger pieces of DNA. Although these characteristics have made phage cloning extremely popular, technological improvements in plasmid cloning methodologies have made plasmid cloning equally or more effective in particular situations. Investigators have also designed cloning vectors such as cosmids and phagemids (see below) that incorporate useful features of both phage and plasmid vectors.

Bacteriophage λ DNA is approximately 50 kb in length and encodes about 60 genes, which are arranged as three general groups: the immediate early, the delayed early, and the late genes. These sets of genes are involved in specific aspects of the life cycle of the virus. Knowledge of the basic steps in the viral life cycle is essential for understanding how phage λ functions as a cloning vector. After the 50 kb linear phage λ DNA genome enters a bacterium, DNA ligase joins the DNA's 12-base cohesive ends to form a circular molecule. Then, depending on a complicated balance of host and viral factors, the virus follows either a lysogenic or a lytic pathway.

If immediate early genes such as *N* and *cro* are not efficiently expressed, the virus enters the lysogenic pathway: the viral genome integrates into the *E. coli* chromosome, and expression of the *cI* gene represses the transcription of almost all the viral genes and thereby maintains the virus in the lysogenic, or dormant, state. On the other hand, if the *N* and *cro* immediate early genes are transcribed, their proteins initiate a cascade of gene transcription leading to the expression of the delayed early genes, which are involved in replication of the viral DNA, and thus the lytic pathway is induced. After expression of the delayed early genes, expression of the late genes begins; they encode proteins involved in construction of the viral capsid, packaging of the viral DNA into the capsid, and lysis of the infected bacterium.

Conversion of this complex bacteriophage into a useful vector for cloning genes has required modification of its genome. Fortuitously, the middle 33 percent of the genome, which is critical for the lysogenic pathway, is not essential for lytic growth, so that one can replace these sequences with a new piece of DNA. In simple terms, phage λ cloning vectors can be thought of as consisting of two pieces of DNA: the left arm and the right arm. The left arm, about 20 kb in length, encodes the late genes, the ones involved in capsid assembly. The right arm, about 10 kb long, encodes the delayed early genes required for replication of the phage DNA and the late genes, which regulate the lysis of the bacterium. The terminal portions of both the left and the right arm are *cos* (cohesive end) sites, which are the signals required for packaging the viral DNA into the capsids.

A versatile phage λ vector called λZAP[10] was extensively engineered to have several important features. First of all, its creators designed a poly-cloning site that has multiple restriction enzyme recognition sequences. The enzymes cut λZAP only in the polycloning site. Also, because their recognition sequences are large (from six to eight bases), they cut DNA infrequently, on average once every 5,000 bases. Such enzymes are helpful for cutting the insert out of the vector without cutting the insert into smaller pieces.

The next special feature of λZAP is that it can make fusion proteins in which the protein encoded by the cloned DNA is covalently linked to the bacterial enzyme β-galactosidase. Fusion proteins are useful for purifying the protein encoded by the cloned gene because antibodies to β-galactosidase can be used to immunoprecipitate the entire fusion protein. The fusion protein can also be injected into animals to create antisera to the cloned gene's product; the antibodies enable one to study many aspects of the protein's biology, such as its localization within tissues and individual cells. Furthermore, some fusion proteins maintain their normal activities, so that they can be used to study the enzymology or binding activities of the protein encoded by the cloned gene. Other types of fusion-protein systems have also been devised in which a specific amino acid sequence links the bacterial protein to the protein encoded by the cloned gene. This linking peptide encodes a site that can be digested by a protease, which cuts the link between the two proteins and allows one to purify the protein encoded by the cloned gene.

The third feature of λZAP is that promoters for two specific RNA polymerases flank its polycloning site. On one side, there is a promoter that is recognized by the RNA polymerase of bacteriophage T3; on the other side, there is a promoter recognized by the RNA polymerase of bacteriophage T7. Because the promoters are on opposite sides of the cloning site, these RNA polymerases transcribe complementary strands of the cloned insert. For instance, the T3 polymerase can make a single-stranded RNA copy of one of the DNA strands of the cloned DNA—either the coding (sense) or the noncoding (antisense) strand, depending on the orientation of the DNA insert. Whichever RNA transcript encodes the coding strand can then be translated to make the protein encoded by the gene. This type of synthetic RNA can also be translated in vitro or in vivo to study the structure and function of the encoded protein.

The most distinctive feature engineered into λZAP is that it encodes a phagemid vector (a hybrid between a filamentous virus and a plasmid) that can be excised in vivo from the λ vector. This is useful because it is technically easier to prepare large amounts of cloned DNA fragments from a phagemid vector than from a λ vector (see below).

The process of ligating a DNA insert into a λ vector is essentially the same as with a plasmid vector [*see Figure 4*]. The critical factor is that the DNA insert must have termini that are compatible with ligation into the λ cloning site. For instance, if the DNA insert has *Eco*RI cohesive ends, the left and right arms of the λ vector must each have *Eco*RI complementary ends. After the ligation step, the DNA is packaged into phage λ as protein capsids with the aid of a complex mixture of structural proteins and enzymes. The recombinant bacteriophages, having been assembled in vitro, are allowed to infect *E. coli*. The infected bacteria are mixed with agarose and poured onto agar plates. Diffusion of the bacteria along the plane of the plate is limited because the bacteria are constrained within the agarose polymeric matrix. Therefore, when an individual infected bacterium is lysed by the recombinant bacteriophage, only neighboring bacteria will be infected by the same virus. Within about five hours, the recombinant bacteriophage will have gone through many rounds of replication and will have lysed bacteria within a 1 mm diameter; the region of cell lysis appears clear when the agar plate is examined visually and is called a plaque. Each plaque contains millions of copies of a single viral clone. In other words, the genotype of each plaque is pure. Just as a bacterial colony corresponds to a clone generated by plasmid vectors, so a plaque corresponds to a clone generated by phage λ vectors.

Individual plaques can be purified, and the phages from within the plaque can be grown on a large scale to isolate the DNA. Furthermore, if a piece of nitrocellulose paper is placed on top of the plaques, some of the phage particles will stick to the nitrocellulose. The phage particles can be disrupted, and the extruded DNA can then be irreversibly attached to the nitrocellulose. Radioactive nucleic acid probes can be used in a hybridization reaction to screen the nitrocellulose filter for the presence of a specific λ clone [*see Figure 5*]. Plaques on the nitrocellulose that contain phage DNA with an insert that is homologous to the probe will become radioactively labeled. Labeled plaques are easily detected by apposing photographic film to the nitrocellulose filter: the plaques appear as black dots on the film. In this manner, one can use nucleic acid probes to identify a gene within a λ gene library.

COSMID VECTORS

Cosmid vectors are hybrids between plasmid and phage λ vectors; they contain elements common to both, and so have more versatility.[3,11] A typical cosmid vector, c2RB,[12] is like a plasmid vector in that it carries an origin of replication and a cloning site. Like pBR322, it has two antibiotic resistance genes (in this case, *amp*^{r} and *kan*^{r}). The feature that distinguishes a cosmid is that it encodes the *cos* sequence, the DNA sequence required

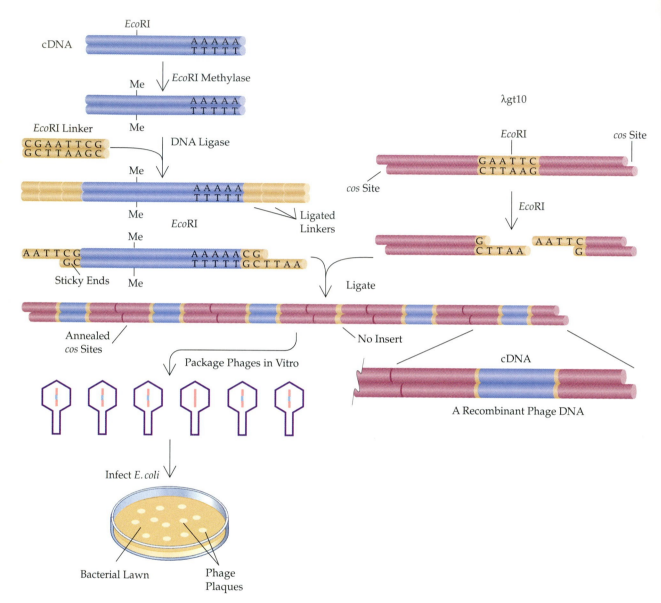

Figure 4   *To clone cDNA in a phage vector, it must be given single-stranded tails complementary to restriction sites on the phage DNA. Phage DNA is usually prepared simply by cleavage with a restriction enzyme, in this case* EcoRI, *and the two phage arms are purified. Meanwhile* EcoRI *ends are atttached to the cDNA. This is done using synthetic oligonucleotide linkers that carry* EcoRI *sites. First, the cDNA is treated with* EcoRI *methylase, which methylates any* EcoRI *sites in the cDNA to protect them from cleavage by* EcoRI *restriction enzyme. Next, the* EcoRI *linkers are attached to the ends of the cDNA with DNA ligase; usually, many linkers become ligated to the ends of each cDNA molecule. The linkered cDNA is exhaustively treated with* EcoRI *to cleave all the linkers, leaving a single* EcoRI *sticky end at each end of the cDNA molecules. Now the cDNA and phage arms have compatible ends. They are covalently joined with DNA ligase, resulting in a tandem array of recombinant phage molecules flanked by* cos *sites. This concatenated DNA is the substrate for packaging into infectious phage paritcles, which is accomplished by adding the DNA to lysates prepared from* λ*-infected* E. coli. *The packaged phages are used to infect fresh* E. coli *cultures, and the infected cells are spread on agar plates to yield plates carrying thousands of individual phage plaques. Each plaque arises from a single recombinant phage molecule, now propagating as a viable phage.*

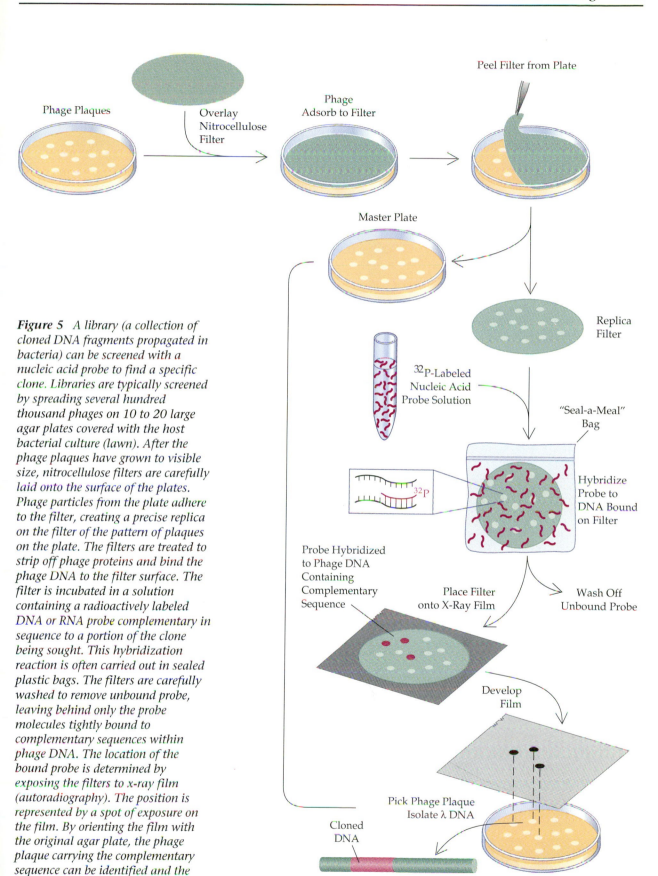

Figure 5 *A library (a collection of cloned DNA fragments propagated in bacteria) can be screened with a nucleic acid probe to find a specific clone. Libraries are typically screened by spreading several hundred thousand phages on 10 to 20 large agar plates covered with the host bacterial culture (lawn). After the phage plaques have grown to visible size, nitrocellulose filters are carefully laid onto the surface of the plates. Phage particles from the plate adhere to the filter, creating a precise replica on the filter of the pattern of plaques on the plate. The filters are treated to strip off phage proteins and bind the phage DNA to the filter surface. The filter is incubated in a solution containing a radioactively labeled DNA or RNA probe complementary in sequence to a portion of the clone being sought. This hybridization reaction is often carried out in sealed plastic bags. The filters are carefully washed to remove unbound probe, leaving behind only the probe molecules tightly bound to complementary sequences within phage DNA. The location of the bound probe is determined by exposing the filters to x-ray film (autoradiography). The position is represented by a spot of exposure on the film. By orienting the film with the original agar plate, the phage plaque carrying the complementary sequence can be identified and the desired clone can be isolated.*

for the packaging of DNA into λ capsids. Any DNA that is between 38 and 52 kb in length and carries *cos* sequences at its ends can be packaged into phage λ particles. (To use the 6.8 kb c2RB as a vector, one must insert into it DNA fragments that are between 31 and 45 kb in length.)

The first step is to digest c2RB with the *Bam*HI and *Sma*I restriction enzymes. This creates two *cos*-containing fragments, which can be thought of as the left and right arms of λ DNA. Next, one prepares the DNA that is to be inserted into the cosmid vector. This can be done in several ways, such as by shearing chromosomal DNA to a length of about 31 to 45 kb and ligating it to *Bam*HI adaptors or by partially digesting the chromosomal DNA with an enzyme called *Mbo*I. *Mbo*I creates cohesive ends that will ligate to *Bam*HI ends. (*Mbo*I is a good choice because it cuts DNA much more frequently than does *Bam*HI, recognizing a four–base pair site in contrast to *Bam*HI's six–base pair site.) By doing a partial digest with *Mbo*I, one can generate an overlapping set of long DNA fragments, which are particularly useful for gene mapping. The chromosomal DNA is treated with phosphatase and then ligated to the cosmid arms. The recombinant DNA is packaged into λ capsids, which are allowed to infect *E. coli*. Because the cosmid does not encode the λ proteins necessary for either the lytic or the lysogenic cycle, it persists and replicates as a plasmid. Because it carries the *cos* sequences, however, if the bacteria are later infected with phage λ, the cosmid is likely to be packaged in vivo during the lytic infection. The bacteria will then produce large amounts of packaged recombinant cosmid, which can serve as a viral stock for storing the cosmid or for infecting new bacteria for other purposes.

Cosmid vectors are specifically designed to clone large pieces of DNA and to propagate their DNA either as a virus or as a plasmid. Cosmids and λ vectors are now the standard vectors for cloning genomic DNA. Cosmids have also been adapted to a wide range of other applications, including homologous recombination between two different plasmids in the same cell and growth in both animal cells and bacteria.

PHAGEMID VECTORS

Phagemid vectors are hybrids between plasmids and a gene from bacteriophage M13.[3,13,14] They are designed for converting a double-stranded plasmid into a single-stranded form. Single-stranded DNA is particularly useful for manipulations such as DNA sequencing, site-directed mutagenesis, and subtractive hybridization (see below).

Bacteriophage M13 is a filamentous DNA virus that infects, but does not lyse, *E. coli*. The viral genome is a circular, single-stranded 6.4 kb DNA molecule. After the single-stranded viral DNA enters the bacterium, it is converted into a double-stranded DNA form, which in turn provides a template for production of the single-stranded viral genomic DNA that is packaged into new phage filaments. A region of the viral genome called the intergenomic domain is responsible for instructing the cell to make these single-stranded DNA copies. Any plasmid growing in *E. coli* that encodes the intergenomic domain will also be converted into a single-stranded circle if the cell becomes infected with M13.[3,13,14] Appreciation of this fact led to the development of the phagemid vectors, which are simply plasmid vectors that carry the M13 intergenomic domain.

The particularly handy phagemid vector called pBluescript SK(–) (the same vector that is part of the λZAP molecule) encodes the pMB1' origin of replication, *amp*[r], T3 and T7 RNA polymerase promoters flanking a polycloning site, the β-galactosidase fusion gene, and the M13 intergenomic domain. New pieces of DNA can be inserted into various cloning sites in the polylinker domain. The recombinant double-stranded DNA molecules are introduced into bacteria. If these bacteria are subsequently infected with M13 bacteriophage, the infected cells will begin to produce phage filaments containing both wild-type M13 and the single-stranded form of the phagemid. The phage can be purified from the supernatant of the infected cells, and the DNA is then isolated from the phage.

YEAST PLASMID VECTORS

Bacteria have been the workhorses for most gene-cloning manipulations and will probably continue to be the host organism of choice in the future. For some operations, however, a eukaryotic host, such as yeast, is clearly preferable. The best example of this has been the development in yeast of artificial chromosomes [*see Chapter 6*], which can carry pieces of DNA as large as a megabase, or 10^6 bases. This is 20 times as much DNA as the most capacious bacterial cloning vectors (cosmids) can propagate. Yeast artificial chromosomes (YACs) are based on YAC vectors.[15] YAC vectors are chimeras of bacterial plasmids and the functional units of eukaryotic chromosomes. A typical YAC encodes a bacterial origin of replication, an antibiotic resistance gene, a cloning site, a yeast centromere, a yeast origin of replication, two telomeres, and a selectable gene for growth in yeast.

A crucial step in the construction of artificial chromosomes is the preparation of very large chromosomal DNA fragments. (DNA that is longer than about 30 kb is relatively fragile; it can easily be broken by shear forces, so that extreme care must be taken to prepare DNA that is longer than 100 kb.) Methods such as flow sorting of chromosomes and pulse-field electrophoresis have been developed that permit the purification of DNA fragments suitable for creating YAC genomic libraries with average insert sizes as large as 430 kb. To achieve this, genomic DNA is partially digested with a restriction enzyme to create cohesive ends. The genomic DNA is then ligated to phosphatase-treated YAC vector DNA, and the recombinant molecules are introduced into yeast. Yeast cells that are transformed by the YAC vector therefore carry an additional chromosome.

YACs are presently the most efficient vectors for cloning large pieces of DNA, which are desirable because they facilitate gene mapping experiments. For instance, if two genes are separated by more than 50 kb, previous cloning methodologies would never be able to show their physical linkage; a YAC clone allows one to show that the genes are linked. This is particularly important in gene mapping experiments in which one is trying to clone a gene on the basis of its physical relation to known genetic markers. Cloning a gene on the basis of its location is a powerful technique that has resulted in the isolation of several disease-causing genes, such as those responsible for cystic fibrosis, neurofibromatosis type 1, and Duchenne's muscular dystrophy. YACs are playing an increasingly important role in these studies.

EUKARYOTIC PLASMID VECTORS

Eukaryotic cloning vectors are used to express cloned genes in animal or plant cells. Like YACs, eukaryotic cloning vectors can express genes in both bacteria and eukaryotic cells, and so they are known as shuttle vectors. They carry a bacterial replicon and an antibiotic-resistance gene, which permit them to be propagated in bacteria. They also carry a eukaryotic enhancer and promoter located 5′ to the coding sequence of a gene and a polyadenylation site located 3′ to the gene. Several vectors also include an intron, either before or after the coding sequence.

Plasmid pSV2*gpt* was one of the first eukaryotic vectors.[16] This plasmid expresses the gene (*gpt*) that encodes the *E. coli* enzyme xanthine-guanine phosphoribosyl transferase, which serves as a selectable marker. The gene is placed under the transcriptional control of several components from the SV40 virus genome: 5′ to the *gpt* gene is the SV40 enhancer and early promoter; 3′ to the gene are the SV40 small T intron and the polyadenylation site.

The function of a eukaryotic expression vector can be evaluated by introducing the plasmid DNA into animal cells by one of several methods, such as electroporation, transfection of precipitated DNA, or microinjection. When pSV2*gpt* is introduced into animal cells, the *gpt* gene is expressed through transcription from the SV40 early promoter to produce an mRNA transcript that can be translated to make the enzyme it encodes. The enzyme can be detected several hours after the plasmid enters the cell. At this stage, most of the pSV2*gpt* molecules are extrachromosomal, but several days after it enters the cell, some of the pSV2*gpt* DNA integrates into the host cell's chromosomes. In general, integration only takes place in a small proportion of the cells, and there is a way to select for cells that stably express the *gpt* gene—a method analogous to those used to select for bacteria expressing antibiotic-resistance genes. At present, there are several other genes that can serve as selectable markers in animal cells. These include aminoglycoside phosphotransferase (*apt*), thymidine kinase (*tk*), dihydrofolate reductase (*dhfr*), hygromycin B phosphotransferase (*hpt*), and adenosine deaminase (*ad*).[3]

Eukaryotic vectors can in theory express any gene, and so these vectors have been used to isolate genes on the basis of their function. This is done by inserting a complementary DNA (cDNA) into the vector between the promoter and the polyadenylation site. The pcD vector was the first eukaryotic vector designed to express a cDNA library in animal cells.[17] It is basically the same as pSV2*gpt*, except that it is designed specifically for the construction of a directional cDNA library using a vector-primer. Entire cDNA libraries constructed in pcD can be introduced into animal cells, and individual cells expressing a specific gene can be isolated, provided there is an assay for the gene product.

Eukaryotic expression vectors can also be used to make a transgenic animal,[18,19] an animal carrying a new gene that was artificially introduced into the embryo. The standard method involves microinjecting a cloned gene, usually in an expression vector, into the female pronucleus of a one-cell embryo. The microinjected DNA integrates into the host chromosome and thereby becomes part of the animal's genome. Genes can also be introduced into embryos with viral vectors (see below). Transgenic animals are powerful systems for studying the effect of mutation or aberrant expression of a gene on an organism.

EUKARYOTIC VIRAL EXPRESSION VECTORS

Just as bacterial viruses have been exploited to clone genes, viruses that infect eukaryotic cells can serve to introduce DNA into animal cells—not, typically, as the primary vector for cloning a gene but rather to demonstrate the expression of a cloned gene in eukaryotic cells. Historically, the first eukaryotic viral vectors were based on the papovavirus SV40.[20] SV40 is a small (5,400 bp) double-stranded DNA virus that can carry only a small amount (2,000 bp) of new DNA.

Two versatile viral vector systems have been developed: retroviral vectors[21] and herpes virus vectors.[22] This discussion will focus on the retroviral vectors. Retroviruses contain a single-stranded RNA genome that is converted into a double-stranded DNA molecule inside the infected cell.[23] The double-stranded DNA integrates into the host cell's chromosome as the proviral genome, which is analogous to the λ provirus in the lysogenic pathway. However, unlike the lysogenic λ provirus, the retroviral provirus continues to transcribe its entire genome, which encodes all the proteins necessary to make new virions; the infected cell therefore continues to make new virus constitutively. Unlike phage λ, however, most retroviruses do not kill the cells they infect.

The retroviral genome is rather simple. Flanking the coding sequence are tandem long terminal repeats (LTRs), which are important for mediating the integration of the provirus into the infected cell's chromosome and for regulating transcription. Just internal to the LTRs are sequences involved in replicating the viral genome and packaging the genomic RNA into the virus. The central 80 percent of the genome comprises three genes: *gag*, *pol*, and *env*.

The *gag* gene encodes several proteins that form the core of the virus. The *pol* gene encodes several enzymes, including reverse transcriptase (the critical enzyme that converts the single-stranded viral genomic RNA into DNA) and an enzyme involved in integration of the proviral DNA into the host chromosome. Finally, the *env* gene encodes the viral envelope glycoprotein, which is required for viral entry into cells. The beauty of retroviral vectors is that all the viral genes can be replaced with new DNA.

Like most eukaryotic vectors, a retroviral vector is a chimera of a bacterial plasmid and DNA sequences that allow it to propagate and express genes in animal cells. In this case, the essential features include a cloning site between two LTRs, the packaging signal, and the sequences necessary for DNA replication [*see Figure 6*]. After ligation of a gene into the cloning site, the vector is grown in bacteria to produce large amounts of the DNA. Then the purified DNA is introduced into an animal cell line in tissue culture. The recombinant DNA integrates into the host chromosome and is transcribed to form recombinant RNA molecules. The RNA transcripts carry the packaging signal and therefore can be packaged into capsids.

Special cell lines are used to accomplish the packaging of the recombinant RNA.[24,25] Packaging cell lines produce all the retroviral gene products but do not produce wild-type virions. Therefore, the packaging cell can be used to encapsidate the recombinant retroviral RNA to produce infectious

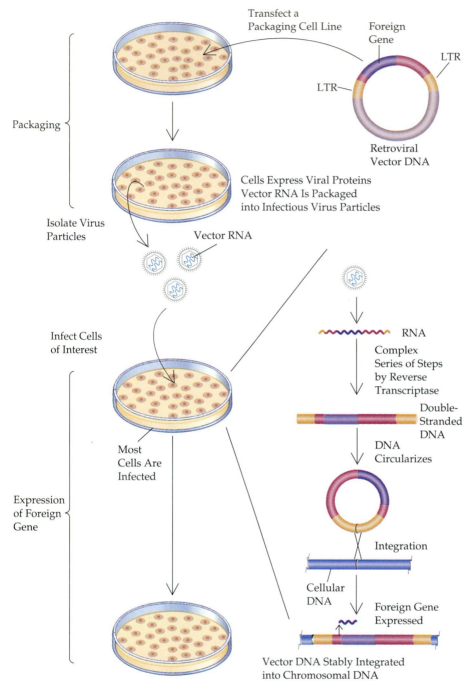

Figure 6 *A retroviral vector can be used for stable, long-term expression of a foreign gene. The gene is cloned into a retroviral vector that lacks most viral genes. The gene is usually expressed under the control of the strong viral promoter in the LTR. The recombinant plasmid is transfected into a special packaging cell line that harbors an integrated provirus. The provirus has been crippled so that, although it produces all the proteins required to assemble infectious viruses, its own RNA cannot be packaged into virus. Instead, RNA produced from the recombinant virus is packaged. The virus stock released from the packaging cells thus contains only recombinant virus. The virus can be used to infect virtually any other cell type, resulting in the integration of the viral genome and the stable production of the foreign gene product.*

virions. The recombinant virions can then infect a target cell and thereby introduce the cloned gene into this new cell. This method has been applied in many ways, including the introduction of genes into preimplantation embryos to make transgenic mice[26-29]; most recently, it has come to be used for gene therapy[30] [*see Chapter 12*].

Genetic Engineering Methods

Along with the techniques directly involved in cloning, such as cutting DNA with restriction enzymes, joining segments of DNA with DNA ligases, insertion of DNA in vectors, and other procedures already described, many additional operations have been developed for modifying DNA to engineer new sequences and new proteins.

MODIFICATION OF THE ENDS OF DNA

For a number of cloning procedures, it is necessary to modify the ends of DNA molecules. As has been noted, restriction enzymes can generate linear DNA molecules having complementary, cohesive ends that greatly facilitate ligation. In many situations, however, one wants to ligate a particular piece of DNA into a cloning vector and the ends of the two molecules are not complementary.

Imagine that the goal is to insert into the *Eco*RI site of a plasmid a DNA fragment whose termini are not complementary to the AATT single-stranded overhang of the *Eco*RI site; its termini were generated by the restriction enzyme *Not*I, which creates single-stranded cohesive ends with the sequence GGCC. The first step in altering the termini is to fill in the *Not*I sticky ends by incubation with DNA polymerase and the nucleosides deoxyguanosine triphosphate (dGTP) and deoxycytidine triphosphate (dCTP). The blunt ends are then converted to sticky ends by ligating onto the blunt ends small so-called adapter oligonucleotides having the *Eco*RI cohesive sequence AATT. The DNA fragment now is compatible for sticky-ends ligation into any *Eco*RI site.

Another useful method for altering the DNA sequence at the end of the molecule depends on the enzyme terminal transferase, which does not require a template to synthesize DNA; it polymerizes DNA in a random sequence onto a DNA primer. If the enzyme is supplied with only one of the four nucleotide substrates, it will add a short stretch of that nucleoside monophosphate at the 3' end of the DNA molecule. For instance, if a DNA fragment is mixed with terminal transferase in the presence of deoxythymidine triphosphate (dTTP), the enzyme will catalyze the addition of thymidines to the 3' end of the DNA, which will anneal to similarly generated poly(A) ends. This method of adding homopolymeric sequences to DNA was, as a matter of fact, one of the first methods developed for creating cohesive ends on DNA fragments.

ALTERATION OF DNA SEQUENCE

The ability to clone specific genes and produce large amounts of them has opened the door to chemical modification of their structure. There are many ways to mutate genes in vitro.

The first method is to make deletions in the gene. The simplest way to do this is to cut out pieces of the gene with restriction enzymes and then to close up the gene with DNA ligase; expression of the gene then produces a modified protein that lacks certain stretches of amino acids. There are also ways to make deletions from an end of a gene with exonucleases. One can also insert new DNA coding sequences into genes. These relatively easy manipulations allow researchers to perform myriad experiments, from testing the function of certain parts of a protein to giving a protein new enzymatic properties. An example is the fusion of one polypeptide with another as in the case, discussed above, of fusions of β-galactosidase with other gene products.

Specific point mutations can even be introduced at particular positions in a gene with the help of M13 phagemid vectors such as pBluescript SK(–). The first step is to insert the gene one wants to mutate into the cloning site of the phagemid vector and convert the vector to a single-stranded form. An oligonucleotide is synthesized that is complementary to a specific region of the gene except for one noncomplementary base, which will become the point mutation. The oligonucleotide is mixed with the single-stranded phagemid; the two molecules hybridize to each other, except at the one–base pair mismatch. DNA polymerase is added to the reaction; with the oligonucleotide as a primer and the single-stranded phagemid as a template, it converts the molecule to a double-stranded form. The double-stranded molecule, which still has the one–base pair mismatch, is introduced into bacteria. During the first round of DNA replication in the bacteria, the two strands of DNA give rise to two different DNA molecules, one with the point mutation and the other without it. These molecules segregate into different bacteria, which give rise to independent colonies when grown on agar plates. Phagemid DNA from several different colonies is then isolated, and DNA sequencing identifies clones carrying the point mutation.

Construction of Gene Libraries

Generally, the first step in the isolation of a gene is the construction of a gene library from a source that contains the gene. There are two general types of gene libraries: genomic libraries and complementary DNA libraries.[3,7,8,31] Genomic libraries are based on chromosomal DNA; for cDNA libraries, mRNA is the original source of the genetic material to be introduced into the cloning vector.

Genomic Libraries

Genomic libraries are constructed from chromosomal DNA isolated from an organism. Chromosomal DNA purified from the tissue is cleaved into smaller pieces with a restriction endonuclease such as *Eco*RI. The next step is to choose a cloning vector. Because the length of genomic DNA fragments tends to be relatively large (> 10,000 bases), phage or cosmid vectors are most effective. The λ DNA is cleaved with the *Eco*RI restriction endonuclease and then mixed with the *Eco*RI-digested chromosomal DNA. DNA ligase is added to the reaction, catalyzing the covalent attachment of the chromosomal DNA to the two arms of the λ vector DNA. The recombinant molecules are packaged into phage λ capsids, which are then allowed to infect *E. coli* bacteria. Several hours after starting the infection, the recombinant phages have replicated several millionfold. The phages can be purified from the bacteria, and the collection of the virions constitutes a phage genomic library.

Phage libraries typically consist of at least 10^7 independent recombinants, implying that 10^7 different recombinant phages productively infected the *E. coli*. If the average length of the genomic DNA insert was 10^4 bases (10 kb), the library is large enough to carry about 10^{11} (10^7 recombinants multiplied by 10^4 bases) bases of genomic DNA. This genomic library of 10^7 recombinants, then, is large enough to incorporate all the sequences found in the human genome (which comprises a total of approximately 2×10^{10} bases).

Genomic libraries constructed in bacteriophages are usually stored as phage particles in solution. To purify an individual recombinant clone, the phage particles are mixed with *E. coli* and plated on agar to create plaques of individual λ clones. Nitrocellulose replicas of the plaques are submitted to hybridization reactions to screen for individual clones having homology to a particular nucleic acid probe.

Methods have been developed to make phage libraries from individual eukaryotic chromosomes. Chromosomes from organisms such as yeast can be separated electrophoretically, so that libraries can be made from the individual chromosomes. Chromosomes from higher organisms are typically much larger, but they can be isolated by fluorescence-activated chromosomal sorting. This procedure has made possible the construction of libraries from individual human chromosomes.

cDNA Libraries

A cDNA library is constructed from mRNA. The first task is to choose the tissue from which the desired mRNA is obtained. For instance, if the goal is to isolate the β-globin gene (which encodes one of the protein subunits of hemoglobin), the mRNA would be purified from cells that express large amounts of this gene, such as reticulocytes (in which globin mRNA accounts for a substantial fraction of total mRNA). Given that the human genome encodes about 10^5 different genes, reticulocyte mRNA is clearly very greatly enriched in globin-coding sequences as compared with genomic DNA. In other words, cDNA cloning helps one to isolate a gene when one can identify cells that contain large amounts of the mRNA corresponding to that gene.

To isolate the mRNA from the cells, the cells are dissolved in a solution that inactivates ribonucleases, and then the RNA is separated from other cellular constituents, typically by density-gradient centrifugation through a solution of cesium chloride. The mRNA is purified from the other types of RNA (rRNA and tRNA) by taking advantage of mRNA's stretch of some 30 to 100 adenines at its 3' end—the so-called poly(A) tail. The adenines can hybridize to a complementary polymer of thymidines. The RNA solution is therefore passed through a chromatography column containing cellulose to which short polymers of thymidine, called oligo(dT) or poly(dT), are covalently attached. The poly(A)+ mRNA binds to the oligo(dT), whereas the poly(A)− RNA flows through the column. When the column is washed with water, the poly(A)+ mRNA detaches from the oligo(dT) and is eluted in pure form.

Now the mRNA must be converted into double-stranded DNA (because current technology is not able to clone RNA directly) by means of a series of enzymatic reactions. In the first reaction, reverse transcriptase makes a single-stranded DNA complement of the mRNA; this single-stranded DNA is the cDNA.

In the reverse transcriptase reaction, the template is the poly(A)$^+$ mRNA, and the primer is supplied in the form of oligo(dT), which hybridizes to the mRNA's poly(A) tail and allows the reverse transcriptase to initiate DNA synthesis. The products of this reaction are double-stranded molecules: one strand is RNA, and the other is DNA. In the next step, the RNA strand is converted into DNA with three different enzymes: *E. coli* DNA polymerase, *E. coli* DNA ligase, and RNase H. The RNase H is an RNA-specific endonuclease that cuts the RNA strand into short pieces, leaving 3′ hydroxyl and 5′ phosphate groups at each site of scission. The 3′ hydroxyl groups serve as primers for the DNA polymerase, which performs two functions: its polymerase activity copies the DNA strand, and its 5′ to 3′ exonucleolytic activity removes RNA and DNA in front of the advancing DNA polymerase. The DNA ligase links the short pieces of DNA. In sum, these enzymes convert the RNA-DNA molecules into double-stranded cDNA. The ends of the cDNA have been modified (as described above) to provide the desired cohesive ends.

The next step is to ligate the cDNAs into one of a variety of cloning vectors, including phagemid, phage λ, and eukaryotic vectors. Finally, the DNA is introduced into bacteria to create the cDNA library. Typically, about 10^6 independent clones of plasmid-containing bacteria can be established when a cDNA cloning experiment is started from about 1 µg of poly(A)$^+$ mRNA. The probability of isolating a desired clone is high when a cDNA library contains one million clones. This is true because even the most complex tissue (in terms of the number of different types of mRNA) has only about 30,000 different mRNA molecules.

Isolation of Genes from Gene Libraries

Once a gene library has been generated, the next step is to search through the millions of clones in the library for the desired gene. The many screening methods now available are based on particular properties of genes and the proteins they encode. One can screen for a gene on the basis of its DNA sequence or the immunoreactivity or function of its product.

PURIFICATION OF THE GRP RECEPTOR GENE FROM A cDNA LIBRARY

A description of the isolation of a specific gene, one encoding the gastrin-releasing peptide (GRP) receptor, will illustrate some of the routes to gene isolation.[32] The GRP receptor is a plasma membrane protein that binds the 27–amino acid gastrin-releasing peptide, an autocrine growth factor for some small-cell carcinoma cells.[33] (Physiologically, the peptide regulates gastric acid secretion, body temperature, carbohydrate metabolism, feeding and grooming behaviors, and pituitary hormone release.[33])

The first step in the isolation of this gene was the construction of a cDNA library from cells known to produce the receptor. The cDNA was inserted into a λ vector. Once a library of several million independent clones was prepared, the search for the GRP receptor gene began.

In very brief summary, the GRP receptor gene was cloned by purifying the GRP receptor protein and obtaining a partial amino acid sequence, which was reverse-translated according to the genetic code to construct a radiolabeled oligonucleotide with which to probe nitrocellulose filters containing replicas of plaques from the cDNA library. Individual radiolabeled plaques harboring the gene were thereby identified. The DNA from their cDNA inserts was sequenced and found to include stretches encoding bits of the purified receptor. Then the cDNA was used to make synthetic mRNA. The mRNA was injected into *Xenopus* oocytes for an expression assay. Binding of the GRP peptide to the GRP receptor on a cell increases the cell's chloride conductance. When the injected oocytes were bathed in a solution containing the peptide, binding of the ligand did increase the cells' chloride conductance. That electrophysiologic result proved that the cDNA encoding the GRP receptor had indeed been isolated. In this case, then, screening with a nucleic acid probe and with an oocyte expression assay were successfully combined to identify the GRP receptor gene.

The general methods for isolation of a gene from a gene library fall into the following categories: screening by homology to nucleic acid probes, screening with antibodies to the gene's product, in vitro and in vivo expression assays, differential screenings, subtractive hybridization, and use of the polymerase chain reaction.

Screening by Homology to Nucleic Acid Probes

The cloning of the GRP receptor gene was, as described above, accomplished in part by probing with a synthesized oligonucleotide probe to detect a cDNA clone within a λ cDNA library. This is the standard method for detecting a cloned gene. In the case of the GRP receptor gene, the probe was based on a partial amino acid sequence of the receptor protein. Often, no amino acid sequence is available for the protein, in which case one usually cannot make a nucleic acid probe. Fortunately, there are exceptions to this limitation. For example, if one suspects that the gene has homology to other genes, one can construct a probe based on the known gene's structure. Imagine that the objective is to isolate the particular IgG gene that is being expressed by a clone of B cells. It would be possible to make a cDNA library from the B cell's mRNA and then to screen the library with a probe homologous to the IgG constant region, a highly conserved domain present on all IgG genes. This general approach takes advantage of the fact that many genes have homologies to other genes that have previously been cloned; it has become an extremely fruitful method of isolating new genes.[3]

Screening for an Immunoreactive Product

In many situations, it is technically easier to make an antibody against a particular protein than to obtain a partial amino acid sequence. Antibodies can be used to screen cDNA libraries for particular genes cloned in expression vectors.[34] For instance, the λZAP and the pBluescript vectors described above can express the cloned gene in bacterial cells as a fusion protein with β-galactosidase. Clones from a cDNA library, in the form of replicas of phage plaques on nitrocellulose filters, can be screened with antibodies against the protein encoded by the desired gene. The antibody will bind to the plaques containing the protein and can be detected by one of a number of methods. The recombinant phage obtained from the plaques that bound the antibody is then purified. The cDNA clone can be further analyzed by DNA sequencing and functional assays to verify that it encodes the desired gene.

Screening with a Functional Assay for the Gene Product

Cloning the GRP receptor gene required verification that the cDNA clone encoded a protein that bound GRP and that could also induce GRP's normal physiologic response. This was done by injecting synthetic mRNA made from the cDNA clone into *Xenopus* oocytes. The method has been very effective for identifying a variety of neurotransmitter receptor genes. The oocyte expression system is one of several methods for assaying a cloned gene's function. These fall into two general classes: in vitro expression and in vivo expression. In vitro expression assays call for making a synthetic mRNA from the cloned gene,[3,35-37] and translating the transcript in vitro.[35] After translation, the presence of the desired protein can be assayed in several ways. If the gene encodes an enzyme, one can measure the enzyme's activity; if an antibody to the protein is available, the protein can be immunoprecipitated and purified for characterization of its structure.

In vivo expression assays call for expressing the cloned gene in cells, as in the oocyte expression system. Other in vivo expression assays depend on such expression vectors as the eukaryotic expression vector pcD and eukaryotic viral vectors. Expression assays are not limited to animal cells: in many situations, yeast and bacteria are excellent organisms in which to test the function of a cloned gene.

Again, there must be a method for detecting the presence of the new gene: an enzymatic (or electrophysiological) assay for the gene product, an antibody against the protein, or an assay in which the cloned gene complements a cellular defect. The complementation assay is a particular strength of in vivo expression. For example, the mutant gene responsible for cystic fibrosis has been cloned.[38] To verify the cloning, a normal copy of the cloned mutant gene was isolated and introduced into cultured cells taken from a patient with cystic fibrosis. It was expressed, and its product corrected the electrophysiological defect associated with the disease,[39,40] confirming that the cloned gene does encode the protein that is defective in patients with cystic fibrosis.

Expression of cDNA libraries in animal cells in tissue culture can also be used to isolate a gene.[41] For example, cDNA clones encoding lymphokines[42,43] and a T cell surface protein[44] have been isolated by expressing a cDNA library in tissue culture cells. A major problem with this approach is that there are not enough mammalian cell lines with well-characterized genetic deficiencies (mutations) in specific genes. Such cell lines would be extremely useful for expression cloning with genetic complementation as the assay. As an alternative to mammalian cells, several research groups are exploring the suitability of other organisms, such as bacteria and yeast, for expression cloning screened by complementation. This approach is reasonable because it is much easier to isolate and characterize mutations in haploid microorganisms. Yeasts have advantages over bacteria because they are eukaryotes and therefore more like animal cells. This is an area of rapid technological change, and progress in it promises to result in the cloning of many more genes.

Differential Screening and Subtractive Hybridization

In many situations, an investigator wants to identify genes of unknown function that are expressed in one type of cell but not in another—in undifferentiated precursor cells and in terminally differentiated cells, for example. Two physical methods for identifying genes whose expression changes in the course of differentiation are differential hybridization and subtractive hybridization. These methods have been employed to isolate genes expressed during differentiation of the brain. The first step is to isolate mRNA from both embryonic and adult brain tissue. The objective is to compare the mRNAs from the two tissues and to isolate transcripts that are found preferentially or exclusively in one of the tissues.

In differential hybridization[45] [*see Figure 7*] (which is easier to perform but less sensitive than subtractive hybridization), after the two mRNAs have been isolated, a cDNA library is made from the target tissue: the tissue from which one wants to isolate the gene. If, for example, the goal is to isolate genes that are expressed after the differentiation of the brain, the target tissue is the adult brain. The mRNA from the adult brain is then cloned into, say, the pBluescript SK(–) phagemid vector to make a cDNA library of 10^6 recombinant clones. Next, 1/1,000 of the library is grown on agar plates as 1,000 discrete colonies. The bacterial colonies are picked individually and replated in a matrix, each colony at one point in a 1,000-point grid. Two replicas of the matrix are made on nitrocellulose filters. The filters are treated chemically to lyse the bacteria and fix their DNA onto the surface of the nitrocellulose.

The next step is to identify bacterial clones that contain cDNAs corresponding to genes that are preferentially expressed in the adult brain. To this end, the mRNAs from the embryonic and from the adult brain are converted into radioactively labeled cDNAs. Then two separate hybridization reactions are performed on the two nitrocellulose filters carrying the target bacterial matrix. One filter is probed with the labeled cDNA made from embryonic brain, the other filter with the adult brain cDNA. Bacterial colonies that harbor cDNAs homologous to the probe mRNA will hybridize to the radioactive probe and can be identified by autoradiography. Finally, one compares the filters from the two samples to find clones that are radioactively labeled by the probe made from the adult brain mRNA but not by the probe made from the embryonic brain mRNA. These clones correspond to genes whose expression is induced in the course of differentiation of the brain. This is a relatively simple procedure that can yield powerful results, but it is seriously limited by the fact that differential hybridization is only sensitive for abundant mRNA molecules. For mRNA molecules less abundant than 0.1 percent, the method is not very effective because of signal-to-noise limitations.

An alternative approach is subtractive hybridization [*see Figure 8*], which in principle should identify any differentially expressed gene. In one subtractive hybridization protocol, cDNA libraries are made from both

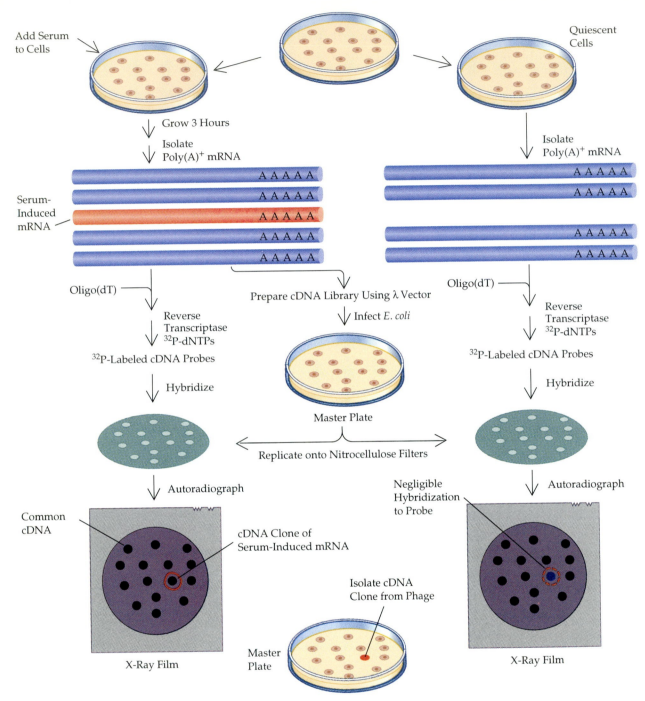

Figure 7 *Shown is an example of the cloning of growth factor–regulated genes by differential hybridization. This strategy was used to clone a family of genes that are rapidly induced when quiescent cells are stimulated to grow by the addition of serum (which contains growth factors). Poly(A)⁺ RNA was isolated from cultures of quiescent cells and from cells stimulated with serum for three hours (the target cells). RNA from the stimulated cells was used to produce a cDNA library in a phage λ vector, which was plated out. Phages from the plaques produced were transferred to duplicate filter replicas. Radioactively labeled probes were generated from the mRNA of quiescent cells and stimulated cells by synthesizing the cDNA strands in the presence of ³²P-labeled deoxynucleotides (dNTPs). One set of filters was hybridized to each cDNA probe. The resulting autoradiographs were carefully compared to identify the position of phage plaques that hybridized to the probe from stimulated cells but not to the probe from quiescent cells. These phages carried cDNAs from genes turned on in the serum-stimulated cells.*

tissues.[46-48] One library is the target, the other the so-called driver. The target is the cDNA library from which one wants to isolate the differentially expressed gene or genes; the driver is a cDNA library that serves to remove from the target library those cDNA clones that are not expressed differentially. Subtractive hybridization has two major phases. In the hybridization phase, one mixes the driver and the target samples and allows cDNAs that are common to both libraries to hybridize to each other. In the subtraction phase, one removes the driver cDNAs and with them any target cDNAs that have hybridized to the driver; the only cDNAs that remain in the sample are the target cDNAs that were not also in the driver sample.

In one such subtractive hybridization procedure, cDNA libraries from adult and embryonic brain are constructed in phagemid vectors, with the cDNAs inserted in opposite orientations in the two libraries. Next, the cDNA libraries are converted into single-stranded form by means of M13 phagemid rescue. Because the cDNA inserts are inserted into the phagemid vectors directionally, complementary strands for a given cDNA will be rescued from the adult and the embryonic libraries. Then, biotin is covalently bound to embryonic single-stranded cDNA; the biotinylated cDNA will serve as the driver in the hybridization reaction. The driver is mixed with the single-stranded adult cDNA library (the target). Complementary sequences in the target and the driver hybridize to each other. After the hybridization step, the protein avidin, which binds to biotin, is added to the reaction. Now the target molecules that have hybridized to the biotinylated driver can be extracted with an organic solvent. Target molecules, which encode cDNAs preferentially expressed in the adult brain, remain in solution and can be recovered by cloning in bacteria.

The Polymerase Chain Reaction

The polymerase chain reaction (PCR) has revolutionized gene cloning because it allows one to isolate a gene from as little as one cell [*see Chapter 6*]. The basis for this procedure is the in vitro amplification of specific pieces of DNA.[49] The first step is to construct two oligonucleotide primers, which must be homologous to some part of the gene one wants to amplify; one oligonucleotide is complementary to the sense strand and the other is homologous to the antisense strand. The primers are mixed with either chromosomal DNA or cDNA. The sample is heated to 95° C to melt the double-stranded DNA and then is allowed to cool. During the cooling process, the oligonucleotides find and anneal to their complementary gene. Typically, the reaction is cooled to 55° C, although other temperatures may be chosen, depending on the melting temperature of the oligonucleotide-DNA hybrid. Next, DNA polymerase is added to the reaction and, with the oligonucleotides as primers and the temperature raised to 72° C, it replicates the DNA. The special DNA polymerase used for this step is purified from a bacterium called *Thermus aquaticus*, an organism that lives in near-boiling water. Unlike most enzymes, this *Taq* DNA polymerase is not denatured at 95° C and is active at 72° C. After the first round of DNA replication, the reaction is again heated to 95° C to melt the DNA; on cooling, the oligonucleotides again anneal to the gene

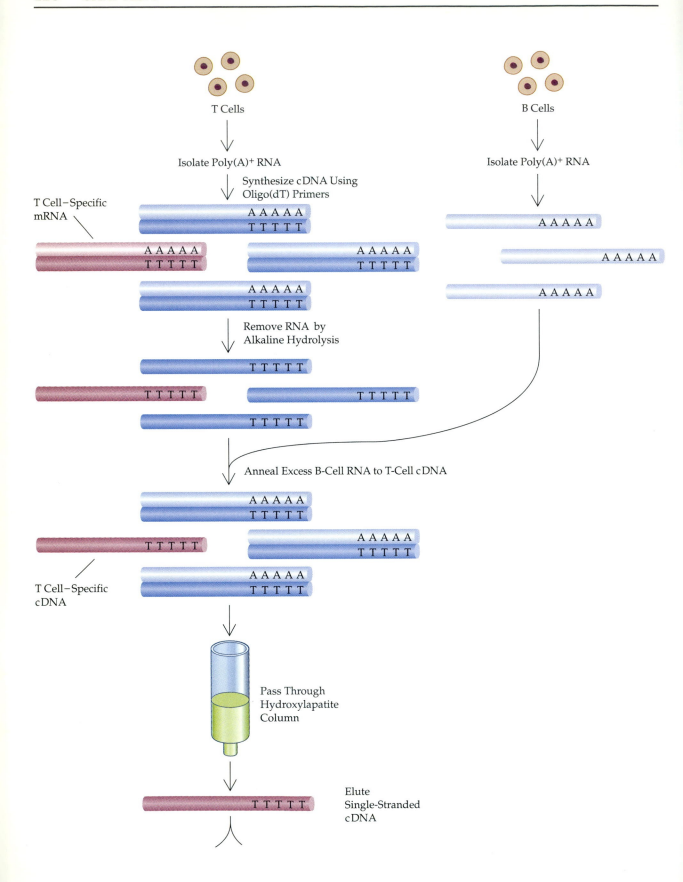

Figure 8 *Shown is an example of the use of subtractive hybridization to isolate cDNAs encoding the T-cell antigen receptor, a gene expressed only in T cells. Poly(A)⁺ RNA was prepared both from T cells and from B cells, which are very closely related to T cells but do not express the T-cell receptor. Using oligo(dT) primers, researchers synthesized the cDNA strands from the T-cell RNA. The RNA was removed from the resulting RNA-DNA hybrids by alkaline hydrolysis. What was left was single-stranded cDNA complementary to T-cell mRNA. The cDNA was incubated with a large excess of B-cell mRNA under conditions that favored DNA-RNA hybridization. All the T-cell cDNAs for genes also expressed in B cells (about 98 percent) hybridized to B cell RNA. T cell–specific cDNAs remained single-stranded. The mixture was passed over a column of hydroxylapatite, which retained the double-stranded molecules and let the single-stranded cDNAs pass through. These cDNAs were recovered, converted to double-stranded cDNAs, and cloned. The library was screened with a subtracted*
³²P-labeled cDNA probe prepared in precisely the same way.

at 55° C, and with reheating to 72° C, the DNA polymerase makes another copy of the gene. The process of melting the DNA, reannealing the oligonucleotide primers, and replicating the DNA is repeated at least 30 times, resulting in an exponential amplification of the gene. A machine called a thermal cycler automates the temperature changes required for the various parts of the reaction. The DNA product of the PCR reaction can be ligated into a vector, cloned, and sequenced.

PCR makes possible the amplification and purification of a gene fragment from a complex mixture of DNA. The only limitation is that to construct the primers one needs to know some of the DNA sequence of the desired gene. Fortunately, many genes have domains that are homologous to other genes, such as genes in the immunoglobulin family. One can therefore design PCR primer oligonucleotides that are complementary to a known gene in an effort to amplify related unknown genes.

PCR is also extremely valuable as a diagnostic and a forensic tool. Because it is such a rapid and sensitive technique, it can easily screen tens of samples simultaneously for the presence of a specific gene. For instance, PCR is used for diagnostic assays to detect pathological alleles of cystic fibrosis.

Isolation of Genes That Cause Human Disease

Application of the methods described in this chapter has led to the isolation and chemical characterization of many genes that, when mutated, cause diseases in humans.[50] The isolation of many of the genes implicated in human disease required some prior information about the molecular nature of the genetic defect. For instance, in sickle cell anemia [*see Chapter 8*], it was recognized that the molecular defect was in the globin protein, and that clue greatly facilitated the isolation of the gene. Unfortunately, for many genetic diseases there is inadequate information about the molecular etiology of the disorder; to isolate genes causing this type of illness, other methods are required.

References

1. Bernard HU, Helinski DR: Bacterial plasmid cloning vehicles. *Genetic Engineering: Principles and Methods*, Vol 2. Setlow JK, Hollaender A, Eds. Plenum Press, New York, 1980, p 133

2. Balbas P, Soberon X, Bolivar F, et al: The plasmid, pBR322. *Vectors: A Survey of Molecular Cloning Vectors and Their Uses*. Rodriguez RL, Denhardt DT, Eds. Butterworths, Boston, 1988, p 5

3. Sambrook J, Fritsch EF, Maniatis T: *Molecular Cloning: A Laboratory Manual*, 2nd ed. Cold Spring Harbor Laboratory Press, 1989

4. Watson JD, Hopkins NH, Roberts JW, et al: *Molecular Biology of the Gene,* 4th ed., Vol 1. The Benjamin Cummings Publishing Company, Menlo Park, California, 1987

5. Singer M, Berg P: *Genes & Genomes: A Changing Perspective*. University Science Books, Mill Valley, California, 1991

6. Lewin B: *Genes IV*. Oxford University Press, New York, 1990

7. Drlica K: *Understanding DNA and Gene Cloning: A Guide for the Curious*. John Wiley & Sons, New York, 1984

8. Watson JD, Tooze J, Kurtz DT: *Recombinant DNA: A Short Course*. W.H. Freeman and Company, New York, 1983

9. Dower WJ, Miller JF, Ragsdale W: High efficiency transformation of *E.coli* by high voltage electroporation. *Nucleic Acids Res* 16:6127, 1988

10. Short JM, Fernandez JM, Sorge JA: Lambda ZAP: a bacteriophage lambda expression vector with in vivo excision properties. *Nucleic Acids Res* 16:7583, 1988

11. Hohn B, Koukolikova-Nicola Z, Lindenmaier W, et al: Cosmids. *Vectors: A Survey of Molecular Cloning Vectors and Their Uses*. Rodriguez RL, Denhardt DT, Eds. Butterworths, Boston, 1988, p 113

12. Bates PF, Swift RA: Double cos site vectors: simplified cosmid cloning. *Gene* 26:137, 1983

13. Vieira J, Messing J: Production of single-stranded plasmid DNA. *Methods Enzymol* 153:3, 1987

14. Mead DA, Kemper B: Chimeric single-stranded DNA phage-plasmid cloning vectors. *Vectors: A Survey of Molecular Cloning Vectors and Their Uses*. Rodriguez RL, Denhardt DT, Eds. Butterworths, Boston, 1988, p 85

15. Hieter P, Connelly C, Shero J, et al: Yeast artificial chromosomes: promises kept and pending. Unpublished paper

16. Mulligan RC, Berg P: Expression of a bacterial gene in mammalian cells. *Science* 209:1422, 1980

17. Okayama H, Berg P: A cDNA cloning vector that permits expression of cDNA inserts in mammalian cells. *Mol Cell Biol* 3:280, 1983

18. Jaenisch R: Transgenic animals. *Science* 240:1468, 1988

19. Palmiter RD, Brinster RL: Transgenic mice. *Cell* 41:343, 1985

20. Hamer DH: DNA cloning in mammalian cells with SV40 vectors. *Genetic Engineering: Principles and Methods*, Vol 2. Setlow JK, Hollaender A, Eds. Plenum Press, New York, 1980, p 83

21. Nicolas JF, Rubenstein JL: Retroviral vectors. *Vectors: A Survey of Molecular Cloning Vectors and Their Uses*. Rodriguez RL, Denhardt DT, Eds. Butterworths, Boston, 1988, p 493

22. Elroy-Stein O, Fuerst TR, Moss B: Cap-independent translation of mRNA conferred by encephalomyocarditis virus 5' sequence improves the performance of the vaccinia virus/bacteriophage T7 hybrid expression system. *Proc Natl Acad Sci USA* 86:6126, 1989

23. Varmus H: Retroviruses. *Science* 240:1427, 1988

24. Watanabe S, Temin HM: Construction of a helper cell line for avian reticuloendotheliosis virus cloning vectors. *Mol Cell Biol* 3:2241, 1983

25. Cone RD, Mulligan RC: High-efficiency gene transfer into mammalian cells: generation of helper-free recombinant retrovirus with broad mammalian host range. *Proc Natl Acad Sci USA* 81:6349, 1984

26. Van der Putten H, Botteri FM, Miller AD, et al: Efficient insertion of genes into the mouse germ line via retroviral vectors. *Proc Natl Acad Sci USA* 82:6148, 1985

27. Huszar D, Balling R, Kothary R, et al: Insertion of a bacterial gene into the mouse germ line using an infectious retrovirus vector. *Proc Natl Acad Sci USA* 82:8587, 1985

28. Stuhlmann H, Cone R, Mulligan RC, et al: Introduction of a selectable gene into different animal tissue by a retrovirus recombinant vector. *Proc Natl Acad Sci USA* 81:7151, 1984

29. Rubenstein JL, Nicolas JF, Jacob F: Introduction of genes into preimplantation mouse embryos by use of a defective recombinant retrovirus. *Proc Natl Acad Sci USA* 83:366, 1986

30. Verma IM: Gene therapy. *Scientific American* 263(5):68, 1990

31. Methods in Enzymology, Vol 152. *Guide to Molecular Cloning Techniques*. Berger SL, Kimmel AR, Eds. Academic Press, Inc, San Diego, 1987

32. Battey JF, Way JM, Corjay MH: Molecular cloning of the bombesin/gastrin-releasing peptide receptor from Swiss 3T3 cells. *Proc Natl Acad Sci USA* 88:1, 1991

33. Cuttitta F, Carney DN, Mulshine J: Bombesin-like peptides can function as autocrine growth factors in human small-cell lung cancer. *Nature* 316:823, 1985

34. Young RA, Davis RW: Efficient isolation of genes by using antibody probes. *Proc Natl Acad Sci USA* 80:1194, 1983

35. Rubenstein JL, Chappell TG: Construction of a synthetic messenger RNA encoding a membrane protein. *J Cell Biol* 96:1464, 1983

36. Mackie GA: Vectors for the synthesis of specific RNAs in vitro. *Vectors: A Survey of Molecular Cloning Vectors and Their Uses*. Rodriguez RL, Denhardt DT, Eds. Butterworths, Boston, 1988, p 253

37. Melton DA, Krieg PA, Rebagliati MR, et al: Efficient in vitro synthesis of biologically active RNA and RNA hybridization probes from plasmids containing a bacteriophage SP6 promoter. *Nucleic Acids Res* 12:7035, 1984

38. Rommens JM, Iannuzzi MC, Kerem B, et al: Identification of the cystic fibrosis gene: chromosome walking and jumping. *Science* 245:1059, 1989

39. Drumm ML, Pope HA, Cliff WH, et al: Correction of the cystic fibrosis defect in vitro by retrovirus-mediated gene transfer. *Cell* 62:1227, 1990

40. Rich DP, Anderson MP, Gregory RJ, et al: Expression of cystic fibrosis transmembrane conductance regulator corrects defective chloride channel regulation in cystic fibrosis airway epithelial cells. *Nature* 347:358, 1990

41. Okayama H, Kawaichi M, Brownstein M, et al: High-efficiency cloning of full-length cDNA; construction and screening of cDNA expression libraries for mammalian cells. *Methods Enzymol* 154:3, 1987

42. Yokota T, Arai F, Rennick LD, et al: Methods for cloning cDNA. *Proc Natl Acad Sci USA* 82:4, 1985

43. Lee F, Yokota T, Otsuka P, et al: Methods for cloning cDNA. *Proc Natl Acad Sci USA* 83:4, 1986

44. Aruffo A, Seed B: Molecular cloning of a CD28 cDNA by a high-efficiency COS cell expression system. *Proc Natl Acad Sci USA* 84:8573, 1987

45. Cochran BH, Zumstein P, Zullo J, et al: Differential colony hybridization: molecular cloning from a zero data base. *Methods Enzymol* 147:64, 1987

46. Rubenstein JR, Brice AE, Ciaranello RD, et al: Subtractive hybridization system using single-stranded phagemids with directional inserts. *Nucleic Acids Res* 18:4833, 1990

47. Duguid JR, Rohwer RG, Seed B: Isolation of cDNAs of scrapie-modulated RNAs by subtractive hybridization of a cDNA library. *Proc Natl Acad Sci USA* 85:5738, 1988

48. Kowalski J, Smith JH, Ng N, et al: Vectors for the direct selection of cDNA clones corresponding to mammalian cell mRNA of low abundance. *Gene* 35:45, 1985

49. *PCR Technology: Principles and Applications for DNA Amplification*. Erlich HA, Ed. M Stockton Press, New York, 1959

50. McKusick VA, Francomano CA, Antonarakis SE: *Mendelian Inheritance in Man: Catalogs of Autosomal Dominant, Autosomal Recessive, and X-linked Phenotypes*, 9th ed. The Johns Hopkins University Press, Baltimore, 1990

Acknowledgments

Figure 1 Adapted from "Medical Genetics," by R. W. Erbe, in SCIENTIFIC AMERICAN *Medicine*, edited by E. Rubenstein and D. D. Federman, Section 9, Subsection IV. Scientific American, Inc., New York, 1994. All rights reserved.

Figures 2, 4 through 8 Adapted from *Recombinant DNA*, 2nd ed., by J. D. Watson, J. Witkowski, M. Gilman, et al. Scientific American Books, New York, 1992. © 1992 James D. Watson, Jan Witkowski, Michael Gilman, Mark Zoller. Used with permission.

Figure 3   Dimitry Schidlovsky. Adapted from "Medical Genetics," by R. W. Erbe, in SCIENTIFIC AMERICAN *Medicine*, edited by E. Rubenstein and D. D. Federman, Section 9, Subsection IV. Scientific American, Inc., New York, 1994. All rights reserved.

CHAPTER 6

The Human Genome Project

Maynard V. Olson, Ph.D.

The Human Genome Project first took clear form in the United States in February 1988, with the release of the National Research Council (NRC) report *Mapping and Sequencing the Human Genome.*[1] To a degree remarkable in Federal science policy, this report has had a clear effect on subsequent programmatic activity. A program is under way, jointly administered by the National Institutes of Health (NIH) and the Department of Energy (DOE), that conforms closely to the recommendations of the NRC committee. It is of both scientific and policy interest to examine how the committee's view toward this project has fared in the field.

Background

The human genome is the genetic material in human egg and sperm cells (i.e., germ cells): 3 billion (3 x 10⁹) base pairs (bp) of DNA. Given the four-letter alphabet of DNA—customarily symbolized with the letters A, G, T, and C—the sequence of 3×10^9 bp corresponds to 750 megabytes of information. If the sequence of the human genome could be determined, it would be possible to store and manipulate it on a desktop computer. The challenge, of course, lies in determining the sequence. Even the dream of acquiring DNA sequence on this scale is of recent origin. Dramatic progress was made during the 1950s and 1960s in understanding the mechanisms by which genetic information specifies biologic structure and function, but the information itself remained nearly inaccessible.

Discovery of Restriction Enzymes

A landmark event in DNA analysis came in 1970 with the discovery of site-specific restriction enzymes.[2-4] These remarkable endonucleases have the ability to scan any source of DNA for every occurrence of a particular string of bases—for example, the enzyme *Eco*RI recognizes the string GAATTC. Restriction enzymes cleave both strands of the double helix at their recognition sites. Since the cleavage events are directed by the DNA sequence, they always occur at the same positions in different samples of genomic DNA extracted from any genetically homogeneous source (e.g., different tissues of the same individual human being or different individuals sampled from an inbred strain of mice).

Restriction enzymes provide a way to develop precise physical maps of DNA simply by determining the coordinates in base pairs of the sites at which particular enzymes cleave.[4,5] Like topographic maps, physical maps of DNA derive their utility through annotation: mapped landmarks provide reference points relative to which functional DNA sequences such as genes can be localized. Restriction enzymes also facilitate a key step in the cut-and-splice procedures by which recombinant DNA molecules (i.e., DNA clones) are constructed [*see Chapter 5*].[4]

The importance of recombinant DNA technology is often attributed primarily to its synthetic dimension. For example, the ability to design and construct a DNA molecule that programs a bacterium to synthesize a mammalian protein provides a route to obtaining large amounts of the pure protein [*see Chapter 11*]. The ability to alter the structure of the protein through site-directed mutagenesis lends genuine novelty to the resultant biosynthetic opportunities.

In contrast to these synthetic applications of recombinant DNA technology, the Human Genome Project is an analytical application. Cloning makes it possible to purify individual recombinant DNA molecules from complex mixtures and then to prepare biochemically useful amounts of the molecules by culturing microbial strains into which they have been introduced.

Genetic Mapping

A less obvious consequence of the discovery of restriction enzymes was the development of the first practical method of genetic mapping in humans.[4,6] Most human cells contain two copies of each DNA sequence, one of maternal and the other of paternal origin. When a new germ cell is produced, it contains only one copy of the genome, a copy that is a unique mosaic of the two genomes from which it was derived. Genetic mapping involves measuring, through actual inheritance studies in families, the probability that two closely spaced segments of the genome will stay together during germ cell formation. The mapping requires an ability to distinguish between the two copies of the genome present in the somatic cells from which the germ cells are derived. Subtle differences in base sequence of particular copies of the human genome sometimes alter restriction sites and, hence, restriction fragment sizes. These alterations are detectable even in complex genomes by a method known as gel-transfer hybridization (the Southern blot), which was developed in 1975.[4,7] In

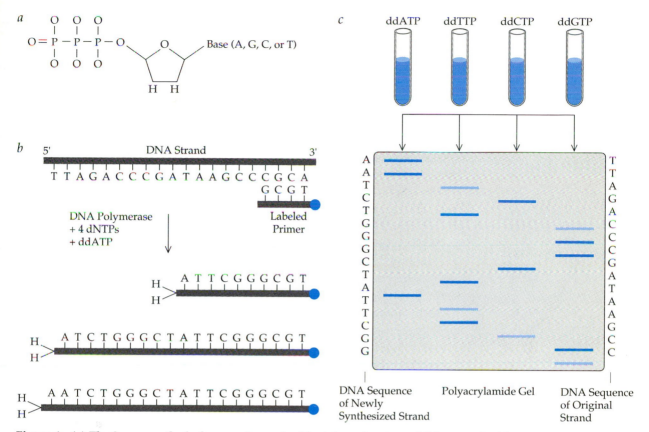

Figure 1 *(a) The Sanger method of sequencing nucleotides takes advantage of dideoxynucleotide triphosphates (ddNTPs). These nucleotides resemble normal deoxynucleotide triphosphates (dNTPs) but terminate, or cap, DNA synthesis because they cannot form a phosphodiester bond with the next dNTP. (b) In the Sanger method, a DNA fragment is mixed with a short primer that is complementary to one end of the unsequenced strand. DNA polymerase is then used to catalyze the synthesis of a complementary strand from a mixture of a ddNTP (in this figure, dideoxyadenosine triphosphate [ddATP]) and the four normal nucleotides (A, G, T, and C). Because the ddATP terminates DNA synthesis, several strands of DNA of different length will be produced, each ending in ddATP and indicating the position of the purine A in the complementary strand. (c) The process is repeated for each of the four nucleotides. Each of the series of DNA fragments is separated by size by polyacrylamide gel electrophoresis; the larger fragments travel least, and the shortest fragments travel farthest. The nucleotide sequence of the unsequenced strand can be read from the relative positions of the fragments on the gel.*

1987, the first global human genetic map, based on such restriction fragment length polymorphisms (RFLPs), was published.[8]

DNA Sequencing Methods

As to the actual determination of DNA sequence, reasonably efficient methods first appeared in 1977.[4,9,10] A technique known as chain-termination sequencing (also termed Sanger sequencing) came to dominate standard practice: it is based on enzymatic DNA synthesis, carried out in vitro in the presence of artificial chain-terminating variants of the normal DNA-precursor molecules [see Figure 1]. By the early 1980s, individual sequences exceeding 10^5 bp had been determined[11]; however, a more common scale of analysis was 10^3–10^4 bp. Most physical mapping was carried out on a similar scale.

Given the gap between the ability to determine 10^5 bp of DNA sequence in a state-of-the-art laboratory and the 10^9 bp size of the human genome, the NRC committee confronted an enormous problem of scale. Partly because of the obvious need for improved technology and also because of a desire to maximize synergy between genome analysis and studies of biologic function, the committee recommended against early emphasis on large-scale sequencing of human DNA. Instead, it advocated comprehensive physical and genetic mapping of the human genome, extensive mapping and sequencing of the smaller genomes of several model organisms, and a systematic effort to develop improved sequencing technology.

Principal Aims of the Human Genome Project

More important than the specific mapping and sequencing objectives of the Human Genome Project are three broader aims that are implicit in these goals:

1. To improve the research infrastructure of human genetics.
2. To help establish DNA sequence as the primary interface between knowledge of human biology and knowledge of the biology of model organisms.
3. To launch an open-ended effort to improve the analytical biochemistry of DNA.

For the purposes of this review, progress in the Human Genome Project will be examined in relation to these three broad aims.

Tools of Genetic Research

In the context of the Human Genome Project, research infrastructure refers to the biologic, informational, and methodological tools with which genetics research is carried out. Intensive genetic analysis of any species is heavily dependent on infrastructure. Particularly important are genetic linkage maps, physical maps of DNA, and characterized DNA clones. Such clones serve as reagents with which to assay for particular short segments of the genome by DNA-DNA hybridization[12] and as the starting points for sequence analysis or functional studies.

Human genetics is uniquely dependent on strong research infrastructure. Although model organisms have been extensively bred for the specific purpose of facilitating genetic analysis,[13] human genetics is limited to the examination of individuals, families, and populations as they are found in contemporary society. The NRC committee therefore set ambitious goals for the construction of detailed physical and genetic maps of the human genome, as well as organized collections of cloned human DNA. By design, the goals were too ambitious for the technology of 1988—so ambitious, in retrospect, that they would probably have overwhelmed the basic methodologies on which the NRC report was based. Fortunately, technical advances since 1988 have exceeded all reasonable expectations.

Polymerase Chain Reaction

Much of this progress was made possible by the development of the polymerase chain reaction (PCR). PCR, which is essentially a method of in vitro cloning, allows the amplification of specific DNA molecules in vitro through cycles of enzymatic DNA synthesis.[4] PCR amplification depends on a pair of short, synthetic primers: single-stranded DNA molecules whose ends can be extended by DNA polymerase under the direction of template molecules. The test sample provides the template molecules, and the primers direct the amplification to a particular segment of the template DNA, typically a region only a few hundred base pairs in length [*see Figure 2*]. If one starts with a minute sample of total human DNA, it is possible to amplify any such region a billionfold while leaving the rest of the genome at its original concentration [*see Table 1*].

Widespread application of the PCR depends on an efficient, automated method for the chemical synthesis of the PCR primers. An approach to DNA synthesis based on phosphoramidite chemistry, which became routine in the early 1980s, meets this need.[4,14-16] The first paper on the PCR appeared in 1985[17] but received little notice; for example, despite its present prominence in genome analysis, it is not mentioned in the NRC report. The explosive growth of PCR applications began with the publication of an important refinement of the PCR protocol in 1989: the use of a thermostable DNA polymerase.[18] This refinement allowed the cycles of DNA synthesis, which are analogous to cellular generations, to be driven by simple thermal cycling with no new addition of reagents at each cycle.

SEQUENCE-TAGGED SITES

By the end of 1989, it was apparent that the PCR provided a practical means of abstracting large-scale physical maps away from the particular methods used to construct them. This capability required a new choice of landmarks called sequence-tagged sites (STSs).[19] An STS is simply a short, unique sequence of DNA that can be amplified with the PCR. STSs are ideal landmarks during map construction because of the ease with which they can be detected by PCR assays. Equally important is their role in map representation and map use.

Complex physical maps based on restriction sites are of little value as experimental tools unless they are supported by a collection of clones that can detect particular segments of the mapped DNA in DNA-DNA hybridization assays. Comprehensive maps of the human genome would have to be supported by tens of thousands of clones, each of which would have to be maintained as a separate microbial strain. In contrast, STSs can be described in an electronic data base in a form that makes them experimentally accessible in any laboratory. The most critical aspect of an STS description is the DNA sequence of the two primers. Laboratory implementation of an STS requires simply that the two primers be synthesized and the appropriate temperature-cycling regime be carried out.

Most large-scale physical maps are constructed through a process called contig building. A contig is an organized set of DNA clones that collectively provide redundant cloned coverage of a region that is too long to clone in one piece.[4,20-22] Typically, the clones have random end points, and

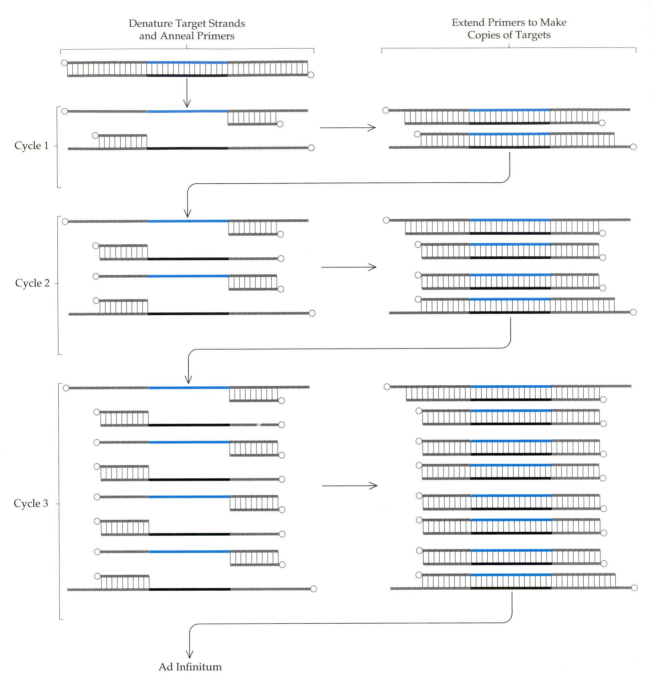

Denature Target Strands
and Anneal Primers

Extend Primers to Make
Copies of Targets

Cycle 1

Cycle 2

Cycle 3

Ad Infinitum

Figure 2 *The polymerase chain reaction is a cyclic process; with each cycle, the number of DNA targets doubles. The strands in each targeted DNA duplex are separated by heating and then cooled to allow single-stranded oligonucleotide primers that are complementary to the end sequences of the opposite strands to bind to them. Next, DNA polymerases extend the primers by adding nucleotides to them. In this way, duplicates of the original DNA-strand targets are produced each cycle, and the quantity of this product increases exponentially.*

the contig is described by specifying the amount of overlap between each clone and its nearest neighbors. A procedure referred to as STS-content mapping provides a convenient method of establishing these overlaps.[4,23] In a step that precedes contig building, the STSs are tested to confirm that they occur in a single copy in the genome; then, if two clones share even a single STS, they can be reliably assumed to overlap.

Yeast Artificial Chromosomes

Although the PCR has had a profound effect on physical mapping, other new developments have also improved the prospects for the construction of large-scale physical maps. One such development has been the introduction of the yeast artificial chromosome (YAC) cloning system [*see Figure 3*], first described in 1987.[4,24] YACs allow large segments of DNA to be cloned as linear, artificial chromosomes into the yeast host *Saccharomyces cerevisiae*. Even some of the earliest YAC clones were 10 times the size of the largest clones that had been constructed previously. Furthermore, the YAC system appears capable of cloning a higher proportion of the genomic DNA of many organisms than could be recovered with earlier systems. This point has been most clearly documented during the physical mapping of the genome of the nematode worm *Caenorhabditis elegans*.[25]

By 1989, YAC cloning technology had evolved to the point where specific segments of the human genome could be recovered efficiently in YAC clones.[26] Soon thereafter, multi-megabase-pair contigs began to appear,[23,27-29] and, in the fall of 1992, complete YAC-based physical maps of human chromosome 21[30] and the human Y chromosome[31] were published. In these projects, contig construction was largely based on STS-content mapping. There is little doubt that the same technology employed on chromosomes Y and 21, as well as on a large segment of the X chromosome,[29] has sufficient power to produce highly connected physical maps of the entire human genome.

Fluorescence in Situ Hybridization

Another important advance in physical mapping has been the development of fluorescence in situ hybridization (FISH) into a routine procedure. In this technique, DNA probes detect segments of the human genome by DNA-DNA hybridization on samples of lysed metaphase cells prepared under conditions that preserve the morphology of the condensed human chromosomes. Attachment of fluorescent molecules to the probe DNA allows one to visualize in the light microscope the position on a chromosome to which the probe binds. The technique is a refinement of previous in situ hybridization methods that depended on labeling of the probes with radioactive isotopes for subsequent autoradiographic detection.[32] The increases in convenience, reliability, and resolution that have accompanied nonisotopic detection have transformed the role of in situ hybridization in physical mapping. The first nonisotopic visualization of single-copy sequences in human chromosomes by in situ hybridization was published in 1985.[33] Fluorescence detection of single-copy sequences was introduced in 1987,[34] after which applications expanded rapidly.[35-37]

FISH contributes to two aspects of long-range physical mapping. First, it allows individual clones to be mapped at a coarse level long before contig building is complete, thereby providing reagents of immediate use in the analysis of targeted regions. Second, contig maps have discontinuities whenever a site in the genome is missing from the available clone collections. FISH provides a way to order and orient contigs along a

Table 1 PCR Amplification of DNA Fragment

Cycle Number	Number of Double-Stranded Target Molecules
1	0
2	0
3	2
4	4
5	8
6	16
7	32
8	64
9	128
10	256
11	512
12	1024
13	2048
14	4096
15	8192
16	16,384
17	32,768
18	65,536
19	131,072
20	262,144
21	524,288
22	1,048,576
23	2,097,152
24	4,194,304
25	8,388,608
26	16,777,216
27	33,544,432
28	67,108,864
29	134,217,728
30	268,435,456
31	536,870,912
32	1,073,741,824

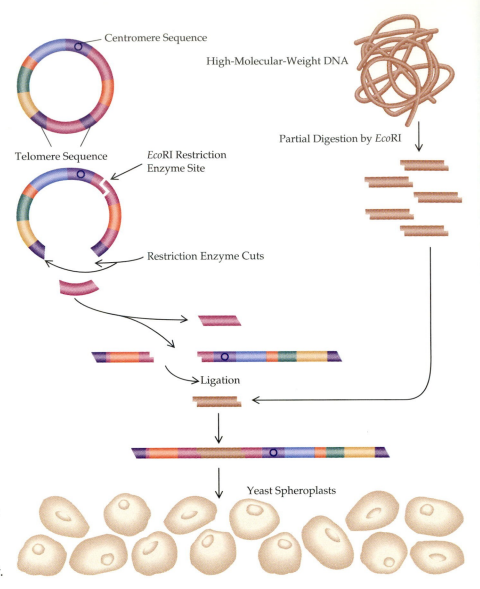

Figure 3 *The cloning vector for a yeast artificial chromosome (YAC) contains the elements needed for its replication as a linear artificial chromosome in yeast cells: a centromere sequence (purple), two telomere sequences (purple), a sequence essential for autonomous replication (blue), two genes for selection of transformed yeast cells (orange), a sequence of bacterial origin that permits replication in bacterial cells (beige), and a gene for antibiotic resistance that permits selection of bacterial cells (green). Two restriction enzymes are used to cut the vector. One deletes the segment between the two telomere genes, and the restriction enzyme EcoRI cuts the vector into two segments. High-molecular-weight DNA is partially digested by EcoRI, and fragments of the right size are isolated by electrophoresis and then ligated with the arms of the YAC. The YACs can then be used to transform yeast spheroplasts (yeast cells that lack cell walls); once the insert DNA has been incorporated, YACs can be replicated in yeast.*

Centromere Sequence

High-Molecular-Weight DNA

Partial Digestion by *Eco*RI

Telomere Sequence

*Eco*RI Restriction Enzyme Site

Restriction Enzyme Cuts

Ligation

Yeast Spheroplasts

chromosome even when occasional discontinuities exist. Early efforts to construct physical maps of human chromosomes, which depended on cosmid clones that are propagated in *Escherichia coli*, yielded relatively small contigs separated by discontinuities.[38,39] YAC-based methods have led to greatly improved continuity, but the need remains for supplementary methods to define the order and orientation of disconnected contigs along chromosomes.

Radiation-Hybrid Mapping

Radiation-hybrid mapping, which involves fragmentation of human chromosomes in cultured cells with high doses of x-rays followed by incorporation of the fragments into stable rodent cell lines by cell fusion [*see Figure 4*], provides still another solution to this problem.[4,40] Current protocols for radiation-hybrid mapping are notable for their abandonment of the traditional goal of isolating a single short segment of the human genome in each rodent cell line. Nearly all of the radiation-hybrid lines produced by these protocols contain many unrelated segments of the human genome. Proximity of two STSs, or other markers, is inferred by statistical analysis of the pattern in which they occur in a large collection of cell lines. Closely spaced markers have a higher probability of occurring together in the same cell line than do pairs of markers that are on different chromosomes or are far apart on the same chromosome.

Genetic Markers Detectable by PCR

While the PCR, together with such new techniques as YAC cloning, FISH, and radiation-hybrid mapping, has led to a surge of success in physical

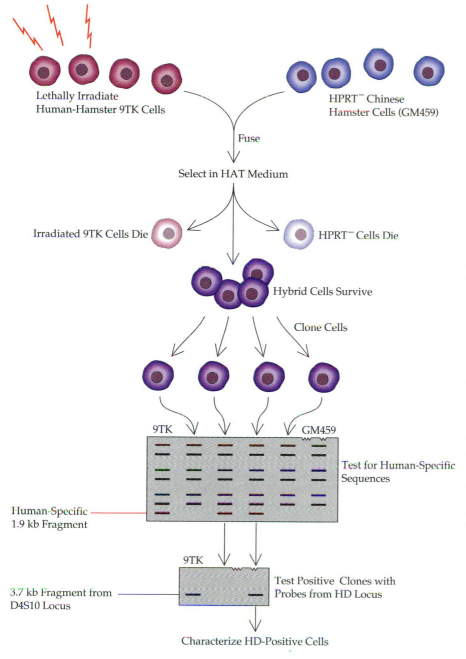

Figure 4 *Shown is an example of the use of x-irradiated hybrids for cloning. 9TK cells are a human-hamster hybrid cell line; the only human DNA present is chromosome 4. These cells are x-irradiated to fragment chromosome 4, and the dosage of radiation is sufficient to kill the cells. The GM459 Chinese hamster cell line is deficient in hypoxanthine phosphoribosyl transferase (HPRT), and these cells are killed when they are grown in medium containing hypoxanthine, aminopterin, and thymidine (HAT). When the parental cells are fused and grown in HAT medium, the only cells that can survive are Chinese hamster cells that have acquired a hamster HPRT gene from the irradiated hamster-human cell line. Clones of surviving cells are first screened for the presence of human DNA by means of probes for Alu or LINE repeat sequences. Clones containing human DNA have a characteristic 1.9 kb fragment. Positive clones were screened with probes mapping close to the Huntington's disease (HD) locus at the tip of chromosome 4. For example, probe pHD2 from the D4S10 locus detects a 3.7 kb band on Southern blots. In this way, other DNA sequences mapping in the HD region were cloned.*

mapping, PCR-based methods have also transformed genetic mapping. In particular, the PCR has made possible the development of a new class of genetic markers that have a particularly high probability of existing in alternate forms in different copies of the human genome.

These markers are based on short, repetitive DNA sequences that are widely distributed in the human genome. A particularly common motif is . . . (CA)$_n$ . . . . At sites where this motif occurs, n, the number of repetitions of the dinucleotide CA, is highly variable from one copy of the human genome to the next.[41,42] When the entire . . . (CA)$_n$ . . . tract is amplified by the PCR with primers that flank the repeat, the size of the amplification product is determined by the value of n. Differences in the product sizes associated with different values of n are readily detected by gel electrophoresis. An attractive feature of PCR-detectable genetic markers is that they are simply a special type of STS. As such, they can be readily included as landmarks in physical maps as well as genetic maps, thereby providing a simple method of interrelating these two types of maps. Many PCR-detectable genetic markers have been integrated into preexisting maps of the human genome, greatly improving the maps.[43] Recently, a human genetic map that is completely based on PCR-detectable markers has been constructed.[44] Markers of the same type have also transformed genetic mapping in the mouse, whose genome is the same size as that of the human.[45]

Positional Cloning of Genes

A key test of the effectiveness of the infrastructure-building features of the Human Genome Project is the extent to which its components are being used even before genome-wide physical maps are available. The most critical test involves projects directed at the positional cloning of genes associated with heritable diseases. Positional cloning is a strategy developed during the 1980s as a way to determine the biochemical basis of the many heritable diseases whose analysis has resisted traditional biochemical approaches based on the analysis of diseased tissue.[46] In general, such analysis is rarely effective unless the genetic defect alters a protein whose metabolic role in normal tissue is already understood. Few of the heritable defects that give rise to mental retardation, psychosis, congenital malformation, malignant tumors, and other similarly complex conditions meet this criterion.

The first step in positional cloning is to localize the "disease" gene by carrying out genetic mapping studies on families with multiple affected members. Studies of the coinheritance of the disease with genetically mapped DNA markers can establish the position of the gene in the genome. Actual biochemical identification of the gene still remains a formidable task, because the resolution of genetic maps in the human is rarely better than one megabase pair (Mbp). Physical mapping and functional studies on the cloned DNA are required to find the gene within the candidate region.

LOCALIZATION OF SPECIFIC DISEASE GENES

Better physical mapping methods, particularly the combination of YAC cloning and FISH analysis, have improved the prospects for positional cloning. An exemplary baseline case, published just before either of these techniques became widely available, is cystic fibrosis [*see Chapter 9*]. Final success in the positional cloning of the cystic fibrosis gene required heroic physical mapping efforts that never achieved any semblance of continuous cloned coverage of the candidate region.[47] Piecemeal cloning and mapping proved adequate only because the gene is large and is in a gene-poor region of the genome.

Subsequent successes with a series of disease genes reveal the influence of improved techniques. Examples in which YACs, FISH, or both figured prominently include the following: fragile X syndrome,[48-50] the most common heritable form of mental retardation; familial adenomatous polyposis,[51,52] a heritable form of colorectal cancer; myotonic dystrophy,[53] an adult-onset disease that affects muscle function; Kallmann syndrome,[54,55] a defect in neuronal development; Lowe syndrome,[56] a developmental defect affecting the lens, brain, and kidney; and Menkes disease,[57-59] a neurologic disease that is lethal in early childhood.

The genes for many other heritable diseases are now under analysis by similar techniques. Particularly impressive is progress on the genetic mapping of diseases such as familial breast and ovarian cancer[60,61] and early-onset familial Alzheimer's disease.[62] The genetic analysis of these diseases is complicated by a set of factors that will be encountered increasingly often as positional cloning is applied to complex, adult-onset genetic disorders: suitable families are rare, small, and incomplete (i.e., few grandparents, parents, or siblings of the affected individuals are available); even family members who remained disease-free throughout a normal life span cannot be reliably categorized as unaffected, because they may have died from other causes before disease developed; the disease is common enough in the general population for cases with genetic and nongenetic causes to occur frequently in the same family. Highly informative genetic markers, such as the PCR-detectable CA-repeat polymorphisms, have helped address these problems: they maximize the likelihood that the segment of the chromosome bearing the disease-causing mutation can be tracked reliably from one generation to the next even when many family members are missing or must be excluded from the study because of their uncertain disease status.

In addition to improved genetic mapping, successful completion of these projects may require further advances in physical mapping and sequencing. Because of the difficulty of the genetic analysis, it is unlikely that disease genes such as the recently described one for early-onset familial Alzheimer's disease on chromosome 14 will be localized even to within 1 Mbp by genetic mapping.[62] Its isolation will place great demands on physical mapping resources and techniques for locating genes within cloned DNA. The case of Huntington's disease, for which ample family resources are available, is instructive: the gene was genetically mapped to a position near the end of the short arm of chromosome 4 in 1983[63] but was not identified in cloned DNA until a decade later.[64,65] Difficulties analogous to those encountered during the 10-year search for the Huntington's disease gene are certain to recur in many similar projects.

Still another class of disease genes whose analysis has been facilitated by the new research infrastructure is genes whose disruption in somatic cells causes cancer. Particularly in leukemias and lymphomas, a common mechanism by which disease-causing mutations arise is translocation, a process of chromosome breakage and rejoining. The combination of YACs and FISH analysis has simplified the mapping of the chromosomal breakpoints and has led to the isolation of genes whose disruption is the initiating event in several forms of neoplasia.[66,67]

DNA Sequencing Reveals Parallels between Human Biology and That of Model Organisms

Central to the NRC committee's recommendations, which emphasized the importance of sequencing the genomes of model organisms, was the belief that DNA sequence offers a potent means of interrelating diverse aspects of biologic knowledge. Events during the past five years have strongly reinforced this concept.

Yeast Genes and Human Genes

Particularly remarkable is the ability of DNA-sequence data to call attention to similarities between biologic phenomena that are superficially unrelated. A typical example involves the successful transfer of information from the study of yeast mating to diverse areas of human biology. Yeast cells have two mating types, commonly referred to as **a** and α. In the yeast life cycle, **a** and α cells are the rough counterparts of mammalian germ cells. The yeast counterpart of fertilization involves the fusion of **a** and α cells, a process that is partly mediated by two peptide hormones, **a** factor and α factor, each named for the cell type that secretes it. The **a**-factor hormone triggers a series of changes in α cells that prepare them for fusion, whereas α factor plays the complementary role for **a** cells.

The mechanisms through which **a** factor and α factor are synthesized and secreted have been studied in detail by genetic techniques that are particularly well developed in yeast.[68] A peculiar feature of **a**-factor secretion is its independence of the pathway through which yeast proteins are normally secreted. A particular gene, *STE6*, encodes a protein that allows **a** factor to leave the cell while bypassing the normal secretory pathway. Sequence analysis of *STE6* revealed unmistakable similarity to the human gene *mdr1*.[69,70] This gene has attracted interest because of its involvement in multiple-drug resistance, a phenomenon in which malignant cells simultaneously become resistant to several of the most commonly used chemotherapeutic agents.[71] Once the relatedness of *STE6* and *mdr1* had been established by sequence comparison, it was quickly shown by gene-transfer experiments that the mouse version of the *mdr1* gene will actually substitute in yeast for the function of *STE6*, correcting the inability of yeast cells with mutations in the *STE6* gene to secrete **a** factor.[72] The availability of the yeast system opens up a powerful new front for the study of this poorly understood transport mechanism.

Studies of α-factor biosynthesis have also provided new insights into human metabolism. Although the secretion of α factor follows the normal pathway, its biosynthesis has a feature that is unusual in yeast but relatively common in human cells: it is produced by proteolytic processing of a precursor peptide at a Lys-Arg linkage. Genetic studies revealed that the gene *KEX2* encodes the protease that carries out this processing step. Comparison of the sequence of *KEX2* with all other known DNA sequences revealed strong similarity to a human gene of previously unknown function, c-*fur*.[73] Subsequent analysis showed that c-*fur* is a member of a family of human genes encoding proteases that process precursors to many important proteins and peptides, including insulin, nerve growth factor, bone morphogenetic protein, and a major component of the AIDS virus.[74] There is a long history of direct, biochemical efforts to identify these proteases because of their potential interest as pharmacological targets. These efforts led to the description of a whole series of proteases that are capable of cleaving Lys-Arg linkages under particular in vitro conditions but that serve other functions in vivo.

These two examples illustrate the strength of the concept, which is fundamental to the Human Genome Project, that DNA sequence provides the key to efficient knowledge transfer between model organisms and human biology. At present, this process requires considerable serendipity, because available DNA sequence data on the genomes of both the human and the major model organisms are fragmentary. There has been enough progress in sequencing the genomes of *E. coli*,[75] *S. cerevisiae*,[76] and the nematode worm *C. elegans*[77] to indicate the value of systematic genomic sequencing, but the real work of determining complete sequences for the genomes of these model organisms still lies ahead.

Sequencing of Human cDNA

In humans, the main new source of systematic data has been the sequencing of complementary DNAs (cDNAs): cloned DNA copies of the messenger RNA (mRNA) molecules that actually direct protein synthesis.[4,78] Sequencing cDNAs is a cost-effective way of discovering new human genes because only a small fraction of genomic DNA directly codes for proteins. However, cDNA sequencing is unlikely to replace genomic sequencing as the definitive method of characterizing the complete set of human genes for several reasons: genes contain critical DNA sequences that regulate their expression but are not included in the mRNA; there are common instances in which one gene produces multiple, substantially different mRNA molecules and in which multiple genes produce nearly identical mRNA molecules, situations that are difficult to sort out without detailed knowledge of the structures of the corresponding genes and gene families; the cost advantages of cDNA sequencing erode when the goal is accurate, full-length sequences rather than one-pass, partial sequences; no adequate solution has been found to the problem that the mRNA products of different genes are present at widely different concentrations, which vary dramatically in different tissues, different developmental stages, and different metabolic states.

Open-Ended Improvements in DNA Analysis

The promise of DNA sequence comparison as a fundamental tool in biologic research emphasizes the need for progressively better methods of DNA analysis, particularly DNA sequencing. A critical feature of this challenge is its open-ended nature. DNA sequencing, like digital computing, is a technology for which there is no obvious point at which further improvements would saturate potential applications. A basic misimpression about the Human Genome Project is that once its narrow goals are met, demands for large-scale DNA sequencing will taper off. DNA sequence data are basically a source of hypotheses, the rigorous testing of which typically requires the acquisition of still more DNA sequence. The determination of a reference human sequence will provide a strong incentive to trace genes through evolution with finer grain than can be provided by the *E. coli*/yeast/worm/fly/mouse/human comparisons on which the NRC committee recommended early emphasis. Finally, the study of individual variation, which plays a central role in both biology and medicine, poses unbounded demands for DNA sequence data.

Efficiency of DNA Sequencing

Juxtaposed to this open-ended need for improvements in the efficiency of DNA sequencing is the reality that there has been no obvious increase in the basic efficiency of DNA sequencing during the past decade. The protocols have become more robust, and the level of skill required for success has been lowered. Fluorescence-based methods with real-time detection of the products of DNA-sequencing reactions during electrophoresis have eased laboratory management of large projects and decreased the subjectivity of data interpretation.[4,79] The practicality of large projects is therefore greater now than it was a decade ago. And yet, it is not apparent that there has been any change in either the efficiency or the accuracy with which an expert DNA sequencer can gather data.

The NRC committee recognized this problem but was overly optimistic about its resolution[1]:

> The technical problems associated with mapping and sequencing the human and other genomes are sufficiently great that a scientifically sound program requires a diversified, sustained effort to improve our ability to analyze complex DNA molecules . . . . Prospects are . . . good that the required advanced DNA technologies would emerge from a focused effort that emphasizes pilot projects and technological development.

The National Institutes of Health and the Department of Energy have both made vigorous efforts to steer a significant portion of the project in the recommended directions, but there is little indication that decisive research momentum has developed in the technology of DNA sequencing. It can be argued that the problem is predominantly cultural rather than technical, relating to the different value systems and research emphases of molecular genetics, on the one hand, and analytical chemistry, applied physics, and engineering, on the other.[80]

An illustration of the magnitude of the technical challenge is provided by the gap between the theoretical and the actual output of the current generation of DNA-sequencing instruments. Standard commercial instruments now have the capacity to produce approximately 30 kilobase pairs (kbp) of raw sequence data per day.[79] Allowing for the desirability of determining the sequence of the two complementary strands of DNA independently and for some oversampling of data for each strand, a ratio of raw sequence data to finished data of 5:1 should be achievable. Hence, a single instrument should be capable of producing 6 kbp of finished sequence per day, or about 2 Mbp per year. In reality, no genome center has yet produced even 1 Mbp of contiguous, finished sequence per year, even though such centers typically have many sequencing instruments.

This paradox reflects the present impossibility of integrating all the steps in DNA sequencing into a continuous process that fully utilizes even the capabilities of current sequencing instruments. Although this experience is universal among DNA sequencing laboratories, there is little consensus about which steps in the process are rate limiting, much less what should be done to improve them.

What is clear is that there is a dramatic gap between the advanced biologic technologies of molecular genetics and the primitive nonbiologic technologies. The latter include the physical manipulation of samples, methods of chemical and physical analysis, process design, quality control, and information handling. These areas are all critical to efforts to scale up bench-top molecular genetics, and most biologists are poorly trained to make the needed innovations. The Human Genome Project has stimulated increased interactions among biologists and the scientists and technologists who have the necessary expertise to solve these problems. However, the difficulties of translating these beginnings into major improvements in DNA analysis continue to pose substantial policy challenges.

Progress Toward Goals

For an effort that has had only a few years of substantial funding, the Human Genome Project in the United States is making good progress toward its central goals. The policy on which it was based has proved farsighted even in the face of rapid technological change. In the mapping phase of the project, which has dominated the first years, the experimental methods that are leading to success have diverged widely from those available when the NRC report was issued, and yet the report's conceptual framework has survived with little alteration.

Examples abound of biologic advances that have benefited directly from the early activities of the Human Genome Project. Precise tracking of the cause-and-effect relation between activities funded through the Human Genome Project in the United States and specific biologic advances is neither possible nor desirable. Human genome analysis is a loosely coordinated international endeavor to which funding agencies and scientists in many countries have already made important contributions. Vigorous research activity funded through other Federal programs, private agencies, and industry has also had a major impact. Nonetheless, the National Institutes of Health and the Department of Energy's programmatic efforts, particularly through productive investment in YACs, FISH, PCR-detectable DNA polymorphisms, and radiation-hybrid mapping, have clearly achieved good progress toward the mapping goals of the NRC report and also contributed directly to the success of many other research projects in the biomedical sciences.

Like other human endeavors, the Human Genome Project has succeeded best when it has aligned itself with broader trends. Examples include its increasing reliance on PCR, yeast genetics, and fluorescence microscopy. It has succeeded least when it has tried to establish new trends such as the importation of high technology from other areas into biology. This tension is healthy and will undoubtedly remain as the project focuses increased attention on its flagship goal of determining the sequence of the 99 percent of the human genome about which we still know almost nothing.

References

1. National Research Council: *Mapping and Sequencing the Human Genome*. National Academy Press, Washington, DC, 1988

2. Smith HO, Wilcox KW: A restriction enzyme from *Hemophilus influenzae*: I. Purification and general properties. *J Mol Biol* 51:379, 1970

3. Smith HO: Nucleotide sequence specificity of restriction endonucleases. *Science* 205:455, 1979

4. Watson JD, Gilman M, Witkowski J, et al: *Recombinant DNA*, 2nd ed. Scientific American Books, New York, 1992

5. Nathans D: Restriction endonucleases, simian virus 40, and the new genetics. *Science* 206:903, 1979

6. Botstein D, White RL, Skolnick M, et al: Construction of a genetic linkage map in man using restriction fragment length polymorphisms. *Am J Hum Genet* 32:314, 1980

7. Southern EM: Detection of specific sequences among DNA fragments separated by gel electrophoresis. *J Mol Biol* 98:503, 1975

8. Donis-Keller H, Green P, Helms C, et al: A genetic linkage map of the human genome. *Cell* 51:319, 1987

9. Sanger F, Nicklen S, Coulson AR: DNA sequencing with chain-terminating inhibitors. *Proc Natl Acad Sci USA* 74:5463, 1977

10. Maxam AM, Gilbert W: A new method for sequencing DNA. *Proc Natl Acad Sci USA* 74:560, 1977

11. Baer R, Bankier AT, Biggin MD, et al: DNA sequence and expression of the B95-8 Epstein-Barr virus genome. *Nature* 310:207, 1984

12. Alberts B, Bray D, Lewis J, et al: *Molecular Biology of the Cell*, 2nd ed. Garland, New York, 1989

13. Fink GR: Anecdotal, historical and critical commentaries on genetics: notes of a bigamous biologist. *Genetics* 118:549, 1988

14. Beaucage SL, Caruthers MH: Deoxynucleoside phosphoramidites—a new class of key intermediates for deoxypolynucleotide synthesis. *Tetrahedron Lett* 22:1859, 1981

15. Caruthers MH: Gene synthesis machines: DNA chemistry and its uses. *Science* 230:281, 1985

16. Hunkapiller MJ, Kent S, Caruthers M, et al: A microchemical facility for the analysis and synthesis of genes and proteins. *Nature* 310:105, 1984

17. Saiki RK, Scharf S, Faloona F, et al: Enzymatic amplification of beta-globin genomic sequences and restriction site analysis for diagnosis of sickle cell anemia. *Science* 230:1350, 1985

18. Saiki RK, Gelfand DH, Stoffel S, et al: Primer-directed enzymatic amplification of DNA with a thermostable DNA polymerase. *Science* 239:487, 1988

19. Olson M, Hood L, Cantor C, et al: A common language for physical mapping of the human genome. *Science* 245:1434, 1989

20. Coulson A, Sulston J, Brenner S, et al: Toward a physical map of the genome of the nematode *Caenorhabditis elegans*. *Proc Natl Acad Sci USA* 83:7821, 1986

21. Olson MV, Dutchik JE, Graham MY, et al: Random-clone strategy for genomic restriction mapping in yeast. *Proc Natl Acad Sci USA* 83:7826, 1986

22. Kohara Y, Akiyama K, Isono K: The physical map of the whole *E. coli* chromosome: application of a new strategy for rapid analysis and sorting of a large genomic library. *Cell* 50:495, 1987

23. Green ED, Olson MV: Chromosomal region of the cystic fibrosis gene in yeast artificial chromosomes: a model for human genome mapping. *Science* 250:94, 1990

24. Burke DT, Carle GF, Olson MV: Cloning of large segments of exogenous DNA into yeast by means of artificial chromosome vectors. *Science* 236:806, 1987

25. Coulson A, Kozono Y, Lutterbach B, et al: YACs and the *C. elegans* genome. *Bioessays* 13:413, 1991

26. Brownstein BH, Silverman GA, Little RD, et al: Isolation of single-copy human genes from a library of yeast artificial chromosome clones. *Science* 244:1348, 1989

27. Anand R, Ogilvie DJ, Butler R, et al: A yeast artificial chromosome contig encompassing the cystic fibrosis locus. *Genomics* 9:124, 1991

28. Silverman GA, Jockel JI, Domer PH, et al: Yeast artificial chromosomes cloning of a two-megabase-size contig within chromosomal band 18q21 establishes physical linkage between BCL2 and plasminogen activator inhibitor type-2. *Genomics* 9:219, 1991

29. Little RD, Pilia G, Johnson S, et al: Yeast artificial chromosomes spanning 8 megabases and 10-15 centimorgans of human cytogenic band X_q26. *Proc Natl Acad Sci USA* 89:177, 1992

30. Chumakov I, Rigault P, Guillou S, et al: Continum of overlapping clones spanning the entire human chromosome 21q. *Nature* 359:380, 1992

31. Foote S, Vollrath D, Hilton A, et al: The human Y chromosome: overlapping DNA clones spanning the euchromatic region. *Science* 258:60, 1992

32. Gall JG, Pardue ML: Formation and detection of RNA-DNA hybrid molecules in cytological preparations. *Proc Natl Acad Sci USA* 63:378, 1969

33. Landegent JE, Jansen in de Wal N, van Ommen G-J, et al: Chromosomal localization of a unique gene by non-autoradiographic in situ hybridization. *Nature* 317:175, 1985

34. Landegent JE, Jansen in de Wal N, Dirks RW, et al: Use of whole cosmid cloned genomic sequences for chromosomal localization by non-radioactive in situ hybridization. *Hum Genet* 77:366, 1987

35. Lawrence JB, Villnave CA, Singer RH: Sensitive, high-resolution chromatin and chromosome mapping in situ: presence and orientation of two closely integrated copies of EBV in a lymphoma line. *Cell* 52:51, 1988

36. Trask B, Pinkel D, van den Engh G: The proximity of DNA sequences in interphase cell nuclei is correlated to genomic distance and permits ordering of cosmids spanning 250 kilobase pairs. *Genomics* 5:710, 1989

37. Lichter P, Tan C-J, Call K, et al: High-resolution mapping of human chromosome 11 by in situ hybridization with cosmid clones. *Science* 247:64, 1990

38. Stallings RL, Torney DC, Hildebrand C, et al: Physical mapping of human chromosomes by repetitive sequence fingerprinting. *Proc Natl Acad Sci USA* 87:6218, 1990

39. Tynan K, Olsen A, Trask B, et al: Assembly and analysis of cosmid contigs in the CEA-gene family region of human chromosome 19. *Nucleic Acids Res* 20:1629, 1992

40. Cox DR, Burmeister M, Price ER, et al: Radiation hybrid mapping: a somatic cell genetic method for constructing high-resolution maps of mammalian chromosomes. *Science* 250:245, 1990

41. Weber JL, May PE: Abundant classes of human DNA polymorphisms which can be typed using the polymerase chain reaction. *Am J Hum Genet* 44:388, 1989

42. Litt M, Luty JA: A hypervariable microsatellite revealed by in vitro amplification of a dinucleotide repeat within the cardiac muscle actin gene. *Am J Hum Genet* 44:397, 1989

43. NIH/CEPH Collaborative Mapping Group. A comprehensive genetic linkage map of the human genome. *Science* 258:67, 1992

44. Weissenbach J, Gyapay G, Dib C, et al: A second-generation linkage map of the human genome. *Nature* 359:794, 1992

45. Dietrich W, Katz H, Lincoln SE, et al: A genetic map of the mouse suitable for typing intraspecific crosses. *Genetics* 131:423, 1992

46. Collins FS: Positional cloning: Let's not call it reverse anymore. *Nature Genet* 1:3, 1992

47. Rommens JM, Iannuzzi MC, Kerem BS, et al: Identification of the cystic fibrosis gene: chromosome walking and jumping. *Science* 245:1059, 1989

48. Verkerk AJ, Pieretti M, Sutcliffe JS, et al: Identification of a gene (FMR-1) containing a CGG repeat coincident with a breakpoint cluster region exhibiting length variation in fragile X syndrome. *Cell* 65:905, 1991

49. Kremer EJ, Pritchard M, Lynch M, et al: Mapping of DNA instability at the fragile X to a trinucleotide repeat sequence p(CGG)n. *Science* 252:1711, 1991

50. Oberle I, Rousseau F, Heitz D, et al: Instability of a 550-base pair DNA segment and abnormal methylation in fragile X syndrome. *Science* 252:1097, 1991

51. Kinzler KW, Nilbert MC, Su LK, et al: Identification of FAP locus genes from chromosome 5q21. *Science* 253:661, 1991

52. Groden J, Thliveris A, Samowitz W, et al: Identification and characterization of the familial adenomatous polyposis coli gene. *Cell* 66:589, 1991

53. Fu YH, Pizzuti A, Fenwick RG Jr, et al: An unstable triplet repeat in a gene related to myotonic muscular dystrophy. *Science* 255:1256, 1992

54. Legouis R, Hardelin JP, Levilliers J, et al: The candidate gene for the X-linked Kallman syndrome encodes a protein related to adhesion molecules. *Cell* 67:423, 1991

55. Franco B, Guioli S, Pragliola A, et al: A gene deleted in Kallman's syndrome shares homology with neural cell adhesion and axonal path-finding molecules. *Nature* 353:529, 1991

56. Attree O, Olivos IM, Okabe I, et al: The Lowe's oculocerebrorenal syndrome gene encodes a protein highly homologous to inositol polyphosphate-5-phosphatase. *Nature* 358:239, 1992

57. Vulpe C, Levinson B, Whitney S, et al: Isolation of a candidate gene for Menkes disease and evidence that it encodes a copper-transporting ATPase. *Nature Genet* 3:7, 1993

58. Chelly J, Tumer Z, Tonnesen T, et al: Isolation of a candidate gene for Menkes disease that encodes a potential heavy metal binding protein. *Nature Genet* 3:14, 1993

59. Mercer JFB, Livingston J, Hall B, et al: Isolation of a partial candidate gene for Menkes disease by positional cloning. *Nature Genet* 3:20, 1993

60. Hall JM, Lee MK, Newman B, et al: Linkage of early-onset familial breast cancer to chromosome 17q21. *Science* 250:1684, 1990

61. Hall JM, Friedman L, Guenther C, et al: Closing in on a breast cancer gene on chromosome 17q. *Am J Hum Genet* 50:1235, 1992

62. Schellenberg GD, Bird TD, Wijsman EM, et al: Genetic linkage evidence for a familial Alzheimer's disease locus on chromosome 14. *Science* 258:668, 1992

63. Gusella JF, Wexler NS, Conneally PM, et al: A polymorphic DNA marker genetically linked to Huntington's disease. *Nature* 306:234, 1983

64. Davies K: Slow search for Huntington's disease gene. *Nature* 357:page following 94, 1992

65. Novel gene containing a trinucleotide repeat that is expanded and unstable on Huntington's disease chromosomes. The Huntington's Disease Collaborative Research Group. *Cell* 72:971, 1993

66. Djabali M, Selleri L, Parry P, et al: A trithorax-like gene is interrupted by chromosome 11q23 translocations in acute leukaemias. *Nature Genet* 2:113, 1992

67. Ziemin-van der Poel S, McCabe NR, Gill HJ, et al: Identification of a gene, MLL, that spans the breakpoint in 11q23 translocations associated with human leukemias. *Proc Natl Acad Sci USA* 88:10735, 1991

68. Botstein D, Fink GR: Yeast: an experimental organism for modern biology. *Science* 240:1439, 1988

69. Kuchler K, Sterne RE, Thorner J: *Saccaromyces cerevisiae* STE6 gene product: a novel pathway for protein export in eukaryotic cells. *Embo J* 8:3973, 1989

70. McGrath JP, Varshavsky A: The yeast STE6 gene encodes a homologue of the mammalian multidrug resistance P-glycoprotein. *Nature* 340:400, 1989

71. Gottesman MM, Pastan I: The multidrug transporter, a double-edged sword. *J Biol Chem* 263:12163, 1988

72. Raymond M, Gros P, Whiteway M, et al: Functional complementation of yeast ste6 by a mammalian multidrug resistance mdr gene. *Science* 256:232, 1992

73. Fuller RS, Brake AJ, Thorner J: Intracellular targeting and structural conservation of a prohormone-processing endoprotease. *Science* 246:482, 1989

74. Barr PJ: Mammalian subtilisms: the long-sought dibasic processing endoproteases. *Cell* 66:1, 1991

75. Daniels DL, Plunkett G 3rd, Burland V, et al: Analysis of the *Escherichia coli* genome: DNA sequence of the region from 84.5 to 86.5 minutes. *Science* 257:771, 1992

76. Oliver SG, van der Aart QJM, Agostoni-Carboni ML, et al: The complete DNA sequence of yeast chromosome III. *Nature* 357:38, 1992

77. Sulston J, Du Z, Thomas K, et al: The C. elegans genome sequencing project: a beginning. *Nature* 356:37, 1992

78. Adams MD, Kelley JM, Gocayne JD, et al: Complementary DNA sequencing: expressed sequence tags and human genome project. *Science* 252:1651, 1991

79. Hunkapiller T, Kaiser RJ, Koop BF, et al: Large-scale and automated DNA sequence determination. *Science* 254:59, 1991

80. Olson MV: A tale of two cities. *Anal Chem* 63:416A, 1991

Acknowledgments

This chapter has been reprinted with minor adaptations from "The Human Genome Project," by M. V. Olson, in *Proceedings of the National Academy of Science of the United States of America* 90:4338, 1993. Used by permission.

Figures 1, 2   Tom Moore. From "Medical Genetics," by R. W. Erbe, in SCIENTIFIC AMERICAN *Medicine*, Section 9, Subsection IV, edited by E. Rubenstein and D. D. Federman. Scientific American, Inc., New York, 1994. All rights reserved.

Figure 3   Dimitry Schidlovsky. From "Medical Genetics," by R. W. Erbe, in SCIENTIFIC AMERICAN *Medicine*, Section 9, Subsection IV, edited by E. Rubenstein and D. D. Federman. Scientific American, Inc., New York, 1994. All rights reserved.

Figure 4   Tom Moore. Adapted from *Recombinant DNA*, 2nd ed., by J. D. Watson, M. Gilman, J. Witkowski, et al. Scientific American Books, New York, 1992. © 1992 James D. Watson, Michael Gilman, Jan Witkowski, Mark Zoller. Used by permission.

Table 1   Adapted from *Recombinant DNA*, 2nd ed., by J. D. Watson, M. Gilman, J. Witkowski, et al. Scientific American Books, New York, 1992. © 1992 James D. Watson, Michael Gilman, Jan Witkowski, Mark Zoller. Used by permission.

CHAPTER 7

Understanding the Human Genome

Douglas L. Brutlag, Ph.D.

There are many compelling reasons to determine the complete genetic information of the human organism. The genome contains the history of human evolution and specifies the mechanism of human development; all humanity's physical capabilities and deficiencies are encoded in the genome. It is no wonder that Walter Gilbert, Nobel laureate and developer of one of the first methods for determining DNA sequence, has said that "sequencing the human genome is like pursuing the holy grail." Less poetically but perhaps more prophetically, Lee Hood has observed, "The sequence of the human genome would be perhaps the most useful tool ever developed to explore the mysteries of human development and disease."

For these promises to materialize, it will be necessary not only to determine the entire sequence of the human genome [*see Chapter 6*] but also to understand it. There is a common misconception that because the genetic code is known, the genetic information in the genome will be immediately understood. The genetic code describes only the relation between the sequences of bases in DNA that encode proteins and the sequence of the amino acids in those proteins [*see Table 1*]. Because less than five percent of the human genome encodes proteins, the genetic code will not help biologists to understand the function of the remaining 95 percent of the genome.

A good example of this dilemma is the recently cloned gene for cystic fibrosis.[1-3] The region of the gene transcribed into RNA is more than 250,000 base pairs long. This large RNA is processed by splicing to yield a contiguous protein-coding region in the mature messenger RNA that is only 6,500 bases long (2.6 percent of the gene). More than 97 percent of the genetic information in the cystic fibrosis gene is discarded during this splicing process, and then only 4,440 bases in the messenger RNA are actually translated into protein. The protein itself is rather large, measuring 1,480 amino acids in length.[4] Another, less extreme example of the difference between gene length and the coding regions is the human α-globin gene and its RNA and protein products [*see Figure 1*].

Even for the five percent of the DNA that encodes protein, one cannot fully predict the structure and function of the protein product merely from

Table 1 The Genetic Code: DNA Codons
Corresponding to Individual Amino Acids

Amino Acid	3-Letter Abbreviation	1-Letter Abbreviation	Codon(s)
Alanine	Ala	A	GCA, GCC, GCG, GCT
Arginine	Arg	R	CGA, CGC, CGG, CGT, AGA, AGG
Aspartic acid	Asp	D	GAC, GAT
Asparagine	Asn	N	AAC, AAT
Cysteine	Cys	C	TGC, TGT
Glutamic acid	Glu	E	GAA, GAG
Glutamine	Gln	Q	CAA, CAG
Glycine	Gly	G	GGA, GGC, GGG, GGT
Histidine	His	H	CAC, CAT
Isoleucine	Ile	I	ATA, ATC, ATT
Leucine	Leu	L	CTA, CTC, CTG, CTT, TTA, TTG
Lysine	Lys	K	AAA, AAG
Methionine	Met	M	ATG
Phenylalanine	Phe	F	TTC, TTT
Proline	Pro	P	CCA, CCC, CCG, CCT
Serine	Ser	S	TCA, TCC, TCG, TCT, AGC, AGT
Threonine	Thr	T	ACT, ACC, ACG, ACT
Tryptophan	Trp	W	TGG
Tyrosine	Tyr	Y	TAC, TAT
Valine	Val	V	GTA, GTC, GTG, GTT
STOP	—	—	TAG, TAA, TGA

```
GCCGCGCCCCGGGCTCCGCGCCAGCCAATG   AGCGCCGCCCGGCCGGGCGTGCCCCCGCGC   CCCAAGCATAAACCCTGGCGCGCTCGCGGC      90


CCGGCACTCTTCTGGTCCCCACAGACTCAG   AGAGAACCCACCATGGTGCTGTCTCCTGCC   GACAAGACCAACGTCAAGGCCGCCTGGGGT     180
    acucuucuggucccacagacucag      agagaacccaccauggugcugucuccugcc   gacaagaccaacgucaaggccgccuggggu
                                             MetValLeuSerProAla       AspLysThrAsnValLysAlaAlaTrpGly

AAGGTCGGCGCGCACGCTGGCGAGTATGGT   GCGGAGGCCCTGGAGAGGTGAGGCTCCCTC   CCCTGCTCCGACCCGGGCTCCTCGCCCGCC     270
aaggucggcgcgcacgcuggcgaguauggu   gcggaggcccuggagaggugaggcucccuc   cccugcuccgacccgggcuccucgcccgcc
LysValGlyAlaHisAlaGlyGluTyrGly   AlaGluAlaLeuGluArg

CGGACCCACAGGCCACCCTCAACCGTCCTG   GCCCCGGACCCAAACCCCACCCCTCACTCT   GCTTCTCCCCGCAGGATGTTCCTGTCCTTC     360
cggacccacaggccacccucaaccguccug   gccccggaccaaaaccccaccccucacucu   gcuucuccccgcaggauguuccuguccuuc
                                                                                   MetPheLeuSerPhe

CCCACCACCAAGACCTACTTCCCGCACTTC   GACCTGAGCCACGGCTCTGCCCAAGTTAAG   GGCCACGGCAAGAAGGTGGCCGACGCGCTG     450
cccaccaccaagaccuacuucccgcacuuc   gaccugagccacggcucugcccaaguuaag   ggccacggcaagaagguggccgacgcgcug
ProThrThrLysThrTyrPheProHisPhe   AspLeuSerHisGlySerAlaGlnValLys   GlyHisGlyLysLysValAlaAspAlaLeu

ACCAACGCCGTGGCGCACGTGGACGACATG   CCCAACGCGCTGTCCGCCCTGAGCGACCTG   CACGCGCACAAGCTTCGGGTGGACCCGGTC     540
accaacgccguggcgcacguggacgacaug   cccaacgcgcuguccgcccugagcgaccug   cacgcgcacaagcuucggguggacccgguc
ThrAsnAlaValAlaHisValAspAspMet   ProAsnAlaLeuSerAlaLeuSerAspLeu   HisAlaHisLysLeuArgValAspProVal

AACTTCAAGGTGAGCGGCGGGCCGGGAGCG   ATCTGGGTCGAGGGGCGAGATGGCGCCTTC   CTCTCAGGGCAGAGGATCACGCGGGGTTGC     630
aacuucaaggugagcggcgggccgggagcg   aucugggucgaggggcgagauggcgccuuc   cucucagggcagaggaucacgcgggguugc
AsnPheLys

GGGAGGTGTAGCGCAGGCGGCGGCGCGGCT   TGGGCCGCACTGACCCTCTTCTCTGCACAG   CTCCTAAGCCACTGCCTGCTGGTGACCCTG     720
gggaggguguagcgcaggcggcggcgcggcu   ugggccgcacugacccucuucucugcacag   cuccuaagccacugccugcuggugacccug
                                                                                   LeuLeuSerHisCysLeuLeuValThrLeu

GCCGCCCACCTCCCCGCCGAGTTCACCCCT   GCGGTGCACGCTTCCCTGGACAAGTTCCTG   GCTTCTGTGAGCACCGTGCTGACCTCCAAA     810
gccgcccaccuccccgccgaguucacccu   gcggugcacgcuucccuggacaaguuccug   gcuucugugagcaccgugcugaccuccaaa
AlaAlaHisLeuProAlaGluPheThrPro   AlaValHisAlaSerLeuAspLysPheLeu   AlaSerValSerThrValLeuThrSerLys

TACCCTTAACCTGGAGCCTCGGTAGCCGTT   CCTCCTGCCCGCTGGGCCTCCCAACGGGCC   CTCCTCCCCTCCTTGCACCGGCCCTTCCTG     900
uaccguuaagcuggagccucgguagccguu   ccuccugcccgcuggggccucccaacgggcc   cuccuccccuccuugcaccggcccuuccug
TyrArg

GTCTTTGAATAAAGTCTGAGTGGGCGGCAG   CCTGTGTGTGCCTGGGTTCTCTCTGTCCCG   GAATGTGCCAACAATGGAGGTGTTTACCTG     990
gucuuugaauaaagucugaguggggcggc

TCTCAGACCAAGGACCTCTCTGCAGCTGCA   TGGGGCTGGGGAGGGAGAACTGCAGGGAGT   ATGGGAGGGGAAGCTGAGGTGGGCCTGCTC    1080


AAGAGAAGGTGCTGAACCATCCCCTGTCCT   GAGAGGTGCCAGCCTGCAGGCAGTGGC                                         1137
```

Figure 1 *The human α-globin gene is 1137 base pairs in length (top line). The primary transcript begins at base 96 and continues to 928 (833 bases) and is shown in lower case below the gene (middle line). The processed messenger RNA is missing two introns, including bases 229 to 345 and 550 to 690 (shaded), and it is only 575 bases long. The α-globin protein is 141 amino acids in length and is shown below its coding region (bottom line, blue).*

its sequence. The goal of this chapter is to show what kinds of information can be derived from genetic sequences and to describe the methods currently available for interpreting the genetic message. Most current methods involve comparing new sequences with preexisting ones, discovering structure and function by homology rather than through a true understanding of the biologic principles underlying structure and function. Before reviewing these methods, it will be useful to consider just why an understanding of gene sequences is critical to medicine.

Medical Benefits from Sequencing the Genome

Many of the immediate medical benefits to be derived from sequencing the human genome do not involve any real understanding of how genes work or of the proteins they encode. Among these benefits is the development of diagnostic DNA probes and therapeutic products for inherited disease. Knowing the difference between the DNA sequence of a normal gene and the gene responsible for a disease, one can design a DNA probe that can detect the difference and thus diagnose the disease. The classic example of this is the gene for the most common form of cystic fibrosis, which differs from its normal counterpart in that it lacks three DNA bases [*see Figure 2*]. In principle, DNA probes can form the basis of a clinical diagnosis for any inherited disease. If the sequence of an infectious agent is known, it is possible to develop a sensitive clinical test for that infectious disease as well.

DNA probes have advantages over such diagnostic tests as radioimmune assays or bacterial cultures. The primary advantage is that the presence of a specific DNA sequence underlying an inherited or infectious disease is the most fundamental indicator of the disease; all other manifestations are secondary. This is the major reason that most biomedical problems are being attacked primarily at the level of the molecular biology. Nowadays, scientists who want to understand, detect, or treat a disease generally attempt first to isolate the gene or genes responsible for that disease: isolation of the defective gene or genes gets at the root of the problem.

Two other major advantages of detecting disease with DNA probes are that the methods are general and that they can readily be automated. Once a probe for a disease is developed, that disease can be detected by the same clinical method as any other disease. This means that a single technology can potentially be applied in the clinic to detect any of the more than 5,000 known inherited diseases—once there is a probe for each of them.[5] Because the methods are general and easily automated, they are ideal for routine analysis of large numbers of samples.

The generality of DNA diagnostics, coupled with the ability to automate the diagnostic tests, means that clinical screens for thousands of diseases can be performed simultaneously.[6] It is the immediate medical value of being able to identify DNA probes for all known medical diseases that primarily motivates the Human Genome Project.

To be sure, the ability to diagnose disease (especially inherited disease) without the ability to cure or treat it leads to numerous social and ethical problems.[7] For example, insurance companies have been free to increase

Figure 2 *Shown is the 3 bp deletion in cystic fibrosis. This mutation consists of the deletion of CTT in the tenth exon of the gene. Loss of 3 bp maintains the reading frame, so that only a single phenylalanine is lost from the protein. The frequency of this mutation in cystic fibrosis patients ranges from as low as 30 percent in parts of southern Europe to 95 percent in Denmark. In Northern Europe it is 75 percent, and in the US population it is about 70 percent.*

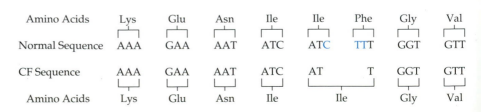

Amino Acids	Lys	Glu	Asn	Ile	Ile	Phe	Gly	Val
Normal Sequence	AAA	GAA	AAT	ATC	ATC	TTT	GGT	GTT
CF Sequence	AAA	GAA	AAT	ATC	AT	T	GGT	GTT
Amino Acids	Lys	Glu	Asn	Ile	Ile		Gly	Val

rates for those in high-risk groups. When insurance companies define high-risk groups on the basis of inheritance, they are in effect holding individuals responsible for their genetic makeup. The social stigma associated with certain genetic differences can also, like more visible phenotypes, lead to discrimination. The most frustrating effects of genetic diagnosis would occur with diseases that have a clearly debilitating or fatal effect but for which there is no hope of a cure or therapy. That is why it is important not only to know the sequence of the human genome but also to understand it well enough to devise cures and rational, inexpensive therapies.

Another early result of having the complete sequence of the human genome will be the general availability of many natural products produced in the human body. Many inherited diseases involve a deficiency of one or more protein products. Having the genetic information in hand for whatever is produced in the body should make it possible to supply any missing products as therapeutic agents. Already many natural therapeutic agents—hormones, antibodies, and so on—can be replaced by products of biotechnology [*see Chapter 11*]. With the complete sequence of the human genome known, the development of these natural products into therapeutic agents will be greatly simplified and accelerated. Given proper licensing policies, it should be possible even to keep the cost of such treatment within the reach of those in need. Another longer-term benefit will be the use of the DNA itself as the therapeutic agent in gene therapy [*see Chapter 12*].

Understanding Genetic Information

Before rational therapies can be developed, one needs to understand the action of the altered gene. A major benefit of determining the complete sequence of the human genome will be in the knowledge it provides about the evolution, development, and functioning of the human organism. Again, the classic example is the level of understanding achieved for cystic fibrosis. Before the isolation of the gene responsible for this most common inherited disease, it was suspected that cystic fibrosis affected the ion balance in secretory cells. That being the case, cystic fibrosis could equally well have resulted from a defect in any gene that affects or controls the expression of any ion-channel gene. The isolation of the gene established that the defect is in the gene encoding an ion channel that regulates the secretion of chloride ions from the apical membrane of secretory cells in a highly regulated fashion. The sequence of the gene revealed that it encodes a membrane protein that apparently can bind the regulatory compound cyclic AMP, which controls the passage of chloride through the membrane.

By introducing the gene for a normal chloride channel into cells from cystic fibrosis patients, scientists have been able to restore normal chloride and water balance to these cells in vitro. This not only proves that the defective gene is the major cause of the disease but also gives hope that it will be possible to introduce the normal gene into the tissues of afflicted individuals to correct the defect. The defective gene for cystic fibrosis has been introduced into laboratory mice, creating an effective animal model of the disease for the first time.[8-10] Clinical trials in which the normal gene is being introduced into patients with cystic fibrosis are under way. ✓

The Flow of Genetic Information

How do molecular biologists determine that a given gene can encode a protein and then how can they deduce the function of that gene or protein from its sequence? Even before it was possible to clone and sequence individual genes, the primary goal of molecular biology was to understand the flow of genetic information from DNA to the phenotype:

$$DNA \rightarrow RNA \rightarrow Protein \rightarrow Function$$

Biologists have studied the maintenance of genetic information, its replication, and its transformation into different forms (RNA, proteins, and phenotype) for more than 40 years. Biophysicists have studied the structures of the various molecules, biochemists have isolated specific proteins and enzymes and studied their functions, and molecular biologists have dissected the mechanisms and regulation of each step in the flow of information.

Now that there is direct access to the genetic information itself, one can investigate just how the genetic information manifests itself during its series of transformations from genome to phenotype. One examines the flow of information from the viewpoint of an information scientist:

$$\begin{array}{cccc} \text{Genetic} & \rightarrow \text{Molecular} \rightarrow \text{Biochemical} \rightarrow \text{Biologic} \\ \text{information} & \text{structure} \quad \text{function} \quad \text{behavior} \end{array}$$

This pathway represents a shift from the classic paradigm of information flow in molecular biology. New procedures are being developed for predicting molecular structure beginning with genetic information. The first step outlined above, converting sequence information into three-dimensional structural information, is a very active field of scientific investigation [see Chapter 3]. There are many methods for performing this prediction. One method involves predicting structure from physical principles. If it is assumed that all the forces between atoms in a molecule, including bond energies and electrostatic attraction and repulsion, are known, then it is possible to calculate the three-dimensional arrangement of atoms that has the lowest energy. This method of predicting molecular structures by minimizing their overall energy is termed molecular dynamics and requires the use of very powerful supercomputers. Other methods of predicting molecular structure involve determining what kinds of amino acid sequences or patterns of amino acids are found in each of the known protein structures. Certain amino acids, such as leucine and alanine, are very common in α-helical regions of proteins, whereas other amino acids, such as proline, are rarely if ever found in α helices. Using patterns of amino acids or rules based on these patterns, one can attempt to predict where helical regions will occur in proteins whose structure is unknown. This method is an example of a larger field of automated learning. The approach involves examining the sequences of many proteins of known structure in an effort to infer rules or patterns that can be applied to novel protein sequences to predict their structure.

Predicting the function of a molecule from its structure has long been the domain of biophysicists, whereas predicting phenotype from biochemical functions has been the domain of biochemists and geneticists. These two steps in the flow of genetic information (i.e., predicting biochemical function and phenotype) are attacked by numerous methods from information science, including simulation.

The transition in molecular biology to the new paradigm for studying the flow of genetic information parallels biology's switch from being an observational science, limited primarily by the ability to make observations, to being a data-bound science limited by its practitioners' ability to understand large amounts of information derived from observations. This change is a natural one in the maturation of scientific fields, which generally progress from observation to theory and simulation as data—and understanding of the data—increase.

Most problems in medicine and biology are now being attacked with molecular methods. More than 60 percent of all National Institutes of Health (NIH) grants depend on molecular methods of cloning, mapping, and sequencing regardless of the problem being addressed. More than 65 percent of all articles indexed by the National Library of Medicine contain molecular biology subject headings. Whether scientists are studying cancer or allergies, aging or infectious disease, they usually apply molecular methods.

The reason for this switch to a molecular approach is obvious from an examination of either pathway for the flow of genetic information outlined above. The fundamental cause of any inherited disease is written in the genome. Even an agent of infectious disease is often best detected by a DNA diagnostic probe, because of its greater sensitivity. Studies at any other level are always secondary and subject to interpretation, whereas DNA diagnostics based on an isolated gene defect are unambiguous. The fundamental nature of the genetic information and the ease with which this information can be obtained make the molecular approach the preferred one in most cases. The benefit of this approach is the accumulation of large amounts of genetic information; the problem is that only a small fraction of this information is understood.

Another way of emphasizing the imperative to interpret the genetic information is to compare the various ways of unraveling the classical pathway of the flow of information. In the past 100 years, biochemists have isolated and characterized about 10,000 enzymes to the point that one can understand their effect on physiology. In the past 50 years, biophysicists have determined the structure of only 1,000 molecules with the degree of accuracy needed to predict their function. Yet in only the past 20 years, scientists have cloned and completely sequenced more than 140,000 genes, of which 20 percent are human. Had all the laboratories of the world been working exclusively on human genes during this period, they would have sequenced the expected number of human genes. This rate of accumulation of genetic information will increase exponentially with the added expenditure of time and money occasioned by the human genome project. To obtain the most benefit from this investment, it will be necessary to predict the structure, function, and behavior resulting from a particular genetic sequence. Hence it is essential to learn from the few examples that are well understood, so that valuable laboratory resources can be focused on novel sequences, structures, and functions.

Challenges in Understanding Genetic Information

There are many challenges in trying to interpret genetic information. The first is that this information is highly redundant: many sequences encode the same function or message. There are more than 650 globin sequences in the protein-sequence databases, all with very similar structure. (It is much like this in the case of languages. The English language is notorious for its numerous synonyms, each with its associated nuances and hidden implications.) Of course, the genetic code itself is highly redundant. On average, three different codons (DNA sequences three bases long) encode each amino acid [*see Table 1*]. (Each triplet in the genetic code, of which there are 64, can represent one of 20 amino acids or the termination of translation; 64 codons divided by 21 meanings is approximately 3.05 codons per meaning. Two amino acids—methionine and tryptophan—are specified by only one codon, but several amino acids can be specified by as many as six codons.) Given the average of three codons per amino acid, one can predict that a protein as short as insulin (51 amino acids) might be encoded by as many as $3^{51} \cong 10^{24}$ different DNA sequences, each encoding precisely the same protein. Fortunately, nature does not fully exploit the available redundancy. Most insulin gene sequences have derived from other insulin sequences in evolution; most natural sequences are related to other preexisting natural sequences rather than being created anew. Molecular biologists can apply this sequence similarity to derive conclusions about structure and function on the basis of homology.

The most important challenge in understanding genetic information is one briefly alluded to above: genetic information is one-dimensional, but biologic molecules are three-dimensional. The information for the three-dimensional nature of DNA, RNA, and proteins must be determined by the one-dimensional sequence of their component nucleotides or amino acids, because when these molecules are denatured (i.e., their native structure completely disrupted) in the laboratory, they can renature and regain their normal three-dimensional structure.[11] The implication is that the tertiary structure of molecules is encoded in their primary sequence. But how? It is this structural code that biologists must next determine in order to understand the genetic message.

Unfortunately, most of the methods described below that are applied to the analysis of gene sequences do not capture the structural information directly. Instead, they look for evolutionarily related sequences and make the assumption that if two DNA segments are related in sequence, they are probably related in structure or function. Although this assumption is usually justified, the methods for detecting similarities at the sequence level are not sensitive enough to detect all structurally or functionally related sequences.

Methods for Understanding Genetic Information

There are three primary methods for analyzing sequences for structure or function: consensus sequences, weight matrices, and sequence alignment.

CONSENSUS SEQUENCES

The first of these methods discovers short, highly conserved sequence patterns. Such sequences, usually called motifs or consensus sequences, are determined by aligning a large number of sequences of common function and looking for conserved positions—that is, for positions at which the same amino acids (or nucleotide bases) are present in most, or at least very many, of the sequences. Once the conserved positions are identified, the motif thus defined can serve as a kind of probe: one can search a database or some new sequence, testing for the presence of the motif.[12]

The concept of a motif is a very powerful one, and databases of motifs have been compiled. The best known is the Prosite database, which currently contains more than 1,000 such patterns.[13] A very useful method for determining the function of a newly sequenced protein is to search it for each and every one of these motifs. With more than 1,000 motifs, there is often one that will match the new protein and thus give a clue as to its structure or function. When this method was applied to the protein sequence of the cystic fibrosis gene product, two motifs were identified that aided in the discovery of two sites on the protein that were involved in binding nucleotides (nucleotide binding folds, or NBFs).

One of the main problems with consensus sequences is the difficulty in striking a balance between their specificity and their precision. In order to eliminate as many false hits (sequences that match the pattern but are known not to be functionally or structurally related) as possible, one often has to make the consensus sequence very specific. Often, however, the motif is made so specific that it misses even many of the known examples of a motif. A motif can often be very specific (finding no matches that are not established examples of the structure or function) but not very precise (missing many other examples). Or it can be very precise (finding all the known examples) but not very specific, in that it also matches many unrelated sequences. One way around this dilemma is to classify a set of protein sequences into narrow subgroups and then to have multiple motifs, one for each subclass or subgroup. Even with this approach, it is often difficult to extract a highly conserved consensus sequence because of the high degree of ambiguity in biologic sequences.

Another fundamental problem with consensus sequences is their discrete nature. A test sequence either matches or does not match the consensus sequence; there is no concept of the degree or probability of matching between a test sequence and a consensus sequence. It is this weakness that has led to the development of probabilistic methods that can generate a more powerful representation of a series of aligned sequences.

WEIGHT MATRICES AND PROFILES

Because of the extreme redundancy of genetic sequences, many proteins having a common structure and function may have very few, if any, amino acids in common. A good example of this is the set of prokaryotic DNA-binding proteins containing a so-called helix-turn-helix motif, 22 amino acids in length, that allows them to bind to DNA in a sequence-specific manner.[14-16] (The motif is called a helix-turn-helix motif because the protein assumes a characteristic structure involving a short α-helix, followed by a 90-degree turn of three amino acids, followed by another short helix.) Examination of the linear amino acid sequences reveals no consensus sequence that could reliably distinguish these proteins from other proteins [*see Table 2*].

The motif is, however, recognizable when a quantitative approach is taken. The frequency with which each amino acid appears at each position is determined [*see Table 3*]. These numbers are then used to calculate the likelihood of finding each amino acid at each position. The frequency matrix is converted to a traditional weight matrix by converting every number in the matrix to a measure of the probability of occurrence of each acid (rather than its frequency). These so-called weight matrices can be applied to measure the likelihood that any given sequence 22 amino acids long is related to the helix-turn-helix family by merely multiplying the likelihoods of each amino acid in a test sequence. A modification of this method, referred to as profiles, allows one to estimate the probability that any amino acid will appear in a specific position—even if a particular amino acid has never been observed at some positions in the set of known examples.[17,18]

These weight matrices or profiles are effective for locating signals in DNA as well as structural motifs in proteins. Indeed, the first application of these probabilistic methods was the detection of promoters and splice sites in DNA by means of weight matrices.[19]

SEQUENCE ALIGNMENT

The most common way to examine a new gene or protein for its biologic function is simply to compare its sequence with all known DNA or protein sequences in the public databases and note any strong similarities.[20-22] The particular gene or protein that has just been determined will of course not be found in the databases, but a homologue from another organism or a gene or protein having a related function may be found. In either case the evolutionary similarity implies a common ancestor and hence a common function. This method becomes more and more successful as the databases grow larger and as the sensitivity of the search procedure increases.

It is for these reasons that it is critical to have available both the most sensitive search procedure and access to the most up-to-date databases possible. Since 1983, the National Institutes of Health has supported the GenBank DNA Database,[23,24] and the European Molecular Biology Laboratory the EMBL DNA Library[25,26]; both databases collect and disseminate all published DNA sequences to the scientific community. These computer resources, together with the younger DNA Database of Japan, accept sequences electronically from the molecular biology community, verify them, and then redistribute them daily to researchers around the world, again via electronic networks. A new sequence is generally on file in these databases within a day or two of its publication. Similar databases of protein sequences are also maintained at various sites.[27,28]

In addition to up-to-date databases, it is critical to be able to compare a query sequence against all the database sequences with methods that allow a flexibility of matching commensurate with the redundancy of the

Table 2   Composition of 22–Amino Acid Sequences
Corresponding to Helix-Turn-Helix Motif
in 37 Prokaryotic Proteins

Name of Sequence	Helix	Turn	Helix
RCRO$LAMBD	F G Q T K T A K D L	G V Y	Q S A I N K A I H
RCRO$BP434	M T Q T E L A T K A	G V K	Q Q S I Q L I E A
RCRO$BPP22	G T Q R A V A K A L	G I S	D A A V S Q W K E
RCP1$LAMBD	L S Q E S V A D K M	G M G	Q S G V G A L F N
RPC1$BP434	L N Q A E L A Q K V	G T T	Q Q S I E Q L E N
RPC2$BPP22	I R Q A A L G K M V	G V S	N V A I S Q W E R
RPC2$LAMBD	L G T E K T A E A V	G V D	K S Q I S R W K R
LACR$ECOLI	V T L Y D V A E Y A	G V S	Y Q T V S R V V N
CRP$ECOLI	I T R Q E I G Q I V	G C S	R E T V G R I L K
TRPR$ECOLI	M S Q R E L K N E L	G A G	I A T I T R G S N
RPC1$BPP22	R G Q R K V A D A L	G I N	E S Q I S R W K G
GALR$ECOLI	A T I K D V A R L A	G V S	V A T V S R V I N
Y77$BPT7	L S H R S L G E L Y	G V S	Q S T I T R I L Q
TER3$ECOLI	L T T R K L A Q K L	G V E	Q P T L Y W H V K
VIVB$BPT7	D Y Q A I F A Q Q L	G G T	Q S A A S Q I D E
DEOR$ECOLI	L H L K D A A A L L	G V S	E M T I R R D L N
RP43$BACSU	R T L E E V G K V F	G V T	R E R I R Q I E A
Y28$BPT7	E S N V S L A R T Y	G V S	Q Q T I C D I R K
IMMRE$BPPH12	S T L E A V A G A L	G I Q	V S A I V G E E T
RFNR$ECOLI	M T R G D I G N Y L	G L T	V E T I S R L L G
MERR$ECOLI	L T I G V F A K A A	C V N	V E T I R F Y N R
IMMRE$BPPH11	L T Q V Q L A E K A	N L S	R S Y L A D I E R
RP32$ECOLI	S T L Q L E A D R Y	G V S	A E R V R Q L E K
LEUO$ECOLI	Q N I T R A A H V L	G M S	Q P A V S N A V A
LYSR$ECOLI	G S L T E A A H L L	H T S	Q P T V S R E L A
AMPR$ECOLI	L S F T H A A I E L	N V T	H S A I S Q H V K
ANTP	M P Q A Q T N G Q L	G V P	Q Q Q Q Q Q Q Q Q
VNU1$LAMBD	V N K K Q L A D I F	G A S	I R T I Q N W Q E
VPB$BPMU	T T F K Q I A L E S	G L S	T G T I S S F I N
DNAB$ECOLI	R S L K A L A K E L	N V P	V V A L S Q L N R
BIRA$ECOLI	H S G E Q L G E T L	G M S	R A A I N K H I Q
BPT7	K Y Q E D L A A L E	G T S	D R I I S D L R S
DBH$RHIME	E L V A A V A D K A	G L S	K A D A S S A V D
CYSB$ECOLI	L N V S S T A E G L	Y T S	Q P G I S K Q V R
CYTR$ECOLI	A M I K D V A L K A	K V S	T A T V S R A L M
MTA1$YEAST	K E K E E V A K K C	G I T	P L Q V R V W V C
RPC$BPP2	L S R Q Q L A D L T	G V P	Y G T L S Y Y E S

genetic code.[29,30] A simple method that merely lines up identical amino acids, for instance, will not detect similarities between similar genes or proteins in organisms as distantly related as plants and animals. (Plant and animal hemoglobins, for example, have less than 10 percent identity of amino acids in such alignments.) By assigning a measure of similarity to each pair of amino acids, however, and then adding up these pairwise scores for the entire alignment, it is possible to detect highly significant similarities between even distantly related proteins. Although related proteins may not have identical amino acids aligned, they usually do have chemically similar or replaceable amino acids in similar positions. In the type of scoring that is usually applied to such alignments,[31] amino acid pairs that are identical or chemically similar are given positive scores, and pairs of amino acids that are not related are assigned negative similarity scores. Negative penalties usually have to be designated for the introduction of insertion/deletion gaps. Use of such matrices markedly improves the sensitivity of a database search.

Many computer programs have been developed for finding the most similar sequences in a database by applying the scoring procedures described above. Because making tens of thousands of alignments of a new sequence with every known sequence is computer-intensive, many methods are mere approximations to the complete alignment method.[32] Other approaches rely on massively parallel computers or supercomputers to carry out database search and alignment programs. The amino acid sequence of the cystic fibrosis transmembrane conductance regulator protein (CFTR) has been compared [*see Figure 3*] with the sequences of

Table 3 Frequency of Occurrence of Each Amino Acid at Each Position in 80 Examples of Helix-Turn-Helix Motif

Amino Acid	Position																					
	1	2	3	4	5	6	7	8	9	10	11	12	13	14	15	16	17	18	19	20	21	22
A	2	1	3	13	10	12	67	4	13	9	1	2	4	3	6	15	4	4	4	11	0	10
R	7	5	8	9	4	0	1	16	7	0	1	0	1	16	6	6	0	11	28	3	0	16
N	0	8	0	1	0	0	0	2	1	1	10	0	7	1	3	1	0	4	8	0	1	11
D	0	1	0	1	13	0	0	12	1	0	4	0	1	2	0	0	0	0	1	1	0	3
C	0	0	1	0	0	0	0	0	0	2	2	1	0	0	0	0	0	0	0	1	0	0
Q	1	1	21	8	10	0	0	7	6	0	0	2	1	17	7	7	0	2	12	5	2	4
E	2	0	0	9	21	0	0	15	7	3	3	0	1	6	11	0	0	2	0	1	13	6
G	9	7	1	4	0	0	8	0	0	0	46	0	6	0	7	1	0	3	1	1	0	4
N	4	3	1	1	2	0	0	2	2	0	5	0	3	3	0	2	0	2	4	5	0	2
I	10	0	11	1	2	10	0	4	9	3	0	16	0	2	0	1	26	1	0	8	16	0
L	16	1	17	0	1	31	0	3	11	24	0	14	0	2	0	1	21	1	1	12	20	0
K	3	4	5	10	11	1	1	13	10	0	5	2	1	4	1	1	0	1	8	4	5	14
M	7	1	1	0	0	0	0	0	5	7	1	8	0	0	2	0	2	0	0	2	0	1
F	4	0	3	0	0	4	0	0	0	10	0	0	0	0	1	0	0	1	1	1	11	0
P	0	6	0	1	0	0	0	0	0	0	0	0	1	12	7	0	0	0	0	0	0	3
S	1	17	0	8	3	1	3	0	2	2	2	0	37	1	24	5	0	29	3	0	1	3
T	5	22	3	11	1	5	0	2	2	2	0	5	16	4	2	38	0	4	1	0	4	3
W	2	0	0	0	0	0	0	0	0	1	0	1	0	0	0	0	0	0	2	10	0	0
Y	1	0	4	2	0	1	0	0	2	4	0	1	1	2	0	2	0	15	5	7	0	0
V	6	3	1	1	2	15	0	0	2	12	0	28	0	5	3	0	27	0	1	8	7	0

```
= = = = = = = = = = = = = = = = = = =
= = = = = = = = = = = = = = = = = = =                    B L A Z E (tm)
              = = = = = =
         = = = = = =          A High-Performance High-Sensitivity Biological
      = = = = = =             Sequence   Similarity   Searching   Program
    = = = = = =               Utilizing a Massively Parallel Implementation
  = = = = = =                 of  the  Dynamic  Programming  Algorithm  of
 = = = = = =                  Smith and Waterman
= = = = =

  = = = = = = = = = = = = = = = = = = = = = = = = = = = = = = = = = = = = = =
= = = = = = = = = = = = = = = = = = Release 1.0 - July 1992 = = = = = = = = - - - =
Copyright  (c)  1992 by IntelliGenetics, Inc. and  MasPar Computer Corporation

INPUT PARAMETERS
DATALIB          SWISS-PROT 23
MATRIX           PAM150
GAPPEN           2.0
GAPSIZPEN        0.5
SCORES           100
MINPERCENTMATCH  0


SEARCH STATISTICS
Number of sequences searched:               26,706
Number of residues in database:          9,011,391
Query sequence length:                       1,480
Score of query vs. itself:                   2,279
Mean score:                                     33
Standard deviation:                          25.47
Time:                                  0:03:40.765
Millions of residues compared per second:   60.428
```

Sequence Name	Description	Length	Score	%Match	Expectation
1. CFTR_HUMAN	CYSTIC FIBROSIS TRANSMEMBRANE COND	1480	2279	100	0.000
2. CFTR_XENLA	CYSTIC FIBROSIS TRANSMEMBRANE COND	1485	1898	83	0.000
3. CFTR_MOUSE	CYSTIC FIBROSIS TRANSMEMBRANE COND	1476	1874	82	0.000
4. CFTR_SQUAC	CYSTIC FIBROSIS TRANSMEMBRANE COND	1492	1798	79	0.000
5. MDR_LEITA	MULTIDRUG RESISTANCE PROTEIN (P-GL	1548	536	24	0.000
6. HETA_ANASP	HETEROCYST DIFFERENTIATION PROTEIN	607	247	11	0.000
7. MDR2_MOUSE	MULTIDRUG RESISTANCE PROTEIN 2 (P-	1276	240	11	0.000
8. STE6_YEAST	MATING FACTOR A SECRETION PROTEIN	1290	231	10	0.000
9. MSBA_ECOLI	PROBABLE ATP-BINDING TRANSPORT PRO	582	230	10	0.000
10. MDR3_CRIGR	MULTIDRUG RESISTANCE PROTEIN 3 (P-	1281	226	10	0.001
11. CYAB_BORPE	CYAB PROTEIN	712	224	10	0.001
12. MDR1_HUMAN	MULTIDRUG RESISTANCE PROTEIN 1 (P-	1280	218	10	0.001
13. MDR1_CRIGR	MULTIDRUG RESISTANCE PROTEIN 1 (P-	1276	216	9	0.002
14. MDR2_CRIGR	MULTIDRUG RESISTANCE PROTEIN 2 (P-	1276	216	9	0.002
15. MDR3_HUMAN	MULTIDRUG RESISTANCE PROTEIN 3 (P-	1279	216	9	0.002
16. MDR1_MOUSE	MULTIDRUG RESISTANCE PROTEIN 1 (P-	1276	214	9	0.002
17. MDR3_MOUSE	MULTIDRUG RESISTANCE PROTEIN 3 (P-	1104	210	9	0.003
18. LKTB_ACTAC	LEUKOTOXIN SECRETION PROTEIN.	707	203	9	0.006
19. HLYB_ECOLI	HAEMOLYSIN SECRETION PROTEIN, PLAS	707	201	9	0.006
20. HLY2_ECOLI	HAEMOLYSIN SECRETION PROTEIN, CHRO	708	201	9	0.006
21. LKTB_PASHA	LEUKOTOXIN SECRETION PROTEIN.	707	199	9	0.008
22. HLYB_PROVU	HAEMOLYSIN SECRETION PROTEIN.	707	194	9	0.013
23. HLYB_ACTPL	HAEMOLYSIN SECRETION PROTEIN (CLYI	707	183	8	0.034
24. PRTD_ERWCH	PROTEASES SECRETION PROTEIN PRTD.	575	178	8	0.055
25. CVAB_ECOLI	COLICIN V SECRETION PROTEIN CVAB.	698	164	7	0.182

Figure 3 *Illustrated is a database search for proteins homologous to the cystic fibrosis transmembrane receptor (CFTR) protein. The human CFTR protein was used as a query and compared to all the known protein sequences via the BLAZE program from IntelliGenetics, Inc., running on a massively parallel computer from MasPar Computer Corporation. The similarity scores for the top 25 protein sequences were printed out. Sequences with an expectation value (far right) of 0.05 or less are considered statistically significant. Notice that match scores as low as eight percent are significant. This is because of the use of an amino acid matching matrix that allows similar amino acids to score highly.*

26,706 proteins in a current protein database by means of a massively parallel computer. An examination of the list of the top 27 similar proteins strongly suggests that the CFTR protein is a membrane protein involved in secretion. There are also highly significant homologies to ATP-binding transport proteins. (Incidentally, some of the most highly significant homologies with this human protein are found for proteins from organisms as remote as *Escherichia coli* and yeast.) It was results such as these that led to an understanding of the function of the CFTR protein.

Toward True Understanding of the Genome

To reap the most benefit from having in hand the human genome, it will be necessary to understand the meaning of the genetic sequences. The methods currently available for interpreting DNA and protein sequences largely utilize evolutionary homology. The consensus-sequence method looks for highly conserved amino acids or bases in specific locations. Weight matrix or profile methods perform the same task quantitatively. With these evolution-based methods, as this chapter has shown, much hypothetical information can be gained from the study of a single gene and protein molecule.

Yet these evolution-based methods do not give much insight into the flow of genetic information from genes to structure and to phenotype, a goal discussed above. What are truly needed are methods that can predict structure and function on the basis of physical and chemical principles. Such methods will have to embody knowledge about how proteins fold, how they mediate catalysis, how they interact, and how they determine phenotype. Research is under way along these lines. Methods based on molecular dynamics aim to predict the structure of DNA, RNA, and proteins from physical principles. Automated learning methods, including some that depend on neural networks, are directed at identifying these physical principles through an analysis of the large amounts of sequence information now available. Probabilistic networks and other statistical methods may also reveal principles of physical structure and function based on examples in the growing public databases.

Even without these sophisticated informatic methods, there is still much to gain from knowing the sequences of the human genome. At the very least it will be possible to design DNA diagnostic probes for many, if not all, inherited diseases. Genome sequences coupled with recombinant DNA technology will make it possible to synthesize and mass produce human proteins having therapeutic value. Eventually, enhanced ability to decode the genetic information will make it possible to understand the nature of disease states and to design more rational therapies in the short term and genetic therapies in the long term.

References

1. Kerem B, Rommens JM, Buchanan JA, et al: Identification of the cystic fibrosis gene: genetic analysis. *Science* 245:1073, 1989

2. Riordan JR, Rommens JM, Kerem B, et al: Identification of the cystic fibrosis gene: cloning and characterization of complementary DNA. *Science* 245:1066, 1989

3. Rommens JM, Iannuzzi MC, Kerem BS, et al: Identification of the cystic fibrosis gene: chromosome walking and jumping. *Science* 245:1059, 1989

4. Collins FS: Cystic fibrosis: molecular biology and therapeutic implications. *Science* 256:774, 1992

5. McKusick VA: Current trends in mapping human genes. *FASEB J* 5:12, 1991

6. Fodor SPA, Read JL, Pirrung MC, et al: Light-directed, spatially adressable parallel chemical synthesis. *Science* 251: 767, 1991

7. Murray TH: Ethical issues in human genome research. *FASEB J* 5:55, 1991

8. Clarke LL, Grubb RR, Gabriel SE, et al: Defective epithelial chloride transport in a gene-targeted mouse model of cystic fibrosis. *Science* 257:1125, 1992

9. Dorin JR, Dickinson P, Alton EW, et al: Cystic fibrosis in the mouse by targeted insertional mutagenesis. *Nature* 359:211, 1992

10. Snouwaert JN, Brigman KK, Latour AM, et al: An animal model for cystic fibrosis made by gene targeting. *Science* 257:1083, 1992

11. Anfinsen CB: Principles that govern the folding of protein chains. *Science* 181:223, 1973

12. Abarbanel RM, Wieneke PR, Mansfield E, et al: Rapid searches for complex patterns in biological molecules. *Nucleic Acids Res* 12:263, 1984

13. Bairoch A: PROSITE: a dictionary of sites and patterns in proteins. *Nucleic Acids Res* 19:2241, 1991

14. Brennan RG, Matthews BW: The helix-turn-helix DNA binding motif. *J Biol Chem* 264:1903, 1989

15. Dodd IB, Egan JB: The prediction of helix-turn-helix DNA-binding regions in proteins: a reply to Yudkin. *Protein Eng* 2:174, 1988

16. Dodd IB, Egan JB: Improved detection of helix-turn-helix DNA-binding motifs in protein sequences. *Nucleic Acids Res* 18:5019, 1990

17. Gribskov M, Homyak M, Edenfield J, et al: Profile scanning for three-dimensional structural patterns in protein sequences. *Comput Appl Biosci* 4:61, 1988

18. Gribskov M, McLachlan AD, Eisenberg D: Profile analysis: dectection of distantly related proteins. *Proc Natl Acad Sci USA* 84:4355, 1987

19. Staden R: computer methods to locate signals in nucleic acid sequences. *Nucleic Acids Res* 12:505, 1984

20. Lipman DJ, Pearson WR: Rapid and sensitive protein similarity searches. *Science* 227:1435, 1985

21. Pearson WR, Lipman DJ: Improved tools for biological sequence comparison. *Proc Natl Acad Sci USA* 85:2444, 1988

22. Wilbur WJ, Lipman DJ: Rapid similarity searches of nucleic acid and protein data banks. *Proc Natl Acad Sci USA* 80:726, 1983

23. Benton D: Recent changes in the GenBank on-line service. *Nucleic Acids Res* 18:1517, 1990

24. Cinkosky MJ, Fickett JW, Gilna P, et al: Electronic data publishing and GenBank. *Science* 252:1273, 1991

25. Cameron GN: The EMBL data library. *Nucleic Acids Res* 16:1865, 1988

26. Stoehr PJ, Omond RA: New nucleotide sequence data on the EMBL File Server. *Nucleic Acids Res* 17:6765, 1989

27. Bairoch A, Boeckmann B: The SWISS-PROT protein sequence data bank. *Nucleic Acids Res* 19:2247, 1991

28. Sidman KE, George DG, Barker WC, et al: The protein identification resource (PIR). *Nucleic Acids Res* 16:1869, 1988

29. Needleman SB, Wunsch CD: A general method applicable to the search for similarities in the amino acid sequence of two proteins. *J Mol Biol* 48:443, 1970

30. Smith TF, Waterman M: Identification of common molecular subsequences. *J Mol Biol* 147:195, 1981

31. Schwartz RM, Dayhoff MO: Matrices for detecting distant relationships. 5(suppl 3):353, 1979

32. Brutlag DL, Dautricourt JP, Maulik S, et al: Improved sensitivity of biological sequence database searches. *Comput Appl Biosci* 6:237, 1990

Acknowledgments

Figures 1, 3   Sal Terillo.

Figure 2   Talar Agasyan. Adapted from *Recombinant DNA*, 2nd ed., by J. D. Watson, M. Gilman, J. Witkowski, et al. Scientific American Books, New York, 1992. © 1992 James D. Watson, Michael Gilman, Jan Witkowski, Mark Zoller. Used by permission.

Table 2   Data from "The Helix-Turn-Helix Binding Motif," by R. G. Brennan and B. W. Mathews, in *Journal of Biological Chemistry* 264:1903, 1989.

CHAPTER 8

Prenatal Diagnosis

Melissa H. Fries, M.D., Mitchell S. Golbus, M.D.

Prenatal diagnosis, the process of obtaining medical information about a fetus before birth, is a rapidly growing part of the work of obstetricians, geneticists, ultrasonographers, and genetic counselors. Its application is potentially universal, given the inevitable question of pregnancy: "Will my baby be healthy?"

Technological advances in molecular biology and ultrasonography have powered the expansion of prenatal diagnosis. As molecular methods elucidate the underlying genetic abnormality in more and more inherited diseases, molecular techniques have been applied to the fetus, greatly extending the repertoire of disorders that can be diagnosed prenatally. Advances in ultrasonography have kept up with those in basic science, making possible the early observation of fetal development and structural abnormalities. Sonography has also allowed physicians to visualize fetal structures when performing various prenatal procedures. This chapter discusses the applications, techniques, and limitations of prenatal diagnosis in characterizing the fetal condition.

The aim of prenatal diagnosis has been to provide accurate fetal information in the safest, least invasive manner. Because the ability to diagnose fetal abnormalities continues to lead the ability to treat them, many diagnostic procedures are performed early enough in gestation so that parents are able to consider the option of terminating a pregnancy if an affected fetus is found. Prenatal diagnosis is provided to those families voluntarily seeking information. The choice to seek information and the choice as to how such information, once obtained, is utilized continue to be the rightful province of the parents. What is critical for physicians who provide care for pregnant women and their families is to be aware of the breadth of conditions that can be diagnosed prenatally and to be ready to offer referrals to patients who desire them.

The provision of prenatal diagnosis offers several benefits. It gives parents at risk for having a child with an abnormality the opportunity to know whether or not the fetus is affected and to make the most informed choices. It reassures and reduces anxiety in high-risk patients. And it allows couples at risk for a defect to attempt pregnancy rather than forgo it, knowing that the presence of the disorder can be identified in the fetus.

Indications for Prenatal Diagnosis

There are multiple indications for prenatal diagnosis, including the following: (1) advanced maternal age at the time of delivery, (2) a previous child with chromosomal abnormalities, (3) a parent who is a carrier for a balanced translocation, (4) a mother who is a carrier for an X-linked disorder, (5) parents who are carriers for an autosomal recessive condition, (6) a previous child or a parent with a multifactorial disorder, (7) a maternal history of teratogenic exposure, (8) certain maternal illnesses, and (9) parental anxiety.

The most common reason for referring a pregnant patient for prenatal diagnostic procedures is advanced maternal age. In the United States this is considered to be 35 years of age or older at the expected time of delivery. This criterion is related to the increased risk of chromosomal aneuploidy with increased maternal age, in particular trisomy of chromosome 21, or Down syndrome. There is a progressive increase in the frequency of Down syndrome live births as a function of maternal age: from a rate of one per 1,250 live births at a maternal age of 15 to 19 years, to one per 350 live births at a maternal age of 35 years, to one per 25 live births at an age of 45 years or greater.[1-3] A similar but greater increase is also noted for the frequency of Down syndrome identified at the time of prenatal diagnosis—consistent with a higher rate of pregnancy loss and stillbirths among chromosomally abnormal fetuses.[2,4] Other aneuploidies, such as trisomy 13 and trisomy 18, also increase in frequency with increasing maternal age. The choice of 35 years of age as a discriminant for prenatal diagnosis is partially based on the potential risk of the procedures for prenatal diagnosis. That is, at 35 years the risk of a chromosomally abnormal fetus (approximately one in 192) equals the risk of losing the fetus as a result of amniocentesis or chorionic villus sampling (approximately one in 200).

A similar increase in chromosomal anomalies is not seen with increasing paternal age. However, an increased rate of spontaneous mutations (i.e., new dominant disorders) has been reported for children born to fathers older than 55 years.[5,6] This is not an indication for prenatal diagnosis, because the risk is nonspecific.

Couples who have had a child with aneuploidy or de novo chromosomal abnormalities are candidates for prenatal diagnosis even if they do not meet criteria based on maternal age. The empiric risk for recurrence of these conditions is approximately one in 100, which may be caused by parental mosaicism or by other factors that predispose to meiotic abnormality.[1]

Carriers of balanced reciprocal, or Robertsonian, translocations or chromosomal inversions are at risk for having a chromosomally abnormal child because atypical chromosomal segregation of gametes may occur at meiosis. The risk is related to the mode of ascertainment (a previous liveborn child or pregnancy loss), the predicted type of segregation leading to possibly viable gametes, and the sex of the parent carrying the chromosomal rearrangement (female carriers of translocations are at greater risk for having trisomic fetuses than male carriers are). The actual risk is variable but is usually put at between five and 30 percent.[7]

Maternal carriers of X-linked disorders are candidates for prenatal diagnosis by two methods. If the nature of the disorder has been characterized genetically, the fetus can be analyzed directly by DNA studies or enzymology (see below). Even if no biochemical analysis is available for the particular disorder, parents may still wish to ascertain the sex of their fetus to further refine the potential risks.

Parents who are carriers of single-gene disorders may want prenatal diagnosis. The list of inheritable diseases characterized by DNA studies [*see Table 1*] continues to expand steadily. In addition, for carriers of metabolic diseases, enzymatic or immunologic studies for known defects can be performed on amniotic fluid or chorionic villi.[8] Direct ultrasonographic diagnosis may be effective in families that are carriers of skeletal dysplasias or conditions with distinctive anatomic findings—such as omphalocele in Beckwith-Wiedemann syndrome [*see Chapter 9*].

Multifactorial disorders—conditions that result from the interaction of environmental factors with genetic factors—have a risk of recurrence in first-degree relatives that is approximately the square root of the population incidence for the condition. For example, neural tube defects, which have an incidence of from one to two per 1,000 live births in North America, have a recurrence risk in first-degree relatives of approximately four percent. For some of these conditions (e.g., cleft lip or palate, congenital heart disease, and neural tube defects), early ultrasonographic diagnosis may demonstrate a recurrence. Population screening for neural tube defects is also available (see below).

A history of maternal exposure to potentially teratogenic agents may prompt referral for prenatal diagnosis. The degree of concern for the fetus may vary depending on the timing, dosage, and particular agent of exposure. For example, early maternal exposure to valproic acid is associated with a one to two percent risk of neural tube defects.[9] Screening for neural tube defects by means of ultrasonography, amniocentesis, or both may be indicated for patients thus exposed. Maternal exposure to other antiepileptics, such as phenytoin or trimethadione, is associated with cleft lip or palate, which can be diagnosed prenatally by means of ultrasonography.[10] Lithium hydrochloride exposure has been associated with cardiac abnormalities (specifically Ebstein's anomaly), which can be diagnosed prenatally by means of fetal echocardiography.[9] The specific method of prenatal diagnosis varies as a function of the characteristic disorder seen with exposure to the particular teratogen and is best determined after referral.

Certain maternal illnesses, such as diabetes mellitus, are associated with a greatly increased risk of fetal congenital anomalies, particularly when

Table 1 Inheritable Diseases Diagnosed by DNA Testing

Disease	Diagnosis Confirmed by Cloned Gene	Diagnosis Confirmed by DNA Linkage
Adenosine deaminase deficiency	—	
Aldolase B deficiency (hereditary fructose phosphorylase intolerance)	—	
α_1-Antitrypsin deficiency	α_1-Antitrypsin	
Congenital adrenal hyperplasia	p450c21	
Cystic fibrosis	Cystic fibrosis transmembrane receptor	
Duchenne's and Becker's muscular dystrophy	Dystrophin	
Ehlers-Danlos syndrome type IV	Procollagen III	
Familial hypercholesterolemia	Low-density lipoprotein receptor	
Fragile X	—	
Glycogen storage disease type VI (Hers disease)	Liver phosphorylase	
Glycogen storage disease type V (McArdle disease)	Muscle phosphorylase	
Hemophilia A	Factor VIII	
Hemophilia B	Factor IX	
Ornithine transcarbamylase deficiency	Ornithine transcarbamylase	
Ornithine aminotransferase deficiency	Ornithine aminotransferase	
Phenylketonuria	Phenylalanine hydroxylase	
Retinoblastoma	Retinoblastoma	
Sickle cell disease	β-Globin	
α-Thalassemia	α-Globin	
β-Thalassemia	β-Globin	
X-linked ichythyosis	Steroid sulfatase	
Von Willebrand's disease	Von Willebrand's factor	
Adult-onset polycystic kidney disease		Yes
Emory-Dreifuss muscular dystrophy		Yes
Huntington's disease		Yes
Myotonic dystrophy		Yes
Neurofibromatosis type 1		Yes
X-linked retinoschisis		Yes

the disease was poorly controlled before conception. The associated anomalies include neural tube defects and cardiac, skeletal, renal, and gastrointestinal disorders, many of which can be diagnosed by means of prenatal ultrasonography.[11] Maternal primary infection with cytomegalovirus, rubella, herpes simplex, varicella, *Toxoplasma gondii*, *Treponema pallidum*, and parvovirus B19 has been associated with distinctive fetal anomalies such as microcephaly, periventricular calcification, and hydrops.[11,12] These features may be seen on prenatal ultrasonography, or direct evidence of fetal infection can be obtained via amniocentesis or fetal blood sampling. Referral for prenatal diagnosis can be very helpful in these cases.

Finally, in the absence of specific indications for prenatal diagnosis, certain couples may still feel a strong need to verify that their fetus is karyotypically normal. Referral of these couples for prenatal diagnosis, ultrasonography, or both may alleviate excessive anxiety that would otherwise persist throughout the pregnancy. Such patients should be made aware, however, that the presence of a normal karyotype in no way excludes all fetal anomalies.

Methods of Prenatal Diagnosis

Prenatal diagnosis can be accomplished by examining the fetus directly, either through inspection (ultrasonography and fetal echocardiography) or through invasive sampling of the fetus to evaluate fetal cells or products for cytogenetic, biochemical, DNA, or histologic abnormalities. Alternatively, one can examine the fetus indirectly, by assaying the mother's blood for fetal proteins or fetal cells. Studies are considered noninvasive if they do not require penetration of the uterus during gestation to sample fetal tissue.

Noninvasive Techniques

The trend in prenatal diagnosis has been away from invasive fetal assay, with its attendant risks, to noninvasive techniques: either the assay of maternal blood for fetal proteins or cells or various advanced ultrasonographic methods.

ASSAYS OF MATERNAL SERUM

Maternal serum is most often examined to screen for fetal neural tube or ventral wall defects by assay of maternal serum α-fetoprotein. α-Fetoprotein is an embryonic glycoprotein similar to albumin with a molecular weight of 70 kilodaltons (kd). It is produced in sequence by the yolk sac, the fetal gastrointestinal tract, and the fetal liver. It is not produced by the mother except in rare cases of maternal tumor or genetically determined persistence of the protein production. Levels are highest in fetal blood, but some α-fetoprotein passes into the amniotic sac in fetal urine or gastrointestinal secretions and from there into the maternal bloodstream. The concentration of α-fetoprotein is highest in the fetal circulation at 12 menstrual weeks (weeks of pregnancy dated from the last menstrual period) and decreases thereafter. This is paralleled by a peak in amniotic fluid α-fetoprotein concentration early in the second trimester, after which the concentration declines. In maternal serum, however, the level continues to increase by approximately 15 percent per week in the second trimester until it peaks at 30 menstrual weeks and then falls.[13]

Normal maternal serum α-fetoprotein levels are established by individual laboratories and vary with maternal weight (higher weight is associated with a lower level), race (levels are higher in African Americans than in Caucasians), and the presence of maternal insulin-dependent diabetes mellitus, or IDDM (levels are lower in IDDM patients than in the general population).

The elevation of maternal serum α-fetoprotein levels in pregnancies with anencephalic fetuses was first described in 1973.[14] Similar elevations were found in pregnancies complicated by open neural tube defects (encephalocele, meningomyelocele, open spina bifida) and open ventral abdominal wall defects (gastroschisis, omphalocele). (These defects are classifed as open because they lack skin covering, so that the amniotic fluid is in direct contact with fetal organs or a thin permeable membrane covering the organs. Amniotic fluid concentrations of α-fetoprotein are increased, and there is a consequent increase in maternal serum levels of this protein.) Elevated maternal serum α-fetoprotein levels also can be seen with multiple gestations, congenital nephrosis, placental abnormalities or cysts, fetomaternal hemorrhage, fetal demise, or parvovirus B19 infection.[13] Some other conditions, such as Turner's syndrome, are typically not associated with elevated maternal serum α-fetoprotein levels, even in the presence of large unruptured cystic hygromas.[13] Maternal serum α-fetoprotein levels are lower than normal in pregnancies in which the fetus has Down syndrome or trisomy 18.

These observations have led to the measurement of maternal serum α-fetoprotein levels at 15 to 20 menstrual weeks to screen (primarily for open neural tube defects, ventral wall defects, and Down syndrome) patients who are younger than 35 years and have no family history of neural tube defects (i.e., those who otherwise would not have been offered prenatal diagnosis during their pregnancy). Such testing is voluntary but widespread; it requires consent for drawing a single tube of blood, which poses minimal risk to the mother.

Results are reported in terms of multiples of the normal median (MoM) as established by each individual laboratory. High levels are those greater than 2 to 2.5 MoM (the exact discrimination point is a function of the desired number of false positives). Low levels are those that, when considered along with age, establish a risk in the midtrimester that is equivalent to the risk in a 35-year-old woman.[15]

The management of pregnancies with elevated maternal serum α-fetoprotein levels involves repetition of maternal blood testing if the pregnancy is still less than 18 menstrual weeks. If the level is still elevated, the patient is referred for ultrasonographic evaluation to ascertain gestational age (a pregnancy more advanced than expected would show spurious elevation of maternal serum α-fetoprotein), a multifetal pregnancy, or fetal demise. If the elevation remains unexplained, the patient can be referred for level II ultrasonography to detect a visible anomaly.[16]

This approach is somewhat controversial because it might fail to detect a small lesion. More conservative management involves amniocentesis for measurement of amniotic fluid α-fetoprotein and acetylcholinesterase (a specific neural protein that is elevated in amniotic fluid in the presence of open neural tube defects). A fetal karyotype is also performed because neural tube defects are associated with some chromosomal abnormalities, particularly trisomy 13, trisomy 18, and triploidy.[17] If a significant abnormality is found, parents then have the choice of continuing or terminating the pregnancy. With these procedures, 80 to 90 percent of fetuses with neural tube defects and significant ventral wall defects can be identified. Pregnancies in which no explanation is found for the elevation of maternal serum α-fetoprotein are managed as "high risk" because adverse obstetric outcomes have been reported in some cases.[18]

Pregnancies with low maternal serum α-fetoprotein levels are managed by referral for ultrasonography without repetition of maternal blood testing. If the original gestational age is confirmed, amniocentesis is performed for karyotyping, specifically for trisomy 21 or 18. Results of the New England Regional collaborative study indicated that one Down syndrome fetus was identified for every 89 amniocenteses performed: chromosomal abnormalities were discovered in one in 65 amniocenteses. This implies that among pregnant women younger than 35 years, maternal serum α-fetoprotein screening identified approximately 25% of the total cases of Down syndrome.[19]

Because 80 percent of the infants with Down syndrome are born to mothers younger than 35 years, other fetal products in maternal serum are being assayed in an effort to refine the criteria for referral for more invasive studies. Two markers that show promise are maternal serum human chorionic gonadotropin and maternal serum unconjugated estriol. Both products are produced uniquely by the fetal-placental unit, not by the mother. In pregnancies complicated by Down syndrome, maternal serum human chorionic gonadotropin levels are elevated,[20] whereas maternal serum unconjugated estriol levels are lower than in control subjects.[21] In conjunction with maternal serum α-fetoprotein, these markers provide additional information regarding the presence of Down syndrome. Preliminary reports have indicated that approximately 60 percent of the cases of Down syndrome could be detected by assessing the measurements of these three proteins in conjunction with maternal age.[22] Large prospective studies are presently under way to evaluate the ultimate utility of these so-called triple markers in predicting fetal chromosomal abnormalities.

FETAL CELLS IN MATERNAL SERUM

In the future, assay of maternal blood may be the only test needed to characterize the fetus fully on the basis of fetal cells present in the maternal circulation during pregnancy. As early as 1893, trophoblast cells were observed in the lungs of women dying of preeclampsia.[23] In 1954, fetal nucleated red blood cells were demonstrated in the maternal circulation after extensive fetomaternal hemorrhage,[24] and such cells were later quantified with an acid elution test.[25] XY cells have been reported in the circulation of women who gave birth to male infants; the cells were thought to be fetal lymphocytes.[26] However, quantification of the number of cells of fetal origin in the maternal bloodstream has been difficult because of their rarity. Before they can be depended on for analysis, special techniques must be applied to enrich this rare cell fraction and to verify that the cells are indeed fetal in origin.

Both verification that cells are of fetal origin and enrichment of fetal cells are feasible if there is a way to identify unique components of such cells. The most common fetal cells entering the maternal circulation include lymphocytes, trophoblastic cells, and nucleated red blood cells. For lymphocytes, no specific fetal HLA marker has yet been identified, but cells with a paternal HLA type have been identified in maternal peripheral blood through the use of antibodies against the paternal HLA type.[27] Mouse monoclonal antibodies against human cytotrophoblast antigens also can select for circulating fetal trophoblast cells.[28] Mouse monoclonal antibodies raised against the transferrin receptor and glycophorin can be used to enrich fetal nucleated red blood cells from the maternal circulation.[29]

In these studies, specific fluorescent monoclonal antibodies to the targeted cell population were attached to the cells, and the fetal cells were then separated from maternal cells by means of fluorescence-activated cell sorting (FACS). This technique involves the passage of a minute stream of cells through the beam of an argon laser, which excites the fluorescence of the antibodies. Any cells coated with the fluorescent antibodies are shunted into a collecting vessel and counted.[30] The process is laborious and time consuming, however. A simpler option for fetal cell selection is to coat magnetic spheres with cell-specific monoclonal antibodies; fetal cells adhere to the antibody-sphere complex and can be attracted out of suspension by cobalt-samarium magnets.[31] Ultimately, a combination of both methods may be required to provide adequate numbers of fetal cells for analysis.

Attempts to culture these fetal cells for full karyotype analysis have not yet been successful. However, fluorescence in situ hybridization for specific chromosomal markers has been utilized to identify the X and Y chromosomes as well as chromosomes 13, 18, and 21.[32] In this technique, probes (specific DNA fragments) for repetitive areas of DNA uniquely found on one or another of those chromosomes are directly hybridized with (that is, bound to the complementary segments of) the DNA of both interphase and metaphase cells. Before hybridization, the probes are labeled with various fluorescent dyes to distinguish which probe has been attached to which chromosome. This method has been applied to identify sex and recognize aneuploidy in cells obtained from the fetus through amniocentesis or chorionic villus sampling (see below),[33] and it could be applied as well to characterize fetal cells obtained from the maternal circulation.

The polymerase chain reaction (PCR), which is a means of amplifying a specific segment of the genome from very small amounts of DNA [*see Chapter 6*], also has been applied to the characterization of fetal cells from the maternal circulation; indeed, it has been the principal method for identifying such cells. A highly repetitive area of the Yq has been amplified to identify male cells from the circulation of patients who were carrying male fetuses, and this method was successful in detecting the Y chromosomal region in 75 percent of male-bearing pregnancies.[29] In another study that used similar PCR primers, the correct sex was assigned to the fetus in 12 out of 13 pregnancies that were analyzed.[28] PCR can be performed with extracted DNA or directly with lysed cells derived from amniocentesis, chorionic villus sampling, or maternal blood. Another study reported that PCR had an efficiency of 94 percent in predicting fetal sex in samples of fetal cells sorted from the maternal circulation by means of FACS.[34] Potentially, PCR could be used to amplify single genes as well as to identify the sex of a fetus.

At present, the isolation of fetal cells from the maternal circulation continues to be experimental, but it is an exciting area of research. The future application of such techniques may make invasive fetal studies less frequent, thereby reducing the anxiety associated with invasive prenatal procedures.

ULTRASONOGRAPHY

Ultrasound is mechanical radiant energy with a frequency above the audible range.[35] In 1952, ultrasound was first used to visualize soft-tissue structures of the body.[36] The usefulness of ultrasonography in obstetrics and gynecology has been demonstrated,[37] and its application to fetal investigation was expanded during the 1960s, when it was first used to study fetal growth.[38]

Ultrasonography involves the generation of a high-frequency signal through electric stimulation of a piezoelectric crystal that vibrates to generate ultrasonic energy at from 3.5 to 7.0 MHz, depending on the characteristics of the crystal. This signal is directed through a transducer into the tissues, which have varying degrees of acoustic impedance. At tissue interfaces, echoes are generated and reflected back along the line of transmission to the transducer, which also acts as a receiver. The signal is amplified and displayed on a video screen as a collection of images in multiple shades of gray. Early scanners utilized B-mode, or static, images that were later arranged to depict the three-dimensional appearance of the tissues. Real-time scanners produce continuous images by two methods: linear scanning and sector scanning. In linear scanning, multiple small transducers in a single probe fire in a predetermined pattern, whereas in sector scanning, a single transducer oscillates to form a continuous picture in cross section.[35] At present, ultrasound diagnoses rely on real-time scanning exclusively because it enables one to visualize various procedures as they occur.

Since the introduction of ultrasonography, efforts have been directed toward assaying the potential hazards of this procedure. The technology has a distinct appeal because it uses no ionizing radiation; however, concerns were initially raised that ultrasonography might cause cavitation ("bubble formation") and thermal side effects.[39] To date, after more than 30 years of use of ultrasonography in pregnancy, no ill effects on fetal development or well-being have been demonstrated.[40]

Typical obstetric ultrasonography is performed by transabdominal scanning with a relatively low sound-wave frequency to achieve deep penetration (2.5 to 5 MHz). Transvaginal transducers, which have a higher sound-wave frequency (5 to 10 MHz) and thus provide better resolution, have been used early in the first trimester. These transducers provide a very clear image because of their proximity to pelvic structures. As the uterus enlarges and moves upward in the abdomen, however, their utility decreases because of the higher attenuation and poor tissue penetration of high-frequency sound waves.[41] Still, in cases of marked maternal obesity or in cases in which the fetal head has descended into the maternal pelvis, vaginal ultrasonography is effective later in pregnancy for the diagnosis of fetal intracranial anatomy or placenta previa.[42,43]

An adjunct to obstetric ultrasonography is Doppler ultrasonography for the assessment of fetal and uteroplacental circulation.[44] Analysis of the wave form of the Doppler flow of the fetal umbilical artery, fetal internal carotid artery, and the uterine arteries has provided information on fetal well-being, particularly for fetuses with intrauterine growth retardation.[45] Such measurements are not specific for any type of fetal anomaly, however, and their efficacy in prenatal diagnosis is not well established. Color flow or Doppler echocardiography does have utility in the diagnosis of fetal cardiac anomalies (see below).

Although prenatal ultrasonography is performed in 90 to 100 percent of pregnancies in some European countries, this level of use has not been the standard of care in the United States, primarily because of financial concerns.[46] Still, it is estimated that more than 50 percent of pregnant women in the United States have undergone at least one ultrasound examination during their pregnancy.[47] For this reason, the National Institutes of Health has established a list of indications for obstetric ultrasonography [*see Table 2*].[48] Significantly absent from this list is routine scanning for fetal anomalies, because this approach would be highly impractical. A targeted approach to identify specific lesions is appropriate when the fetus is known to be at risk for a certain malformation.[49] The ability of the ultrasonographer to detect abnormalities is a function of operator experience, the type of equipment utilized, gestational age at the time of examination, and the indication for examination.

A full discussion of the anomalies detectable by ultrasonography and their appearance is beyond the scope of this chapter. It should be pointed out, however, that in each trimester of pregnancy, there are particular malformations that are likely to be recognized. In the first trimester, scanning may reveal central nervous system defects, including fetal

---

Table 2   Indications for Ultrasonographic Examination: NIH Consensus Meeting

Estimation of gestational age for confirmation of clinical dating

Estimation of gestational age for late registrants for prenatal care

Evaluation of fetal growth

Vaginal bleeding of undetermined etiology in pregnancy

Determination of fetal presentation if this cannot be adequately confirmed clinically

Suspected multiple gestation

Adjunct to amniocentesis and prenatal diagnosis procedures

Significant uterine size/clinical dates discrepancy

Pelvic mass detected clinically

Suspected hydatidiform mole

Adjunct to cervical cerclage placement

Suspected ectopic pregnancy

Suspected fetal death

Suspected uterine anomaly

IUD localization

Ovarian cyst development surveillance

Biophysical profile for fetal well-being

Observation of intrapartum events

Suspected abruptio placentae

Adjunct to external version from breech to vertex

Estimation of fetal weight and/or presentation in premature rupture of membranes and/or preterm labor

Abnormal serum α-fetoprotein value requiring fetal age determination

Follow-up observation of identified fetal anomaly

History of previous congenital anomaly

Serial evaluation of fetal growth in multiple gestation

acrania (absence of the calvarium) and choroid plexus cysts, which in one or two percent of cases are associated with trisomy 18.[50] Cystic hygromas—thin-walled, fluid-filled masses on the posterior neck—are visible and may be associated with chromosomal abnormalities in more than 50 percent of cases.[51] Severe skeletal dysplasias, such as thanatophoric dwarfism, may be detectable before 13 menstrual weeks, whereas in other growth disorders, such as achondroplasia, osteogenesis imperfecta, or Jeune thoracic dystrophy, the limb measurements may be normal until the second trimester. In addition, one diagnosis of conjoined twins has been made as early as 10 menstrual weeks.[41]

The second trimester is the optimal time for sonographic identification of fetal anomalies, and it is then that a targeted examination for a specific malformation is usually performed. Scanning can reveal neural tube defects such as encephalocele, meningomyelocele, spina bifida, anencephaly, and other CNS abnormalities, including hydrocephalus, hydranencephaly, holoprosencephaly, and porencephalic cysts. Renal agenesis can be recognized on the basis of profound oligohydramnios and the absence of a dilated urinary collecting system. Skeletal dysplasias such as thanatophoric dwarfism, osteogenesis imperfecta, and hypophosphatasia can be recognized on the basis of characteristic calvarial, vertebral, and long bone abnormalities. Significant cardiac defects are recognizable, but further evaluation by fetal echocardiography may be necessary.

Other, less severe anomalies, such as cleft lip and palate, ventral abdominal wall defects (e.g., omphalocele or gastroschisis), diaphragmatic hernia, cystic adenomatoid malformation of the lung or other intrathoracic masses, obstructive uropathy, and placental abnormalities, can be noted on careful scanning.[52] Specific malformations of multiple gestations, including conjoined twins, twin-to-twin transfusion syndrome, and twin reversed-arterial-perfusion syndrome (acardiac twin) are likewise recognizable. The discovery of a single anomaly prompts a full ultrasonographic search for other abnormalities; often, further prenatal testing for karyotype analysis is recommended because of the frequent association of multiple malformations with chromosomal disorders.[53] The early discovery of a potentially lethal condition gives parents the option of terminating the pregnancy.

Some conditions, however, evolve slowly and may not be clearly visible until the third trimester. Such defects include some cases of hydrocephalus, hydranencephaly, closed neurologic disorders such as Dandy-Walker cysts, cardiovascular disorders, duodenal or jejunal atresia, meconium peritonitis, kidney dysplasia, cloacal anomalies, and such nonlethal skeletal dysplasias as heterozygous achondroplasia and osteogenesis imperfecta type I or III.[33] (Often, these conditions might indeed have been seen earlier in gestation, but the patients were not referred for evaluation until a distinct alteration in fetal growth or amniotic fluid quantity was recognized.) In the case of multiple anomalies, karyotypic evaluation is still helpful in the third trimester in order to guide obstetric management. In addition, when a potentially correctable abnormality is found, parents and physicians are able to plan neonatal management, including options for surgery and referral to high-risk centers.

FETAL ECHOCARDIOGRAPHY

Fetal echocardiography is the study of the fetal heart with high-resolution real-time ultrasonography. Although the heart can be seen clearly on routine ultrasonography, details of its structure and function are better revealed by precise imaging with M-mode, pulsed Doppler, continuous-wave, and color-flow Doppler ultrasonography.[54] Fetal echocardiography is largely practiced through high-risk centers by appropriately trained pediatric cardiologists. Typical indications for referral are the following: (1) a family history of congenital heart disease, (2) maternal disease (such as diabetes mellitus or systemic lupus erythematosus) affecting the fetus, (3) maternal ingestion of drugs (such as lithium or alcohol), (4) other detected fetal anomalies (5) hydrops fetalis, (6) fetal arrhythmias, and (7) polyhydramnios.[55] Studies are optimally performed at 18 to 22 menstrual weeks with 5 or 7.5 MHz sector-scan transducers and M-mode echocardiography, which can visualize valvular opening and closure, atrial contraction, and changes in muscle thickness or cavity size. Pulsed Doppler shows the direction and quality of the blood flow in the heart and the great vessels and, along with color-coded flow mapping, can show flow disturbance.[54] Optimal benefit from these studies requires careful orientation of the fetal heart relative to the body of the fetus and may require alterations of maternal position from prone to lateral. A typical scan may take an hour of detailed study.

Not all cardiac anomalies can be diagnosed prenatally, in part because of the specific cardiac anatomy of the fetus. A patent foramen ovale and ductus arteriosus are normal in the fetus, so that one cannot predict whether these conditions will exist after birth. Small ventricular septal defects and discrete aortic coarctation may not be visualized.[56] On the other hand, congenital heart lesions that can be diagnosed include tetralogy of Fallot, transposition of the great vessels, atrioventricular canal defects, large ventricular septal defects, intracardiac tumors, valvular lesions, Ebstein's anomaly of the tricuspid valve, the presence of only a single ventricle, hypertrophic cardiomyopathy, endocardial fibroelastosis, ectopia cordis, hypoplastic right or left heart syndrome, double-outlet right ventricle, tricuspid atresia, truncus arteriosus, and large coarctations.[56] Once cardiac anomalies are discovered, follow-up evaluation may be needed to assess the full prognosis of the condition and to direct the parents' actions in the remainder of the pregnancy.

Invasive Techniques

Although maternal serum assays and sonographic visualization provide much information about the fetus, most present technologies require some fetal tissue for analysis of karyotype, DNA, metabolic assay, or pathologic review. The principal methods for obtaining this tissue are amniocentesis, chorionic villus sampling, cordocentesis, and direct fetal tissue biopsy.

AMNIOCENTESIS

Amniocentesis is the most widely practiced method of invasive prenatal diagnosis [see Figure 1]. The procedure dates from 1952, when Bevis first described the assay of amniotic fluid for fetal erythroblastosis.[57] In the

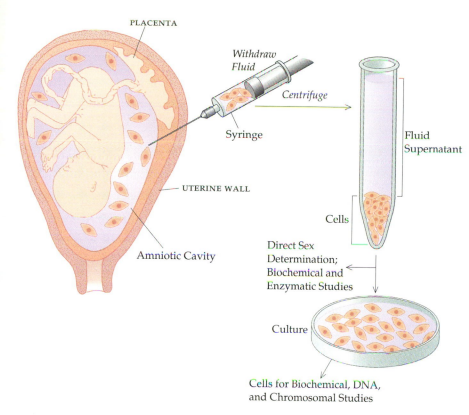

PLACENTA

Withdraw Fluid

Centrifuge

Syringe

UTERINE WALL

Amniotic Cavity

Fluid Supernatant

Cells

Direct Sex Determination; Biochemical and Enzymatic Studies

Culture

Cells for Biochemical, DNA, and Chromosomal Studies

Figure 1 In amniocentesis, a sample of amniotic fluid (mostly fetal urine and other excretions) is taken by inserting a needle into the amniotic cavity, typically between the 15th and the 20th menstrual week (although it has been done between nine and 14 menstrual weeks). The fetal cells are separated from the fluid by centrifugation. They can either be used immediately or, as is more common, cultured so that biochemical, enzymatic, and chromosomal analyses can be made. The cultured cells can also be a source of DNA.

1960s, as human karyotyping developed, amniotic fluid cells were first cultured and studied in women at risk for fetal chromosomal abnormalities.[58] As evidence of the association of advancing maternal age with aneuploidy accumulated,[2-4] the practice was expanded to include Down syndrome and other trisomies.

The demand for this prenatal information prompted most diagnostic centers to begin performing amniocentesis in the early 1970s. Because real-time ultrasonography was not available at that time, amniocenteses were performed blind, without knowledge of the position of the placenta or the fetus. Once real-time ultrasonography was developed, it was combined with amniocentesis to enable the operator to place the needle in a precisely determined spot.[59] Much of the skill required for other prenatal diagnostic invasive procedures has been derived from the extensive practice of ultrasound-guided amniocentesis.

Classically, amniocentesis is performed at from 15 to 20 menstrual weeks. The procedure includes a level I ultrasound scan to determine fetal viability, fetal position, and placental placement; to ascertain whether multiple gestations are present; to assess the appearance of the fetal spine and abdomen; to provide a four-chamber view of the heart; and to allow measurement of the fetal biparietal diameter and femur length. The maternal abdomen is then sterilely prepared and draped, and under ultrasonographic guidance (either linear or sector array), the operator inserts a 22-gauge spinal needle through the maternal abdomen and uterus into the amniotic sac and aspirates from 20 to 24 ml of amniotic fluid. Local anesthesia for the needle insertion site may be used; it may reduce maternal anxiety and does not seem to affect the outcome of the procedure. The patient may experience slight uterine cramping during and after the procedure; many women do not feel any ill effects, however, and can resume their usual activities immediately after the procedure.

The amniotic fluid, which largely represents fetal urine, contains cells sloughed from the fetal skin, trachea, esophagus, and uroepithelium. At best, only 10 percent of these cells are viable and able to divide. The cells are cultured in tissue culture for some five to 10 days and then are treated with colchicine to stop cell division in metaphase. The cells are treated with hypotonic solution, fixed, and stained with chromosomal stains. The time from procedure to results is 10 to 20 days. The amniotic fluid is also assayed for α-fetoprotein. In addition to karyotyping, the lysed amniotic cells can be subjected directly to the polymerase chain reaction to determine fetal sex in X-linked disorders or tested for disorders such as sickle-cell anemia or hemophilia A. If the results are inconclusive with direct amniocytes or PCR tests, DNA is extracted from the cultured amniocytes and then tested. The cell-free fluid can also be subjected to direct hormonal assay; for example, amniotic fluid measurement of tetrahydrocortisone, tetrahydro-11-deoxycortisone, and tetrahydrocortisol is used for prenatal diagnosis of 11-hydroxylase deficiency, which is one cause of congenital adrenal hyperplasia.[60]

The major risk of amniocentesis is the risk of fetal loss. Studies of amniocenteses performed in Canada and the United States have indicated an increased fetal loss rate of 0.5 percent or less in comparison with pregnancies in control (untested) subjects.[61,62] Other studies in the United Kingdom reported loss rates closer to one percent,[63] and this rate was confirmed by a large randomized Danish study in 1986.[64] The explanation for the increased loss rate observed after amniocentesis in these studies is still not clear. The Danish study did note a larger increase in fetal loss (2.1 percent) when the amniocentesis needle penetrated an anterior placenta, compared with a loss of 1.2 percent when there was no placental penetration; this finding, however, has not been substantiated in further reviews. Many institutions that perform large numbers of amniocenteses will have a sufficiently broad data base to generate their own statements of fetal loss, which may be the most reliable estimates to cite in prenatal counseling.

Other potential risks include an increased rate of respiratory complications in neonates born after amniocentesis. Reports from Denmark and the United Kingdom imply an increase in respiratory distress syndrome (1.1 percent versus 0.5 percent in control subjects) and infant pneumonia (0.7 percent versus 0.3 percent in control subjects) after amniocentesis. These findings have not, however, been confirmed in other studies.[65]

Because of the desire for earlier diagnosis, amniocentesis has been performed late in the first trimester at nine to 14 menstrual weeks. Such procedures are termed early amniocenteses and differ from second-trimester amniocenteses in that less amniotic fluid is withdrawn (generally, 1 ml for every week of gestation). Earlier in gestation, fewer cells are found in the amniotic fluid, and this fact, together with the decrease in total fluid volume aspirated, may make cell culture more difficult. In addition, the risks of amniocentesis at this gestational age may not be derived by downward extrapolation from that of second-trimester amniocentesis.

The broad range of timing of early amniocentesis potentially includes the period from nine to 12 weeks, when amniotic fluid volume does not yet have a significant component of fetal urine.[66] At this gestational age, it may be considerably more difficult to replenish amniotic fluid than it is in the second trimester.

Many recent reports have described the outcome of early amniocentesis. An increase in number of complications with early amniocentesis has been reported (seven cases out of 42) compared with midtrimester amniocentesis (one out of 140); complications included ruptured membranes, oligohydramnios, intrauterine hematoma, and fetal demise.[67] One group of investigators described a fetal loss rate of 1.8 percent with early amniocentesis at nine to 14 menstrual weeks,[68] whereas another group reported a 4.1 percent fetal loss rate for early amniocentesis that was performed primarily at a mean age of 14.0 menstrual weeks.[69] One study compared fetal losses after early amniocentesis at nine to 14 menstrual weeks with fetal losses after transabdominal chorionic villus sampling.[70] This study found that seven fetal losses occurred in 150 early amniocenteses, whereas only two fetal losses occurred in 150 chorionic villus samplings (see below). On the other hand, another study reported a loss rate with early amniocentesis comparable to that of midtrimester amniocentesis and better than the rate observed with chorionic villus sampling (see below).[71] In addition, the analysis of acetylcholinesterase activity in early amniotic fluid has not been reliable in predicting open neural tube defects.[72] It is apparent that early amniocentesis is an experimental procedure whose risks are not yet well established.

CHORIONIC VILLUS SAMPLING

The timing of second-trimester amniocentesis is late enough in gestation that terminating the pregnancy may be physically difficult and emotionally wrenching. That is why other prenatal procedures have been attempted earlier in gestation. Aside from early amniocentesis, the major invasive procedure is chorionic villus sampling (CVS) [*see Figure 2*]. CVS was initially done in the early 1970s by Chinese investigators who, in the interests of sex selection, sampled the placental bed with transcervical catheters. They worked without ultrasonographic guidance, and yet their overall loss rate was only six percent.[73] The procedure was not widely publicized until 1982, when a report appeared on its use for prenatal diagnosis of inherited diseases.[74] Since that time, more than 100,000 samplings have been performed.[75]

CVS can be performed as early as seven to eight menstrual weeks but is more typically performed at nine to 12 weeks. It can be accomplished either transcervically or transabdominally. The route depends on the position of the placenta (posterior placentas are typically sampled transcervically, anterior and fundal placentas transabdominally); on gestational age (almost all CVS after 12 menstrual weeks is performed transabdominally because of the increased distance from cervix to placental bed); on the presence of cervical infection (patients with active herpes simplex virus 2 lesions are sampled transabdominally); and on the discretion of the operator. Patients receive a preliminary level I ultrasound scan to assess fetal viability and determine gestational age by crown-to-rump length and sac size, placental location, and the presence of multiple gestations. Some operators have considered a finding of an empty second sac or a multiple pregnancy to be a contraindication for CVS because it may not be possible to delineate the limits of each placenta.

For transcervical sampling, either a soft polyethylene catheter 1.5 mm in diameter with a metal stylet (Portex) or a 16-gauge long angiocatheter with a metal stylet is used. A speculum is placed in the vagina, the vagina and cervix are sterilely prepared, and the catheter and stylet are inserted—under continuous ultrasonographic guidance—through the cervical opening into the placental bed. The stylet is removed, and a 20 ml syringe is attached to the catheter; some eight or 10 aspiration movements of the syringe at 10 to 15 ml of negative pressure serve to collect the sample as the catheter is withdrawn.

For transabdominal sampling, the maternal abdomen is sterilely prepared and draped, and a local anesthetic is applied to the needle site. Under sterile ultrasonographic guidance, a 6-in 20-gauge needle is directed through the abdominal wall and uterus into the placental bed. A 20 ml syringe is attached, and 15 ml of steady pressure is maintained while the tip of the needle is delicately moved about within the placenta. The patient is instructed to rest after either procedure and to refrain from vigorous activity for 48 hours; some mild postprocedural cramping is not uncommon, and approximately 20 to 30 percent of patients may experience vaginal spotting or bleeding after transcervical CVS.[76]

Immediately after collection of the tissue sample and before the patient leaves the procedure room, the placental tissue is placed in tissue culture

Figure 2 *Chorionic villus sampling is typically performed between the ninth and the 12th menstrual weeks, although it has been done as early as seven to eight menstrual weeks. It can be accomplished either transcervically or transabdominally; a transcervical approach is shown here. A catheter is introduced into the uterus, and a small sample of chorionic villi is drawn into a syringe. DNA can be isolated directly from the tissue, or cell cultures can be established.*

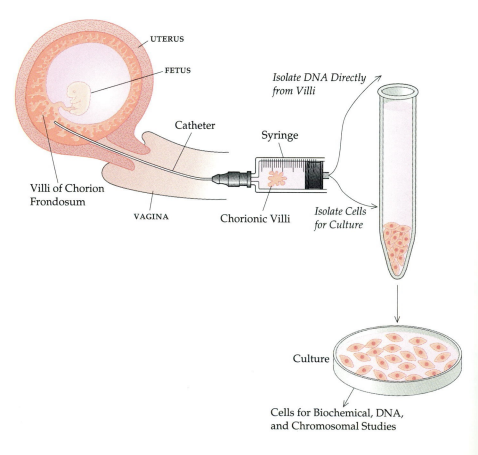

medium and analyzed under a dissecting microscope for the presence of an adequate amount of villi. If insufficient tissue (less than 2 to 3 mg) was obtained, the sampling is repeated.[77] (Repetition may be necessary in some 10 to 30 percent of procedures.) The specimen is cleaned of maternal decidua both mechanically and with the enzyme pronase (which inactivates surface proteins of maternal origin) and is placed in tissue culture medium. If a sufficient volume of tissue is obtained, part of the sample can be studied directly for trophoblast mitoses, allowing rapid determination of karyotype (in 24 to 48 hours). For cultured tissue, the medium is replaced at 48- to 72-hour intervals, and when adequate growth is achieved, the cultured cells are treated in the same manner as amniotic fluid cells to obtain a karyotype. Villi are composed of three distinct types of cells: syncytiotrophoblast, cytotrophoblast, and mesenchymal core. Unlike amniocytes, many of which are sloughed dead cells, these cells are actively growing and dividing. Their growth in culture is therefore more rapid than that of amniocytes, so that results may be obtained in 10 to 12 days. Maternal cell contamination of cultured chorionic villus cells is rare once a laboratory is experienced in CVS analysis.

Chorionic villus can serve for karyotyping in the case of advanced maternal age or as a direct trophoblast preparation for enzyme or PCR analysis to determine sex or detect single-gene disorders. Confirmatory biochemical or DNA studies are performed on DNA extracted from the cultured cells. (For enzyme analysis, it is important to ascertain before sampling whether the enzyme in question is normally expressed in villus tissue at measurable levels and if it is better expressed in direct or in cultured tissue.[8])

Mosaic cytogenetic results (reflecting the presence of two or more cell lines) are obtained in CVS with an incidence of one to two percent. Such a finding is significant because if the fetus is truly mosaic, there may be associated fetal anomalies and mental retardation. The frequency is greater in karyotypes done with a direct cytotrophoblast preparation of chorionic villi than in those done with cultured mesenchymal core cells. Such cases may represent mosaicism confined to the placenta, and the results are frequently not confirmed in cultured tissue or the fetus. Because of the relative unreliability of results from direct preparations, most centers performing CVS rely exclusively on results from cultured cells. Mosaicism is, however, seen even in cultured mesenchymal cells, with an incidence of approximately one percent. Most of these abnormalities are confined to the placenta and not found in the fetus.

Because of the difficulty in knowing whether mosaicism found on CVS actually reflects the true fetal situation, patients with mosaicism usually undergo further prenatal testing, such as amniocentesis or percutaneous umbilical blood sampling (see below). If the mosaicism is for a lethal genetic defect, the presence of a normal-appearing fetus on ultrasonography and normal results from amniocentesis are reassuring. If the mosaicism is for a potentially viable condition, however, such as Down syndrome or trisomy 13, the patient is referred for both amniocentesis and percutaneous umbilical blood sampling to inspect at least two fetal tissue lines for the presence of the chromosomal abnormality.

Although few CVS-determined mosaics are confirmed in the fetus, some data suggest that even confined placental mosaicism may be associated with a poor perinatal outcome. A 16.7 percent fetal loss rate has been reported for cases identified as confined placental mosaics, compared with a 2.7 percent loss rate in nonmosaics; in addition, a 24 percent fetal loss rate has been noted in cases in which the mosaicism was found only in the cytotrophoblast.[78] In another study, three pregnancy losses were reported in eight cases of confined placental mosaicism in which the fetal karyotype was normal.[79]

Complications of CVS include a risk of fetal loss that exceeds the spontaneous loss rate for the gestational age at which the procedure is performed.[80] The degree of this risk has been assessed in several large multicenter collaborative studies comparing the safety of CVS with that of second-trimester amniocentesis. The first, conducted by the National Institute of Child Health and Development (NICHD), compared 2,278 patients who underwent transcervical CVS with 671 control patients who underwent amniocentesis, all of whom were referred because of advanced maternal age. CVS was found to carry a 0.8 percent greater risk of fetal loss than amniocentesis, with the increased risk coming in the first 16 weeks of pregnancy.[81] A randomized study performed by the Canadian Medical Research Council showed a 0.6 percent increase in fetal loss rate with transcervical CVS compared with amniocentesis, with the increase occurring in the second half of pregnancy.[82] Neither increase was statistically significant. However, a recent Medical Research Council European trial comparing chorionic villus sampling with amniocentesis showed that fetal loss was increased by 2.9 percent in CVS over amniocentesis and that there was a 4.6 percent overall reduction in successful pregnancy outcome after first-trimester CVS versus second-trimester amniocentesis.[83] A comparison of transcervical and transabdominal CVS by the NICHD group showed that the spontaneous miscarriage rate for cytogenetically normal pregnancies up to 28 menstrual weeks was 2.5 percent for transcervical CVS and 2.6 percent for transabdominal CVS.[81] Our recent data at the University of California, San Francisco, indicate that the addition of transabdominal CVS to the prenatal armamentarium has reduced the CVS risk to that of amniocentesis.

Other complications of CVS include the rare risk of severe oligohydramnios without amnion rupture, which may be related to altered chorion permeability after CVS.[79] A recently recognized serious complication is the risk of severe limb abnormalities after very early CVS. This complication was described in a review of 289 pregnancies in which CVS was performed at 56 to 66 days (eight to somewhat less than ten menstrual weeks). Five infants were found to have severe limb abnormalities, four of which were consistent with oromandibular limb hypogenesis syndromes.[84] Other investigators have also found an increase in this very rare condition after CVS that was performed before nine menstrual weeks; the incidence was one in 500 neonates. Still other series, in which the procedure was performed between 10 and 12 weeks' menstrual age, showed no increase in the incidence of such abnormalities.[85] The etiology of these transverse limb-reduction defects is not clear; it is possible that the initiating cause may be a vascular disruption after CVS, leading to alteration in fetal perfusion and subsequent limb hypogenesis. Most centers performing CVS limit the procedure to between 9.5 and 12 weeks.

FETAL BLOOD SAMPLING

Although amniocentesis and chorionic villus sampling provide fetal cells for analysis, in many conditions fetal blood is the optimal or even the only diagnostic tissue. Early attempts to obtain fetal blood involved aspirating blood from the placenta, but this approach frequently resulted in a mixed maternal-fetal specimen.[86] The technique of fetoscopy was subsequently developed, whereby the fetus and placenta could be visualized endoscopically through a percutaneously placed device termed a needlescope.[87] This technique permitted direct observation of the puncture site in a fetal vessel and allowed aspiration of pure fetal blood.[88] Fetoscopy was found to be technically demanding, however, and was limited in its timing to 18 to 20 menstrual weeks, with a three to five percent rate of fetal loss.[89] In 1983, a method was introduced for sampling umbilical blood by ultrasonographically guided aspiration through a percutaneously placed spinal needle.[90] This is the current method of choice because of its relative simplicity and good fetal tolerance.

Percutaneous umbilical blood sampling, also referred to as cordocentesis or funipuncture, can be performed at any gestational age from 18 menstrual weeks to term. The procedure has been carried out earlier in gestation, although it is more technically demanding at that time and is associated with a higher fetal loss rate. Typically, the procedure is performed on an outpatient basis. The mother is prepared and sterilely draped, and a local anesthetic is applied at the needle insertion site. Under sterile ultrasonographic guidance, a 22-gauge 9 cm spinal needle is directed through the abdomen and uterus and into the umbilical vessels. The optimal site for blood aspiration is at the insertion of the cord into the placenta, a site that is relatively immobile. If this preferred site is obscured or hard to reach, blood can be aspirated from the site at which the cord is inserted into the fetus or even from a free loop of cord. (Alternative routes for obtaining blood are percutaneous cardiac puncture and intrahepatic vein aspiration.[91]) Blood is collected in heparinized 3 ml plastic syringes and is verified as fetal by comparision with a previously collected maternal specimen analyzed on a red-cell channelyzer (Coulter Counter). After the procedure, the mother is observed for one or two hours and then sent home; if the sampling is performed later in gestation (from viability to term), it is done in an operating room in the labor and delivery area to facilitate management of possible fetal distress; at these later gestational ages, the patient fasts before the sampling and an anesthesiologist is available.

The greatest risk of percutaneous umbilical blood sampling is that of fetal loss. In a review of 1,320 pregnancies in which fetal blood sampling was carried out, the overall fetal loss rate was 1.6 percent.[92] Other sources have confirmed a fetal loss rate of one to two percent.

At present, the most common indication for percutaneous umbilical blood sampling is to provide rapid karyotyping of a fetus found on ultrasonography to have an anatomic anomaly. The procedure also may be necessary when an amniocentesis culture fails or if there is evidence of mosaicism from an amniocentesis or CVS. Because of the rapid results attained by karyotyping from blood cells (48 to 72 hr), the procedure also has utility for patients who are too late in gestation for amniocentesis but wish to maintain their option for pregnancy termination (typically at 22 to 24 menstrual weeks). Rapid karyotyping also may be helpful in the obstetric management of a fetus in whom multiple malformations are discovered late in gestation and whose delivery is imminent. An additional cytogenetic indication is the ascertainment of fragile X status when amniocentesis or CVS studies have been inconclusive.[91,92]

Umbilical blood sampling is also used to determine the degree of fetal anemia in cases of red-cell alloimmunization, maternal parvovirus B-19 infection, or unexplained hydrops fetalis. In these circumstances, rapid measurement of fetal hemoglobin or hematocrit is obtained, and if indicated, an intravascular transfusion of packed red cells can be done through the sampling needle itself. A similar approach is taken for platelet counts in cases of alloimmune thrombocytopenia.[93]

Fetal blood sampling can be diagnostic for fetal infection in the event of maternal primary infection with toxoplasmosis and, less frequently, rubella and varicella.[94,95] The fetal sample is analyzed for specific fetal IgM and an attempt is made to culture the organism from the blood and amniotic fluid. (Multiple studies may be necessary, particularly when only one of the battery of tests has been positive in an infected individual.[94]) Evidence of fetal infection with toxoplasmosis in early gestation can be treated by the administration of pyrimethamine to the mother.[92]

As it has become possible to diagnose hematologic disorders such as α- and β-thalassemia via DNA analysis of fetal cells, fetal blood assay for hematologic parameters has become less frequent. Yet there are still families with these disorders for whom full genetic characterization either does not exist or does not provide an informative or timely result. Percutaneous umbilical blood sampling for globin-chain synthesis may be the most rapid method of diagnosis in cases of previously undescribed mutations for β-thalassemia. Similar constraints may affect the evaluation of such coagulation disorders such as hemophilia A or B, for which factor VIII, factor IX, and factor VIII antigen are studied if DNA methods are unavailable. In addition, percutaneous umbilical blood sampling may be used to diagnose immunodeficiency syndromes, such as severe combined immunodeficiency syndrome.[91] Through studies of lymphocyte stimulation, other conditions including chronic granulomatous disease[96] and bare-lymphocyte syndrome[97] have been diagnosed by their unique hematologic findings. Recently, Chédiak-Higashi syndrome was diagnosed in an 18-week-old fetus through visualization of the characteristic large lysosomal granules in fetal neutrophils obtained by umbilical blood sampling.

Some investigators have also used fetal blood sampling to determine fetal stress in cases of growth retardation by assessing chronic fetal anoxia and to evaluate fetal metabolism of certain drugs.[92] The utility of such studies is not yet clear.

FETAL TISSUE SAMPLING

For many genetic conditions, DNA analysis is still unavailable, precluding dependence on amniocentesis or CVS for diagnosis. If the condition is expressed in a particular tissue, however, it may be possible to sample that fetal tissue for enzyme analysis, pathological review, or immunofluorescence studies. At present, this methodology has been applied to prenatal biopsy of fetal liver, skin, and muscle.

Certain enzymes of the glycogen storage pathway or urea cycle are found exclusively in liver and duodenum. These include glucose-6-phosphatase, the enzyme whose deficiency leads to von Gierke's disease (glycogen storage disease type Ia), and ornithine transcarbamylase, a vital enzyme for the production of urea, whose deficiency leads to fatal hyperammonemic encephalopathy in male neonates. Glycogen storage disease type Ia is still not fully characterized by DNA analysis, and although the disease is compatible with life, it poses a significant burden of care on parents. Ornithine transcarbamylase deficiency is an X-linked disorder mapped to Xp2.1. Prenatal diagnosis is possible through analysis of restriction fragment length polymorphisms (RFLPs), but DNA studies in parents are informative in only 70 to 80 percent of cases. Because of the severity of the disorder, noninformative parents carrying a male fetus at risk for ornithine transcarbamylase deficiency have been eager to determine the enzyme status of their fetus. For these reasons, percutaneous fetal liver biopsy has been performed in families at risk for these two disorders.[98]

Fetal liver biopsy involves the passage of a Lee soft-tissue biopsy needle through the maternal abdomen and uterus after sterile preparation. With ultrasonographic guidance, the needle is directed into the most accessible lobe of the fetal liver. A core specimen with a weight of 3 to 5 mg is obtained, and the tissue is analyzed for enzymatic function, using an internal control (a different enzyme from the sampled fetus that is not predicted to be deficient) and an external control (from another person) for the specific enyzme in question. The procedure is performed at 18 to 22 weeks, and results are typically available in two to three days. Risks of the procedure include significant hepatic injury or bleeding leading to fetal loss, skin scarring, and the obstetric risks of preterm rupture of membranes or preterm labor; there is also the possibility that inadequate sampling will require rebiopsy. Although the number of cases have been few, for the most part these risks have been only potential ones.[99]

Fetal skin biopsy has been undertaken for the prenatal diagnosis of severe hereditary skin disorders that lack DNA characterization. These disorders include harlequin ichthyosis, an autosomal recessive hyperkeratosis syndrome that frequently leads to early neonatal demise; epidermolysis bullosa lethalis, another autosomal recessive fatal disorder remarkable for intraepidermal blisters produced by minimal trauma; and epidermolytic hyperkeratosis, an autosomal recessive condition of severe bullous lesions that progress to disfiguring ichthyosis.[100]

Originally, the procedure was performed by fetoscopy alone, but skin sampling is now guided by real-time ultrasonography. The procedure is usually done at 19 to 22 menstrual weeks. Again, the patient is sterilely prepared and draped, and mild sedation with intravenous benzodiazepine has been helpful. The fetoscope cannula is inserted through the maternal abdomen and uterus into the amniotic cavity. A flexible biopsy forceps is then threaded through the cannula and directed against the fetal skin surface, preferably at the back or gluteal region. A series of samples are taken, providing a total biopsy mass of 1 to 2 mg. The tissue is then fixed and evaluated pathologically, usually by light and electron microscopy. Because of the immaturity of the fetus, a false negative diagnosis may be reached, reflecting the fact that significant skin pathology may not develop until later in gestation. A false negative finding has occurred once in a reported series of 15 cases.[99] Other risks include the potential for fetal scarring or injury, the possible need for multiple sampling attempts, and obstetric risks of preterm rupture of membranes, preterm labor, or chorioamnionitis.

A recent application of direct fetal biopsy has been for the diagnosis of Duchenne's muscular dystrophy. This is an X-linked disorder in which absence or dysfunction of the protein dystrophin leads to progressive muscle wasting and atrophy in males, with death in the second or third decade [*see Chapter 9*]. The dystrophin gene has been fully cloned,[101] and prenatal diagnosis is typically accomplished by means of a PCR search for specific gene deletions (which occur in approximately 60 percent of cases) or by restriction fragment length polymorphism (RFLP) analysis. Because of the large size of the gene, however, recombination within the gene can occur at a rate of two to four percent. If recombination occurs in a patient without a deletion, or if RFLP analysis is noninformative, the diagnosis of an affected fetus cannot be made via DNA methodology. The absence of dystrophin can, however, be accurately determined through immunofluorescence assay, even in fetal muscle. Direct fetal muscle biopsy has been performed in four cases at 19 to 22 menstrual weeks.[102,103] Continuous ultrasonographic guidance was used to direct a 14-gauge biopsy needle through the sterilely prepared and anesthetized maternal abdomen and uterus into the fetal gluteal region. The sample was analyzed for dystrophin, which was present in three of the four cases and absent in one case (which was confirmed by tissue analysis at the time of pregnancy termination). All three of the unaffected pregnancies were carried to term, and normal male babies were delivered. No significant fetal scarring was found. This method holds promise for future diagnosis of Duchenne's muscular dystrophy as well as other neuromuscular disorders that can be recognized on the basis of pathological findings in fetal tissue.

Preimplantation Embryo Analysis

In addition to prenatal diagnosis involving an already established pregnancy, another option is that of preimplantation diagnosis, in which the cell material of a conceptus is analyzed in vitro before being implanted into the uterus. For couples at risk for genetic disorders, this is done in association with in vitro fertilization in order to evaluate postfertilization embryos and transfer only those embryos that are unaffected with the disease. Such a technique would avoid later termination of a pregnancy in which the fetus was affected and thus reduce maternal physical and psychological trauma. It also would offer reproductive options to a couple at risk for genetic disease who would not consider pregnancy termination.

To provide effective preimplantation analysis, the very early post-fertilization embryo must be sampled. Such sampling has obvious limitations. The biopsy method must not compromise the developmental capacity of the preimplantation embryo; the in vitro and in vivo viability of the embryo must remain unchanged from what it was before biopsy; and the biopsy material must be suitable for diagnosis (i.e., assayed material should reflect embryonic function and activity, not residual maternal responses).

Biopsy techniques have been developed with mouse preimplantation embryos because of their similarity in cell number to the human preimplantation embryo. Embryos are biopsied at the four-cell stage (day 2 after fertilization) or the eight-cell stage (day 3 after fertilization). At these stages, a single blastomere is removed from the embryo with suction and micromanipulation.[104] An alternative technique involves the removal of from five to 10 trophoblast cells by aspiration from day 3 to day 5 postfertilization blastocysts.[106] The removed cells and residual embryos are maintained in cell culture during the analysis.

Although these techniques are still experimental, preimplantation biopsy has been applied to sex analysis by in situ hybridization with Y chromosome probes.[106] Sex was also determined by Y chromosome–specific PCR amplification of DNA in human female embryos biopsied at the eight-cell stage in five families at risk for X-linked disorders. Two female embryos were transferred to each of the five women on the same day as the biopsies. Two of the women were subsequently confirmed as carrying normal female twins.[107]

PCR has also been used to analyze single cells from eight-cell embryos obtained through in vitro fertilization of three couples at risk for cystic fibrosis.[108] In all three cases, the embryos were successfully analyzed, but in only two cases could unaffected embryos be transferred. One pregnancy resulted, and a healthy female infant unaffected by cystic fibrosis was born. It is hoped that this technology can be applied to the identification of many genetic disorders in the preimplantation embryo, and it is an exciting area of research at this time.

Embryoscopy

A prenatal diagnostic technique that straddles the categories of observational and invasive is the newly developed procedure of embryoscopy of the first-trimester fetus.[109] A narrow fiberoptic endoscope is inserted through the maternal abdomen or the uterine cervix (under ultrasonographic guidance) into the chorionic cavity—an embryonic space between the amniotic sac and the uterine decidual wall that is later obliterated as the amniotic sac enlarges (beyond 12 menstrual weeks). Fetuses as early as five menstrual weeks can be directly observed with this method, and access can be obtained to their umbilical circulation.[110] Congenital anomalies of the face, the abdomen, and the digits have been observed, with resolution far beyond that achievable with ultrasonography. Because this technique was developed only recently, relatively few ongoing pregnancies have been described, and the associated risks have not been established. The technique does, however, have great potential for very early identification of fetal anomalies as well as elucidation of the process of embryonic development.

Prenatal Diagnosis by DNA Analysis: Four Examples

So far, this chapter has been devoted to the indications, methodology, and applications of various procedures of prenatal diagnosis. This section addresses the specific methods of DNA analysis by means of which four distinct genetic disorders—phenylketonuria, sickle cell anemia, cystic fibrosis, and Huntington's disease—have fairly recently been characterized. The analytic principles underlying these diagnoses are typical of standard molecular methods and thus provide illustrative examples of the approach to DNA analysis in prenatal diagnosis.

Phenylketonuria

Phenylketonuria is an autosomal recessive condition resulting from defective metabolism of the enzyme phenylalanine hydroxylase [*see Chapter 9*]. If dietary phenylalanine restriction is not initiated very early in life, there is significant cognitive and neuropsychological delay leading to severe mental retardation. If adequate dietary control is achieved, however, patients may retain good function and achieve near-normal productivity.[111] Phenylketonuria is one of the diseases tested in neonatal screening, which makes early diagnosis and treatment possible.

Although dietary therapy seems to provide simple medical management of this disorder, full compliance may be difficult to achieve. In extensive phenylketonuria screening programs, wide variations in clinical phenotype and disease severity have been recognized. Benign hyperphenylalaninemia is characterized by a persistent elevation in plasma phenylalanine that is well tolerated without treatment and does not lead to cognitive loss.[112] Clinical phenylketonuria, with its potential for severe retardation, is at the opposite end of the clinical spectrum. The recurrence risk for families that have had one child affected with phenylketonuria is 25 percent, which often prompts a desire for prenatal diagnosis in subsequent pregnancies.

The gene for phenylalanine hydroxylase was mapped to 12q22–24.2 in 1984,[113] and the DNA nucleotide sequence was cloned in 1985.[114] With this cDNA as a probe, eight RFLPs in the phenylalanine hydroxylase gene were identified, and their genotype has defined a distinctive RFLP haplotype. (The haplotype is the appearance of the RFLP patttern on each chromosome. Since each chromosome is of either maternal or paternal origin, this corresponds to identifying the origin of each chromosome.[115]) By comparing the RFLP haplotypes of the known mutant phenylalanine hydroxylase genes in a child who has phenylketonuria with those of the parents, a mutant and a normal haplotype could be distinguished in each parent. Forty-three specific haplotypes have been detected, as defined by differences in eight RFLP patterns.[116] Four prevalent haplotypes were noted in the European population (haplotypes 1, 2, 3, and 4), with the classical phenylketonuria phenotype found in haplotype combinations of 2 and 3. Haplotypes 1 and 4 were associated with a milder clinical presentation.[115]

Haplotype analysis has been used extensively for prenatal diagnosis. Initially, RFLP haplotypes are ascertained for the parents seeking diagnosis and for their affected child. Total genomic DNA derived from peripheral-blood nucleated white cells is cleaved with seven restriction endonucleases, and the haplotype pattern is found through Southern blot analysis.

DNA is then isolated from fetal cells (obtained by means of either amniocentesis or CVS) and is cleaved with whichever endonucleases provided informative fragments in the parental analysis. Comparison of the fetal Southern blot banding patterns with those of the parents and an affected sibling distinguishes between an affected and an unaffected fetus.[117]

Such prenatal diagnosis can be applied effectively to approximately 90 percent of Caucasian families with previously affected children; the reliability of haplotype analysis may be lower in other populations that are more heterogeneous for these RFLP sites.[118] Because RFLP patterns simply reflect the presence or absence of an endonuclease cleavage site, they typically do not represent the actual mutated area of DNA in a gene. More than 18 distinct mutations in the phenylalanine hydroxylase gene have now been identified. Particular mutations appear to occur only in particular haplotypes; two of these—the splice 12 mutation, which leads to the deletion of exon 12, and the 408 mutation, which causes an amino acid change from arginine to tryptophan—lead to the production of an unstable protein and are found in haplotypes 2 and 3 alone.[118] Classical phenylketonuria may result from homozygosity (the presence of two copies of the same mutation) or compound heterozygosity (the presence of two different mutations) for these specific mutations, whereas benign hyperphenylalaninemia may arise from compound heterozygosity for less serious mutations.[112]

Direct mutation analysis for phenylketonuria is now also possible. Oligonucleotide primers for 13 exon-containing regions of the phenylalanine hydroxylase gene are used, the regions are individually amplified through PCR, and the DNA is sequenced.[119] Such mutation analysis can be accomplished with fetal cells for prenatal diagnosis, provided that antecedent studies of parents and the affected child have been performed. This method is specific and is replacing haplotype analysis for prenatal diagnosis of phenylketonuria.

Sickle Cell Anemia

Sickle cell anemia is an autosomal recessive hemoglobinopathy of variable severity. It is associated with a single-base change (adenine to thymine) in the β-globin gene, which is mapped to chromosome 11 at 11p15.5. This change results in the substitution of the amino acid valine (encoded by GTG) for the intended amino acid glutamic acid (encoded by GAG) at position 6 in the β-globin molecule, thus altering its surface charge. Under conditions of reduced oxygen tension, the abnormal globin molecule forms rodlike polymers, which become aligned and thus confer a distinct sickle shape on erythrocytes. A patient with sickle cell anemia experiences hemolytic anemia, early splenomegaly and later splenic infarction, chronic infection, and vaso-occlusive "pain" crises affecting bones, joints, and periosteum. The frequency of carrier status (heterozygosity for the mutation) in African Americans is approximately 1 in 12, or eight percent.[120]

Testing for sickle cell heterozygotes (i.e., persons with the sickle trait) can be accomplished with a simple chemical test of peripheral blood. Couples in which both members carry the sickle trait are at a 25 percent risk of having a child who is homozygous for the mutation and develops severe sickle cell anemia. The fact that parents with the sickle trait may know their carrier status before conception represents a somewhat uncommon circumstance in genetics. Some couples may wish to have prenatal diagnosis because of their concern about having an infant with severe sickle cell disease.

The β-globin gene has been extensively mapped and sequenced on the basis of RFLPs.[121] The mutation of sickle cell anemia can be detected by several restriction endonucleases, including *Mst*II [*see Figure 3*], *Dde*I, *Mnl*I, and *Cvn*I. *Mst*II has been especially effective in diagnosis of sickle cell disease because it recognizes the sequence CCTNAGG (N designates any nucleotide), which is present in codons 5, 6, and 7 of the normal β-globin gene but is altered by the sickle mutation (A to T) at codon 6.[122] This gives rise to the fortuitous circumstance in which an RFLP pattern is associated with a specific mutation and thus provides a rapid option for prenatal diagnosis.

Blood samples from parents at risk for having fetuses with sickle cell disease are obtained at the time of prenatal testing by CVS or amniocentesis. DNA is obtained by extraction from parents' peripheral blood cells and from lysis of fetal cells (without extraction). It is amplified by PCR with primers that flank the sickle mutation site. The amplified DNA is then digested with *Mst*II (or the equivalent endonuclease *Dde*I), and the resultant fragments are electrophoretically separated on an agarose gel, stained with ethidium bromide, and examined for the distinctive band patterns found with normal β-globin and with sickle globin. The results of this process are highly accurate and can be obtained in 48 hours.

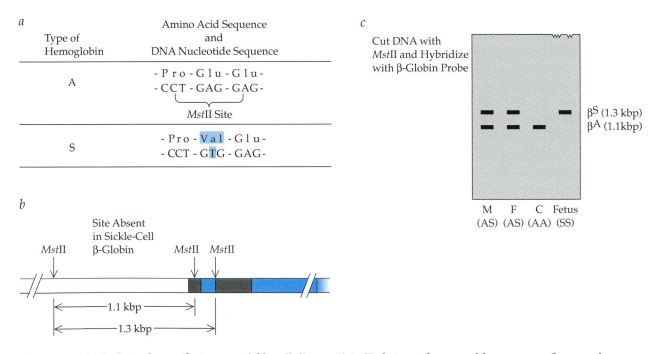

Figure 3 (a) The base change that causes sickle cell disease (A to T) destroys the recognition sequence for several restriction enzymes, including MstII. (b) MstII cuts the normal globin gene and yields two fragments of different sizes (1.1 kbp and 0.2 kbp), which can be detected with a probe from the 5' end of the β-globin gene. (c) Prenatal diagnosis of sickle cell disease using the MstII polymorphism. The mother (M) and father (F) are carriers because they have 1.3 kbp and 1.1 kbp fragments. Their unaffected child (C) is homozygous for the normal 1.1 kbp fragment. The fetus (Fe) has inherited a β^S allele from each parent and will be affected by sickle cell disease.

Cystic Fibrosis

Cystic fibrosis is an autosomal recessive disorder of the epithelium of all exocrine glands [*see Chapter 9*]. It is characterized by the production of dense, viscous glandular secretions whose altered viscosity predisposes patients to severe lower respiratory tract infections as well as to pancreatic and liver impairment. Children become affected in early infancy. Treatment is inadequate for this condition, and the prognosis is usually poor, varying with the severity of the pulmonary involvement. Death often occurs in the second or third decade of life.[123] Experimental gene therapy trials have been mounted.

This condition is the most common inherited disease in the Caucasian population. Disease frequency has been estimated at one in 2,500 births, but this value may be too low. The results of neonatal screening suggest an incidence of one in 1,800,[124] placing the carrier frequency in the Caucasian population at appproximately one in 20 to one in 25.

Initial attempts at prenatal diagnosis for cystic fibrosis depended on ultrasonographic identification of meconum ileus, a characteristic finding in 10 percent of affected newborns that results from intestinal obstruction caused by inspissated meconium.[125] This abnormality is not specific for cystic fibrosis but is highly suggestive in a fetus suspected of having the disorder. Measurement of microvillar enyzmes at the time of second-trimester amniocentesis was also utilized for diagnosis, with low levels found to be predictive of cystic fibrosis. This method is more reliable in couples at risk for cystic fibrosis than in others, but it has a false positive rate of one to four percent and a false negative rate of six to eight percent.[125]

Attempts to improve the reliability of diagnosis were aided by the discovery of specific DNA markers close to the putative cystic fibrosis site. By using these markers as probes and using five different endonucleases to cleave the DNA, investigators were able to derive distinctive RFLP haplotypes for families at risk for cystic fibrosis.[126] Prenatal diagnosis then could be accomplished via RFLP analysis of the parents and a known affected child, followed by fetal sampling by CVS or amniocentesis.

In 1989, the cystic fibrosis gene was identified at chromosome 7q3.1,[127] and the cDNA was cloned. The structure of the protein involved in the disorder was predicted to be membrane spanning, with sites capable of binding ATP. A deletion of three base pairs, resulting in the omission of a phenylalanine residue, was the first specific cystic fibrosis mutation described; it was designated delta 508.[128] This mutation turns out to account for 70 percent of the cystic fibrosis mutations in the Caucasian population in the United States;[129] it and the additional mutations G551D, G542X, R553X, and N1303K account for some 85 percent of the known cystic fibrosis alleles in the United States.

Identification of distinct mutations has made possible prenatal diagnosis by means of a direct mutation analysis [*see Figure 4*] similar to that used to diagnose phenylketonuria. An exciting new method of diagnosis is provided by color PCR and reverse dot-blot hybridization.[130]

Direct mutational study holds promise for the future prenatal diagnosis of cystic fibrosis, although RFLP haplotype analysis may continue to be needed in the case of previously undefined family-specific mutations.

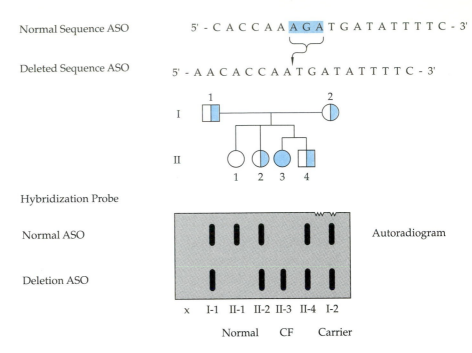

Figure 4 *Illustrated is diagnosis of cystic fibrosis by means of PCR, with allele-specific oligonucleotides (ASOs) used as probes. DNA spanning the region of the 3 bp sequence deleted in many cystic fibrosis patients was amplified with PCR. The fragments were not separated by electrophoresis; a vacuum device was used to apply the DNA in narrow bands to a nitrocellulose filter. A sample from each patient was tested with two ASOs to determine whether the normal sequence, the deleted sequence, or both had been amplified. One ASO was complementary to the normal sequence; the other lacked the AGA nucleotides complementary to the deleted 3 bp sequence. The amplified sequence from the patient (II-3) hybridized only to the deletion ASO. Her parents (I-1 and I-2) must be heterozygotes; indeed, both ASOs annealed to their DNA. Two of the patient's siblings (II-2 and II-4) are also heterozygotes; the third (II-1) inherited a normal allele from each parent, so her DNA anneals only to the normal ASO. (The first lane, x, was a PCR with no DNA to check for contamination of the PCR reagents.)*

Huntington's Disease

Huntington's disease is an autosomal dominant disorder of the basal ganglia of the brain that is characterized by premature neuronal cell death and a decline in neurotransmitters. Fortunately, it is rare, with a disease prevalence of 50 to 60 cases per million in English-speaking countries. Patients typically are in good health until between 30 and 40 years of age, when they develop behavioral changes, dementia, and choreiform movements. Mental deterioration progresses, with marked loss of function. Life expectancy is reduced, and patients typically die of cardiovascular disease and pneumonia, completely unable to care for themselves and wasted by unceasing choreiform activity. Treatment for the disorder is minimally effective, and the pathophysiology of the cerebral changes is not known.[131]

For the initial case in a family, prenatal diagnosis would not be considered at all, because there would be no indication of risk. Given the late onset of Huntington's disease, patients may well have completed childbearing before the disorder manifests itself. Yet the children born to an affected parent have a 50 percent chance of developing Huntington's disease and, if affected, a 50 percent chance of passing the disease on to their children. (If the father is the carrier, the onset of the condition may be earlier and may be marked by rigidity or a parkinsonian appearance.[131])

Appropriate genetic counseling with regard to Huntington's disease is critical. For example, consider the case of a 30-year-old woman whose father died of Huntington's disease. She has a 50 percent chance of being affected, but if she is symptom-free at the age of 30, she may see no need to consider prenatal diagnosis at the time of childbearing. Her partner, however, may weigh the need differently, considering that he would assume the burden of care if she and an affected child should acquire the disease. The woman also might be unwilling to undergo prenatal diagnosis because the identification of an affected child would a priori identify her as being affected. These and other psychological and ethical issues are complex, and approaches to their management at the time of prenatal diagnosis must be clearly discussed.

Prenatal diagnosis can be accomplished in three ways. First, exclusion testing is resorted to when the disease status of the parent at risk is not determined; the fetus is examined at the molecular level to ascertain whether it has inherited a chromosome (not necessarily the mutated one) from the affected grandparent. Second, definitive testing involves analysis of the parents and the fetus to determine their specific disease status. Finally, stepwise testing initially involves exclusion testing; if this is found to place the fetus in a high-risk category (i.e., it has inherited a chromosome from the affected grandparent), definitive testing of the parent at risk is done to prevent the termination of an unaffected fetus. The choice of approach is individual and requires extensive counseling.[132]

The gene for Huntington's disease was first mapped to chromosome 4 distal to 4p16.3[133]; more recently, it has been cloned. However, certain DNA markers are tightly linked to the disorder, implying close proximity to the gene. These markers can serve as probes of DNA that has been digested with multiple restriction endonucleases. As with phenylketonuria, the distinct pattern of RFLP fragments is termed the haplotype and allows one to characterize the fetus in comparison to its parents. Because these markers are not for the Huntington's disease gene itself, the reliability of such studies is affected by the possibility of recombination between the marker site and the true Huntington's disease gene.[134]

For prenatal testing, preliminary studies of parents and grandparents are accomplished by means of Southern blot analysis of DNA extracted from peripheral blood cells. The digested DNA is probed with disease-linked markers.[134] The use of a large number of endonuclease and probe combinations greatly increases the possibility of informative studies. DNA extracted from chorionic villus tissue or amniocytes is then analyzed in a similar manner, and the haplotype patterns of the fetus and the parents are compared. This process is lengthy, and several weeks of effort may be required before results are available.

The gene for Huntington's disease was very recently identified and found to contain an expandable trinucleotide repeat site.[135] This places the disorder in a category similar to that of fragile X mental retardation,[136] myotonic dystrophy,[137] and spinal-bulbar muscular atrophy,[138] all of which display an expanded number of nucleotide repeats in affected persons. In those unaffected by Huntington's disease, the number of trinucleotide repeats ranges from 11 to 33. In affected persons (or in presymptomatic persons who will eventually be affected), this number rises to between 42 and 66 copies or more. Just how this expansion leads to the expression of Huntington's disease is still being investigated. To date, no prenatal diagnoses of Huntington's disease based on the trinucleotide repeat number have been reported, but PCR has been used with primers flanking the trinucleotide repeat site to identify affected persons.[135] Further studies in this area may speed the DNA analysis of this disorder, but unfortunately, they are not likely to solve the complexities of prenatal counseling for this debilitating condition.

References

1. Thompson MW, McInnes RR, Willard HF: *Genetics in Medicine*, 5th ed. WB Saunders Co, Philadelphia, 1991, p 411

2. Hook EB, Cross PK, Jackson L, et al: Maternal age-specific rates of 47 +21 and other cytogenetic abnormalities diagnosed in the first trimester of pregnancy in chorionic villus biopsy specimens: comparisons with rates expected from observations at amniocentesis. *Am J Hum Genet* 42:797, 1988

3. Hook EB: Rates of chromosome abnormalities at different maternal ages. *Obstet Gynecol* 58:282, 1981

4. Hook E, Cross PK: Rates of mutant and inherited structural cytogenetic abnormalities detected at amniocentesis: results on about 63,000 fetuses. *Ann Hum Genet* 51:27, 1987

5. Karp LE: Older fathers and genetic mutation. *Am J Genet* 7:405, 1980

6. Riccardi VM, Dobson CE 2d, Charkraborty R, et al: The pathophysiology of neurofibromatosis: IX: paternal age as a factor in the origin of new mutations. *Am J Med Genet* 18:169, 1984

7. Gardner RJM, Sutherland GR: *Chromosome Abnormalities and Genetic Counseling*. Oxford University Press, New York, 1989, p 43

8. Grabowski GA, Desnick RJ: Antenatal metabolic diagnosis: a compendium. *Human Prenatal Diagnosis*, 2nd ed. Filkins K, Russo JF, Eds. Marcel Dekker, Inc, New York, 1990, p 109

9. Briggs GG, Freeman RK, Yaffe SJ: *Drugs in Pregnancy and Lactation*. Williams and Wilkins, Baltimore, 1990, p 638

10. Jones KL: *Smith's Recognizable Patterns of Human Malformation*, 4th ed. WB Saunders Co, Philadelphia, 1988, p 495

11. Nyberg DA, Mahony BS, Pretorius DH: *Diagnostic Ultrasound of Fetal Anomalies: Text and Atlas*. Mosby Year Book, St. Louis, 1990, p 27

12. Humphrey LO, Magoon M, O'Shaughnessy R: Severe non-immune hydrops secondary to parvo virus B-19 infection: spontaneous reversal in utero and survival of a term infant. *Obstet Gynecol* 78:900, 1991

13. Haddow JE: Alpha-fetoprotein. *The Unborn Patient*, 2nd ed. Harrison MR, Golbus MS, Filly RA, Eds. WB Saunders Co, 1991, p 65

14. Leek AE, Ruoss CF, Katau Mi, et al: Raised alpha-fetoprotein in maternal serum with anencephalic pregnancy. *Lancet* 2:385, 1973

15. American College of Obstetricians and Gynecologists Technical Bulletin. Alpha-Fetoprotein. 154, April 1991

16. Nadel AS, Green JK, Holmes LB, et al: Absence of need for amniocentesis in patients with elevated levels of maternal serum alpha-fetoprotein and normal ultrasonographic examinations. *N Engl J Med* 323:557, 1990

17. Romero R, Pilu G, Jeanty P: *Prenatal Diagnosis of Congenital Anomalies*. Appleton & Lange, Norwalk, Connecticut, 1988, p 37

18. Robinson L, Grau P, Crandall BF: Pregnancy outcomes after increasing maternal serum alpha-fetoprotein levels. *Obstet Gynecol* 74:17, 1989

19. Haddow JE: Prenatal screening for open neural tube defects, Down's syndrome and other major fetal disorders. *Semin Perinatol* 14:488, 1990

20. Bogart MH, Pandian MR, Jones OW: Abnormal maternal serum chorionic gonadotropin levels in pregnancies with fetal chromosome abnormalities. *Prenat Diagn* 7:623, 1987

21. Canick JA, Knight GJ, Palomaki GE, et al: Low second trimester maternal serum unconjugated oestriol in pregnancies with Down's syndrome. *Br J Obstet Gynaecol* 95:330, 1988

22. Wald NJ, Cuckle HS, Densen JW, et al: Maternal serum screening for Down's syndrome in early pregnancy. *BMJ* 297:883, 1988

23. Andrew LB: Newborn screening for sickle cell disease and other hemoglobinopathies: overview of legal issues. *Pediatrics* 83:886, 1989

24. Chown B: Anemia from bleeding of the fetus into the mother's circulation. *Lancet* 1:1213, 1954

25. Kleihauer E, Braun H, Betke K: Demonstration von fetalem Hemaoglobin in den Erythrocyten eines Blutausstrichs. *Klin Wochenschr* 35:637, 1957

26. Walknowska J, Conte FA, Grumbach MM: Practical and theoretical implications of fetal-maternal lymphocyte transfer. *Lancet* 1:1119, 1969

27. Yeoh SC, Sargent IL, Redman CWL, et al: Detection of fetal cells in maternal blood. *Prenat Diagn* 11:117, 1991

28. Mueller UW, Haves CS, Wright AE, et al: Isolation of fetal trophoblast cells from peripheral blood of pregnant women. *Lancet* 336:197, 1990

29. Bianchi DW, Flint AF, Pizzimenti MF, et al: Isolation of fetal DNA from nucleated erythroctyes in maternal blood. *Proc Natl Acad Sci USA* 87:3279, 1990

30. Bianchi DW, Harris P, Flint A, et al: Direct hybridization to DNA from small numbers of flow-sorted nucleated newborn cells. *Cytometry* 8:197, 1987

31. Lea T, Vartdal F, Nustad K, et al: Monosized magnetic polymer particles: their use in separation of cells and subcellular components, and the study of lymphocyte function in vitro. *J Mol Recognit* 1:9, 1988

32. Golbus MS: Prenatal diagnosis using fetal cells in the maternal circulation (abstr). *Am J Hum Genet* 49(suppl):24, 1991

33. Lebo RV, Flandemeyer RR, Diukman R, et al: Prenatal diagnosis with repetitive insitu hybridization probes. *Am J Med Genet* 43:848, 1992

34. Wachtel S, Wachtel G, Phillips O, et al: Fetal cells in the maternal circulation: isolation by multiparameter flow cytometry and confirmation by polymerase chain reaction. *Hum Reprod* 6:1466, 1991

35. Thompson HE: Diagnostic ultrasound in gynecology. *Gynecology and Obstetrics*, Vol 1. Droegemuller W, Sciarra JJ, Eds. Harper and Row, Philadelphia

36. Howry DH, Bliss WR: Ultrasonic visualization of soft tissue structures of the body. *J Lab Clin Med* 40:579, 1952

37. Donald I, MacVicar J, Brown TG: Investigation of abdominal masses by pulsed ultrasound. *Lancet* 1:1188, 1958

38. Thompson HE: Studies of fetal growth in utero by ultrasound. *Diagnostic Proceedings of the First International Conference*. Grossman CC, Holmes JH, Joycer C, et al, Eds. University of Pittsburgh, Plenum Press, New York, 1965, p 416

39. Hohler CW: Ultrasound bioeffects for the perinatologist. *Gynecology and Obstetrics*, Vol 3. Depp R, Eschenbach DA, Sciarra JJ, Eds. Harper and Row, Philadelphia, 1984

40. American Institute of Ultrasound in Medicine: Safety statements. *J Ultrasound Med* 2:519, 1983

41. Vats S, Filkins K, Elejalde BR: First trimester ultrasound evaluation. *Human Prenatal Diagnosis*, 2nd ed. Filkins K, Russo JF, Eds. Marcel Dekker, Inc, New York, 1990, p 63

42. Monteagudo A, Reuss ML, Timor-Tritsch E: Imaging the fetal brain in the second and third trimesters using transvaginal sonography. *Obstet Gynecol* 77:27, 1992

43. Farine D, Fox HE, Jakobsen S, et al: Vaginal ultrasound for diagnosis of placenta previa. *Am J Obstet Gynecol* 159:566, 1988

44. Campbell S, Pearce JM, Hackett G, et al: Qualitative assessment of uteroplacental blood flow: early screening test for high risk pregnancies. *Obstet Gynecol* 68:649, 1986

45. Beattie RB, Doran JC: Antenatal screening for intrauterine growth retardation with umbilical artery Doppler ultrasonography. *BMJ* 289:631, 1989

46. Nyberg DA, Mahony BS, Pretorius DH: *Diagnostic Ultrasound of Fetal Anomalies: Text and Atlas*. Mosby Year Book, St. Louis, 1990, p 1

47. Wade RV, Smythe AR, Walt GW, et al: Reliability of gynecologic sonographic diagnoses, 1978-1984. *Am J Obstet Gynecol* 153:186, 1985

48. The Use of Diagostic Ultrasound Imaging in Pregnancy: US Department of Health and Human Services, Public Health Service, National Institutes of Health, NIH publication no. 84-667, 1984

49. Callen PW: *Ultrasonography in Obstetrics and Gynecology*, 2nd ed. WB Saunders Co, Philadelphia, 1988, p 9

50. Achiron R, Barkai G, Katznelson M, et al: Fetal lateral ventricle choroid plexus cyst: the dilemma of amniocentesis. *Obstet Gynecol* 78:815, 1991

51. Bernstein HS, Filly RA, Goldberg JD, et al: Prognosis of fetuses with a cystic hygroma. *Prenat Diagn* 11:349, 1991

52. Bennett MJ, Wass DM: Ultrasonography for detection of fetal disorders in the second trimester of pregnancy. *Human Prenatal Diagnosis*. Filkins K, Russo JR, Eds. Marcel Dekker, Inc, New York, 1990, p 375

53. Filkins K, Hadlock FP: Ultrasonography for detection of fetal disorders in the third trimester of pregnancy. *Human Prenatal Diagnosis*, Filkins K, Russo JR, Eds. 2nd ed. Marcel Dekker, Inc, New York, 1990, p 425

54. Silverman NH, Schmidt KG: Fetus with a cardiac malformation. *The Unborn Patient*, 2nd ed. Harrison MR, Golbus MS, Filly RA, Eds. WB Saunders Co, Philadelphia, 1990, p 264

55. Schmidt KG, Silverman NH: Evaluation of the fetal heart by ultrasound. *Ultrasonography in Obstetrics and Gynecology*, 2nd ed. Callen PW, Ed. WB Saunders Co, New York, 1990, p 165

56. Friedman DM: Fetal echocardiography and Doppler flow studies. *Human Prenatal Diagnosis*, 2nd ed. Filkins K, Russo JR, Eds. Marcel Dekker, Inc, New York, 1990, p 407

57. Bevis DCA: The antenatal prediction of hemolytic disease of the newborn. *Lancet* 1:395, 1952

58. Steele MW, Breg WR Jr: Chromosome analysis of human amniotic fluid cells. *Lancet* 1:383, 1966

59. Jeanty P, Rodesch F, Romero R, et al: How to improve your amniocentesis technique. *Am J Obstet Gynecol* 146:593, 1983

60. Rosler A, Wesler N, Leiberman E, et al: 11 Beta hydroxylase deficiency congenital adrenal hyperplasia: update of prenatal diagnosis. *J Clin Endocrinol Metab* 66:830, 1988

61. Diagnosis of Genetic Disease by Amniocentesis During the Second Trimester of Pregnancy. Medical Research Council, report no. 5, 1977

62. Low CU, Alexander D, Bryla D, et al: *The NICHD amniocentesis registry*. The safety and accuracy of midtrimester amniocentesis. US Dept. of Health, Education and Welfare: DHEW Publication (NIH) 1978, p 78

63. An assessment of the hazards of amniocentesis: report to the Medical Research Council by their Working Party on Amniocentesis. *Br J Obstet Gynecol* 85:1, 1978

64. Tabor A, Madsen M, Obel EB, et al: Randomized controlled trial of genetic amniocentesis in 4606 low risk women. *Lancet* 1:1287, 1986

65. Crandall B, Howard J, Lebher TB, et al: Follow-up of 2000 second trimester amniocenteses. *Obstet Gynecol* 56:625, 1980

66. Elder JS, Duckett JW: Management of the fetus and neonate with hydronephrosis detected by prenatal ultrasonography. *Pediatr Ann* 17:19, 1988

67. Knight AB, Gold WR, Pohodich AJ, et al: Implications for counseling based on comparison of incidence of complications in undergoing early vs. mid-trimester amniocentesis. *Am J Hum Genet* (suppl 49):228, 1991

68. Nevin J, Nevin NC, Dorman JC, et al: Early amniocentesis: clinical and cytogenetic evaluation of 500 cases. *Am J Hum Genet* 49(suppl):226, 1991

69. Sato M, Witl D: Early amniocentesis: prospective follow up of 604 cases. *Am J Hum Genet* 49(suppl):230, 1991

70. Shulman LP, Elias S, Simpson JL, et al: Early amniocentesis: complications in initial 150 cases compared to complication in initial 150 cases of transabdominal chorionic villus sampling. *Am J Hum Genet* 49(suppl):231, 1991

71. Eljalde BR, de Eljalde M: Prospective study of early amniocentesis and comparison with chorionic villus sampling. *Am J Hum Genet* 49(suppl):12, 1991

72. Burton BK, Nelson LH, Pettenati MJ: False positive acetylcholinesterase with early amniocentesis. *Obstet Gynecol* 74:607, 1989

73. Fetal sex prediction by sex chromatin of chorionic villi cells during early pregnancy. *Chin Med J* 1:117, 1975

74. Kazy Z, Rozovosky IS, Bakharev VA: Chorion biopsy in early pregnancy: a method of early prenatal diagnosis for inherited disorders. *Prenat Diagn* 2:39, 1992

75. Jackson LG: *CVS Newsletter No. 30*, May 1990

76. Jackson LG, Wapner RJ, Grebner EE, et al: Fetal genetic diagnosis by chorionic villus sampling. *Human Prenatal Diagnosis*. Filkins K, Russo JR, Eds. Marcel Dekker, Inc, New York, 1990, p 37

77. Silver RK, MacGregor SN, Waldec JK: Percutaneous transvesical chorionic villus sampling: an alternative approach to the retroverted uterus. *Obstet Gynecol* 7:798, 1991

78. Johnson A, Wapner RJ, Davis GH, et al: Mosaicism in chorionic villus sampling: an association with poor perinatal outcome. *Obstet Gynecol* 75:573, 1990

79. Hogge WA, Schonberg SA, Golbus MS: Chorionic villus sampling: experience of the first 1000 cases. *Am J Obstet Gynecol* 154:1249, 1986

80. Rhoads GG, Jackson LG, Schlesselman SE, et al: The safety and efficacy of chorionic villus sampling for early prenatal diagnosis of cytogenetic abnormalities. *N Engl J Med* 320:609, 1989

81. Transcervical and transabdominal chorionic villus sampling are comparably safe procedures for first trimester prenatal diagnosis: preliminary analysis. USNICHD Collaborative CVS Study Group. *Am J Hum Genet* 47(suppl):A278, 1990

82. Multicentre randomized clinical trial of chorion villus sampling and amniocentesis. Canadian Collaborative CVS-Amniocentesis Clinical Trial Group. *Lancet* 1:1, 1989

83. MCR working party on the Evaluation of Chorion Villus Sampling (1991): Medical Research Council European Trial of chorion villus sampling. *Lancet* 1:1491, 1991

84. Firth HV, Boyd PA, Chamberlain P, et al: Severe limb abnormalities after chorion villus sampling at 56-66 days' gestation. *Lancet* 337:762, 1991

85. Firth HV, Boyd PA, Chamberlain P, et al: Limb abnormalities and chorion villus sampling. *Lancet* 338:51, 1991

86. Kan YW, Valenti C, Carnazza V, et al: Fetal blood sampling in utero. *Lancet* 1:79, 1974

87. Hobbins JC, Mahoney MJ: In utero diagnosis of hemoglobinopathies: technique for obtaining fetal blood. *N Engl J Med* 290:1065, 1974

88. Rodeck CH, Campbell S: Umbilical cord insertion as a source of pure fetal blood for prenatal diagnosis. *Lancet* 1:1244, 1979

89. The status of fetoscopy and fetal tissue sampling: the results of the first meeting of the International Fetoscopy Group. *Prenat Diagn* 4:79, 1984

90. Daffos F, Capella-Pavlovsky M, Forestier E: A new procedure for fetal blood sampling in utero: preliminary results of fifty-three cases. *Am J Obstet Gynecol* 146:985, 1983

91. Goldberg JD, Antasaklis AJ: Fetal blood sampling. *Human Prenatal Diagnosis*. Filkins K, Russo JR, Eds. Marcel Dekker, Inc, New York, 1990, p 389

92. Daffos F: Fetal blood sampling. *The Unborn Patient*, 2nd ed. Harrison MR, Golbus MS, Filly RA, Eds. WB Saunders Co, Philadelphia, 1990, p 75

93. Bussel JB, Berkowitz RL, McFarland JG, et al: Antenatal treatment of neonatal alloimmune thrombocytopenia. *N Engl J Med* 319:1374, 1988

94. Desmonts G, Daffos F, Forestier F, et al: Prenatal diagnosis of congenital toxoplasmosis. *Lancet* 1:500, 1985

95. Daffos F, Forestier F, Grangeot-Keros L, et al: Prenatal diagnosis of congenital rubella. *Lancet* 2:1, 1984

96. Newburger PE, Cohen HJ, Rothchild SB, et al: Prenatal diagnosis of chronic granulomatous disease. *N Engl J Med* 300:178, 1979

97. Durandy A, Dumez Y, Griscelli C: Prenatal diagnosis of severe inherited immunodeficiencies: a five year experience. *Progress in Immunodeficiency. Research and Therapy 11*. Elsevier, Amsterdam, 1986

98. Golbus MS, Simpson TJ, Koresawa M, et al: The prenatal determination of glucose-6-phosphatase activity by fetal liver biopsy. *Prenat Diagn* 8:401, 1988

99. Golbus MSG, McGonigle KF, Goldberg JD, et al: Fetal tissue sampling: the San Francisco experience with 190 pregnancies. *West J Med* 150:423, 1989

100. Elias S, Esterly NB: Prenatal diagnosis of hereditary skin disorders. *Clin Obstet Gynecol* 24:1069, 1981

101. Keening M, Hoffman EP, Bertclson CJ, et al: Complete cloning of the Duchenne muscular dystrophy (DMD) CDNA and preliminary genomic organization of the DMD gene in normal and affected individuals. *Cell* 50:509, 1987

102. Evans MI, Greb A, Kunkel LM, et al: In utero fetal muscle biopsy for the diagnosis of Duchenne muscular dystrophy. *Am J Obstet Gynecol* 165:728, 1991

103. Kuller JA, Hoffman EF, Fries MH, et al: Prenatal diagnosis of Duchenne muscular dystrophy by fetal muscle biopsy. *Hum Genet* 90:34, 1992

104. Wilton LJ, Trounson AO: Biopsy of preimplantation mouse embryos: development of micromanipulated embryos and proliferation of single blastomeres in vitro. *Biol Reprod* 40:145, 1989

105. Monk M, Muggleton-Harris AL, Rawlings E, et al: Preimplantation diagnosis of HPRT-deficient male and carrier female embryos by trophoectoderm biopsy. *Hum Reprod* 3:377, 1988

106. West JD, Grosden JR, Angell RR, et al: Sexing whole human preembryos by in-situ hybridization with a Y chromosome specific DNA probe. *Hum Reprod* 3:1010, 1988

107. Handyside AH, Kontogianni EH, Hardy K, et al: Pregnancies from biopsied human preimplantation embryos sexed by Y-specific DNA amplification. *Nature* 344:768, 1990

108. Handyside AH, Lesko JG, Tarín JJ, et al: Birth of a normal girl after in vitro fertilization and preimplantation diagnostic testing for cystic fibrosis. *N Engl J Med* 327:905, 1992

109. Cullen MT, Reece EA, Whetham J, et al: Embryoscopy: description and utility of a new technique. *Am J Obstet Gynecol* 162:82, 1990

110. Reece EA, Rotmensch S, Whetham J, et al: Embryoscopy: a closer look at first trimester diagnosis and treatment. *Am J Obstet Gynecol* 166:775, 1992

111. Scriver CR, Kaufman S, Woo SLC: The hyperphenylalaninemias. *The Metabolic Basis of Inherited Disease*, 6th ed. Scriver CR, Beaudet AL, Sly WS, et al, Eds. McGraw-Hill Information Services Co, New York, 1989, p 495

112. Avigad S, Kleiman S, Weinstein M, et al: Compound heterozygosity in non-phenylketonuria hyperphenylalanemia: the contribution of mutations for classical phenylketonuria. *Am J Hum Genet* 19:393, 1991

113. Lidsky A, Ledley FO, DiLella AG, et al: Molecular genetics of phenylketonuia: extensive restriction site polymorphisms in the phenylalanine hydroxylase locus. *Am J Hum Genet* 37:619, 1985

114. Kwok S, Ledley FD, DiLella AG, et al: Nucleotide sequence of a full-length complimentary DNA clone and amino acid sequence of human phenylalanine hydroxylase. *Biochemistry* 24:556, 1985

115. Guttler F, Ledley FD, Lidsley AS, et al: Correlation between polymorphic DNA haplotypes at phenylalanine hydroxylase locus and clinical phenotypes of phenylketonuria. *J Pediatr* 110:68, 1987

116. Woo SLC: Collation of RFLP haplotypes at the human phenylalanine (PAH) locus. *Am J Hum Genet* 43:781, 1988

117. Wulff K, Wehnert M, Schutz M, et al: Prenatal diagnosis of phenylketonuria by haplotype analysis. *Prenat Diagn* 9:421, 1989

118. Cotton RGH: Heterogeneity of phenylketonuria at the clinical, protein and DNA levels. *J Inherit Metab Dis* 13:739, 1990

119. Okano Y, Want T, Eisensmith RC, et al: Missence mutations associated with RFLP haplotypes 1 and 4 of the human phenylalanine hydroxylase gene. *Am J Hum Genet* 46:18, 1990

120. Phillips JA, Kazazian HH: Haemaglobinopathies and thalassemias. *Principles and Practice of Medical Genetics*, 2nd ed. Emery AEH, Rimoin DL, Eds. Churchill Livingstone, Edinburgh, 1990, p 1324

121. Bunn HF, Forglt BG: *Hemoglobin: Molecular, Genetic and Clincial Aspects*. WB Saunders Co, Philadelphia, 1986

122. Driscoll MC, Lerner N, Anyane-Yeboa K, et al: Prenatal diagnosis of sickle hemoglobinopathies: the experience of the Columbia University Comprehensive Center for Sickle Cell Disease. *Am J Hum Genet* 40:548, 1987

123. McCrae UM, Williamson R: Cystic fibrosis. *Principles and Practice of Medical Genetics*, 2nd ed. Emery AE, Rimoin DL, Eds. Churchill Livingstone, Edinburgh, 1990, p 1165

124. Stephan U, Busch EW, Kolberg H, et al: Cystic fibrosis: detection by means of a test-strip. *Pediatrics* 55:35, 1975

125. Christian CL: Prenatal diagnosis of cystic fibrosis. *Clin Perinatol* 17:779, 1990

126. Cutting GR, Antonarakis SE, Beutow KH, et al: Analysis of DNA polymorphism haplotypes linked to the cystic fibrosis locus in North American Black and Caucasian families supports the existence of multiple mutations of the cystic fibrosis gene. *Am J Hum Genet* 44:307, 1989

127. Rommens JM, Iannuzzi MC, Kerem B, et al: Identification of the cystic fibrosis gene: chromosome walking and jumping. *Science* 245:1059, 1989

128. Riordan JR, Rommens JM, Kerem B, et al: Identification of the cystic fibrosis gene: cloning and characterization of complementary DNA. *Science* 245:1066, 1989

129. Strong T, Smut L, Cole J, et al: Identification of 3 CF mutations by chemical mismatch cleavage including a missense mutation in 2 mildly affected sisters without elevated sweat sodium levels. *Am J Hum Genet* 49(suppl):493, 1991

130. Chehab FF, Wall J, Evans ME, et al: The molecular diagnostics of cystic fibrosis in the clinical laboratory by color PCR and an improved method of reverse dot blot hybridization. *Am J Hum Genet* 49(suppl):206, 1991

131. Conneally PM: Huntington disease. *Principles and Practice of Medical Genetics*, 2nd ed. Emery AEH, Rimoin DL, Eds. Churchill Livingstone, Edinburgh, 1990, p 373

132. Spurdle A, Kromberg J, Rosendorff J, et al: Prenatal diagnosis for Huntington's disease: a molecular and psychological study. *Prenat Diagn* 11:177, 1991

133. Gusella JF, Wexler NS, Conneally PM, et al: A polymorphic DNA marker genetically linked to Huntington's disease. *Nature* 306:234, 1983

134. Skraastad MI, Verseest A, Bakker E, et al: Presymptomatic, prenatal and exclusion testing for Huntington disease using seven closely linked DNA markers. *Am J Med Genet* 38:217, 1991

135. The Huntington's Disease Collaborative Research Group: A novel gene containing a trinucleotide repeat that is unstable on Huntington's disease chromosomes. *Cell* 72:971, 1993

136. Oberle I, Rousseau F, et al: Instability of a 550 base pair DNA segment and abnormal methylation in fragile X syndrome. *Science* 252:1711, 1990

137. Suthers GK, Huson SM, Davies KE: Instability versus predictability: the molecular diagnosis of myotonic dystrophy. *J Med Genet* 29:761, 1992

138. La Spada AR, Wilson EM, et al: Androgen receptor gene mutations in X-linked spinal and bulbar muscular atrophy. *Nature* 352:77, 1991

Acknowledgments

Table 1 Data from "Defining DNA Diagnostic Tests Appropriate for Standard Clinical Care," by R. V. Lebo, G. Cunningham, M. J. Simons, et al, in *American Journal of Human Genetics* 47:583, 1990.

Figures 1 and 2 Tom Moore. Adapted from "Medical Genetics," by R. W. Erbe, in SCIENTIFIC AMERICAN *Medicine*, edited by E. Rubenstein and D. D. Federman, Section 9, Subsection IV. Scientific American, Inc., New York, 1994. All rights reserved.

Figures 3 and 4 Adapted from *Recombinant DNA*, 2nd ed., by J. D. Watson, J. Witkowski, M. Gilman, et al. Scientific American Books, New York, 1992. © 1992 James D. Watson, Jan Witkowski, Michael Gilman, Mark Zoller. Used with permission.

CHAPTER 9

Hereditary Disorders

Gregory S. Barsh, M.D., Ph.D.

The revolution in molecular biology over the past two decades has led to a detailed understanding of many well-known hereditary disorders. Moreover, it has become clear that understanding the molecular basis of inherited disease is relevant to many aspects of human phenotypic variation. Common multifactorial conditions frequently exhibit pathophysiological similarities with rare single-gene disorders: the lessons learned from familial hypercholesterolemia and Gardner syndrome, for example, are relevant to the diagnosis, prevention, and treatment of atherosclerosis and colon carcinoma, respectively. In addition to identifying genes and the protein products that are responsible for a variety of inherited disorders, the tools of molecular biology have also uncovered data that raise new questions about diseases other than the ones they were focused on initially. For example, although the retinoblastoma (Rb) and p53 genes responsible for retinoblastoma and Li-Fraumeni syndrome, respectively, have been identified, isolated, and studied in detail, it is still not clear to what extent mutations in these genes account for isolated cases of osteosarcoma and how such mutations are acquired.

Discussions of clinical genetics generally take a problem-based approach in which, for example, disorders of the cardiovascular, musculoskeletal, and gastrointestinal systems are all considered as separate groups. This approach may be helpful in differential diagnosis, but many heritable disorders affect multiple organ systems. Furthermore, this approach can obscure fundamental pathogenetic principles. For example, the causes of congenital interrupted aortic arch include such conditions as a deletion of a small portion of chromosome 22 that occurs sporadically, with little or no chance of recurrence; single-gene disorders such as X-linked DiGeorge syndrome, which will affect one half of the male children born to female carriers; and multifactorial conditions in which the familial recurrence risk lies somewhere between that of the two preceding examples.

This chapter will focus on recent advances in the understanding of human genetic diseases and their impact on diagnosis and therapy. First, a group of single-gene disorders will be considered: Duchenne's and Becker's muscular dystrophy, cystic fibrosis, neurofibromatosis type 1, and phenylketonuria. Passed from one generation to the next according to probabilities defined by the characteristics of meiosis, these so-called mendelian disorders are relatively infrequent and easily distinguished from the distribution of phenotypic variation in the general population. Each of these conditions accounts for a significant fraction of inherited disease, illustrates an important principle of human genetics, or both. Because the gene responsible for each of these disorders has been identified, particular attention will be focused on the pathogenesis of the disease and how an understanding of pathogenesis may guide diagnosis, prevention, and treatment.

Next, two examples of disorders with unusual features or inheritance patterns will be considered. In the Beckwith-Wiedemann syndrome, some cases are associated with a normal amount but an abnormal origin of chromosome 11 material: two copies are inherited from the father and none from the mother. In the X-linked mental retardation condition associated with a fragile site at Xq27.3, most males are affected more severely than females, but some males who pass the syndrome on to their grandchildren are phenotypically normal. Isolating the genes responsible for these conditions will yield immediate rewards: more fundamentally, these exceptions to the laws of Mendel may point the way toward fundamental aspects of mammalian biology revealed only by their effects on human genetic disease.

Duchenne's and Becker's Muscular Dystrophies

The identification of dystrophin as the gene product mutated in the most common forms of muscular dystrophy is often cited as the paradigm for positional cloning: the isolation of a gene on the basis of its genetic map position. Despite a large body of work over several decades based on biochemical analysis of affected tissues, the substantial progress in understanding the molecular basis of Duchenne's muscular dystrophy made over the past five years has depended on identification of the dystrophin gene.[1,2] Consideration of this progress provides a reminder, however, that success in isolating a gene responsible for an inherited disease is really just a beginning in understanding the condition. Indeed, the normal function of dystrophin is still not fully understood, and it is not at all clear why lack of dystrophin leads to muscular dystrophy.

Clinical, Pathological, and Molecular Aspects of Duchenne's Muscular Dystrophy

The natural history and X-linked recessive inheritance pattern of Duchenne's muscular dystrophy were recognized more than a century ago.[3] The disease is usually brought to the attention of the general pediatrician as a delay in gross motor milestones between 12 and 24 months of age; its characteristic clinical findings, which may not be evident initially, include global hypotonia, calf pseudohypertrophy, and proximal muscle weakness as manifested by the Gower sign (using the lower legs as a fulcrum when attempting to rise). Early suspicion of the diagnosis may be confirmed by elevated serum levels of creatine kinase, pedigree analysis, analysis of a muscle biopsy specimen for reduced or absent dystrophin, and DNA analysis for deletions of the dystrophin gene, which is seen in approximately two thirds of all cases. The course of Duchenne's dystrophy in early childhood is characterized by progressive deterioration of newly acquired motor skills, and most individuals are nonambulatory by the age of 11. Myocardial tissue is universally affected, but symptoms of heart failure are usually not predominant. Instead, cardiac conduction abnormalities and respiratory problems are the major source of morbidity, resulting in a mean lifespan less than 20 years. Aside from problems arising from the involvement of skeletal, cardiac, and occasionally smooth muscle, the central nervous system is sometimes also involved (see below), and approximately one fifth of affected patients exhibit a significant degree of cognitive impairment.[4]

Muscle biopsies of patients with Duchenne's dystrophy show variation in muscle fiber size and nuclear location, degradation and phagocytosis of muscle fibers, and fatty and fibrous infiltration. This appearance is similar but not identical to that of other muscular dystrophies and to inflammatory conditions of muscle, although the leukocyte infiltration that accompanies polymyositis is absent in the dystrophies. An early pathogenetic step in Duchenne's dystrophy may be abnormal regulation of Ca^{+2} or stretch-gated Ca^{+2} channels, because electrophysiological studies have demonstrated elevated levels of free Ca^{+2} in myotubules from affected patients or in animal models, which correlate with the amount of protein degradation.[5]

Early attempts to understand the pathogenesis of Duchenne's dystrophy focused on contractile proteins of muscle, muscle enzymes, or more general abnormalities in the cell membrane or microvasculature.[2] These studies failed to identify dystrophin, in part because it accounts for only a small fraction of total muscle protein. Ultimately, the dystrophin gene was isolated solely on the basis of its genetic map position on the short arm of the X chromosome. The gene was initially suspected to lie in this position because a group of unusual female patients affected with Duchenne's dystrophy were found to have X;autosome translocation breakpoints within Xp21.[6,7] A breakthrough came with the recognition that a male patient (designated BB) affected with multiple X-linked conditions, including Duchenne's dystrophy, chronic granulomatous disease, and the McLeod red blood cell phenotype, suffered from a small but cytogenetically detectable deletion of Xp21 [*see Figure 1*].[8,9] Application of subtractive hybridization, a clever technique for isolating anonymous DNA sequences present in one sample but missing from another [*see Chapter 5*], to DNA derived from patient BB and DNA from a cell line carrying multiple normal X chromosomes yielded seven molecular clones that had been deleted from the X chromosome of patient BB.[10] One of these, pERT87, was deleted in about 10 percent of patients with

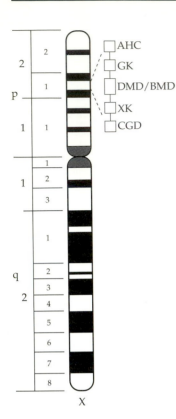

Figure 1 *Shown is an idiogram of an X chromosome from the mother of a male patient with an interstitial deletion that removes the AHC, GK, and DMD loci (del 1). The order of several genes and the relative location of the deletion responsible for DMD in the patient BB (del 2) are also shown. AHC is the locus for congenital adrenal hypoplasia, GK is the locus for glycerol kinase, XK is the locus for the Kell blood group precursor (its absence produces the McLeod phenotype), CGD is the locus for chronic granulomatous disease, and DMD/BMD is the locus for Duchenne's and Becker's muscular dystrophy.*

Duchenne's dystrophy.[11] Concurrently, a female patient with Duchenne's dystrophy and an X;autosome translocation was found to have an autosomal breakpoint within ribosomal DNA, for which molecular probes had previously been isolated.[12] Juxtaposition of these autosomal sequences with Xp21 made possible the isolation of molecular clone XJ, which lay on the X side of the translocation breakpoint and between the centromere and pERT87.[13]

Using pERT87 and XJ as starting points, investigators isolated adjacent genomic DNA and evaluated it for the presence of mRNA coding sequences, which ultimately led to the identification of the dystrophin cDNA.[14,15] Analysis of many patients with Duchenne's dystrophy with probes derived from the dystrophin cDNA indicated that about two thirds of mutations in this disorder were caused by deletions or duplications.[16] The end points of these deletions and duplications were often found to lie in clusters, suggesting that certain areas of the dystrophin gene were mutation hotspots for genomic rearrangements leading to Duchenne's dystrophy.[17,18]

Perhaps the most startling finding surrounding the isolation of the dystrophin gene was its tremendous size. More than two megabases in length, the gene is larger than most entire yeast chromosomes, accounts for almost 0.1 percent of the human genome, and is roughly 100 times as long as most human genes.[19] Two factors contribute to this immensity: the size of the protein itself (approximately 400 kilodaltons, with a 14 kilobase cDNA) and a high ratio of noncoding to coding sequences compared with most other human genes.[15] Evolutionary factors that led to this arrangement are still a matter of considerable discussion, but the size of the dystrophin gene has provided an answer to several genetic puzzles.

First, estimates of the mutation rate for Duchenne's dystrophy are among the highest for any single-gene disorder and are in the range of 10^{-4} per generation per chromosome compared with 10^{-6} to 10^{-5} for most single-gene disorders.[1,20] If most of the dystrophin gene is subject to mutations that produce Duchenne's dystrophy (which seems to be true in retrospect[18,21]), the high mutation rate is at least partly a result of increased target size. Second, in families that did not exhibit deletion of pERT87 or XJ, pedigree analysis had indicated about a five percent recombination frequency between the gene for Duchenne's dystrophy and the two molecular markers.[22] This finding seemed to indicate either a particularly high rate of meiotic recombination close to or within the gene or genetic heterogeneity, whereby two different genes for the disorder might lie close together, with only one of them marked by pERT87 and XJ. The former alternative turns out to be correct; indeed, a careful analysis of meiotic exchange points using markers at the end of the dystrophin gene indicated a 12 percent frequency of intragenic recombination.[23,24] The ratio of genetic to physical distance is therefore 12 recombination units/2 megabases, or 6 recombination units/megabase, compared with the average of about 1 recombination unit/megabase for the entire human genome. It is not yet clear whether this indicates a generalized increase in recombination over the entire Xp21 area or (as seems to be the case for breakpoints leading to deletion or duplication) a small number of recombination hotspots within the dystrophin gene, which serve as preferred sites of normal meiotic exchange.[15,18,21,25,26]

Isolation of the dystrophin gene has had a remarkable impact on genetic counseling for Duchenne's dystrophy, but some problems remain unsolved. The two thirds of cases of this disease caused by DNA rearrangements can be detected by the absence or abnormal size of products when genomic DNA is amplified by the polymerase chain reaction (PCR) with sets of oligonucleotide primers that cover most of the rearrangement-prone regions.[27] Although this approach allows prenatal diagnosis of the disease in affected males in informative families, it cannot be applied to the one third of cases caused by point mutations rather than deletions or duplications. Prenatal diagnosis by restriction fragment length polymorphism (RFLP) linkage analysis [*see Figures 2 and 3*] is possible in these families,[28] but it generally requires unaffected male relatives to establish which of two polymorphisms lies on the same X chromosome as the Duchenne's mutation, and it suffers from the attendant complications of intragenic recombination. A potential solution may lie in using peripheral blood lymphocytes, which contain extremely low but nonetheless detectable levels of dystrophin RNA, to produce the entire cDNA, followed by PCR amplification.[29] More sophisticated methods, such as denaturing gradient gel electrophoresis or automated direct sequencing, can then be applied to detect subtle point mutations within the cDNA.

Diagnosis of female carriers of the defective gene remains a problem in the one third of cases not caused by DNA rearrangement. Also, in situations in which the PCR product is absent rather than being of abnormal size in affected males, carrier females cannot be diagnosed reliably because a product of normal size arises from the nonmutant X chromosome. This state of affairs is, however, greatly improved over the situation that obtained before there was any molecular information, when a probability-based approach was taken to estimate the likelihood that female relatives of affected patients were gene carriers.[30] The principal tenet of that approach, based on population genetic theory, was that one third of apparently new cases of Duchenne's dystrophy represented new mutations and that gonadal mosaicism accounted for only a small fraction of the mutations.[31] In fact, it now appears that gonadal mosaicism is quite frequent in this disease, to the extent that the recurrence risk to mothers of apparently new cases of Duchenne's dystrophy may be as high as 10 percent, even when the mother's somatic tissues lack the mutation.[32]

The Dystrophin Protein

The dystrophin cDNA was identified after such molecular clones as pERT87 and XJ were found to lie in the region of the X chromosome thought to contain the defective gene. Proof that dystrophin represented the actual defect in Duchenne's dystrophy came when antibodies generated against an artificially synthesized protein coded for by the cDNA were found to react with a real protein that was reduced or missing in all patients with Duchenne's dystrophy.[33]

Clues to the normal function of dystrophin have come from information about its subcellular distribution, its appearance in the electron microscope, the similarities between its sequence and those of myofibrillar and cytoskeletal proteins, and biochemical analyses.[34,35] Dystrophin contains domains at the amino terminus and close to the carboxyl terminus that are similar in sequence to the amino and carboxyl termini of α-actinin. The internal portion of dystrophin is also related to that of α-actinin but is much longer. In dystrophin there are 24 segments, each

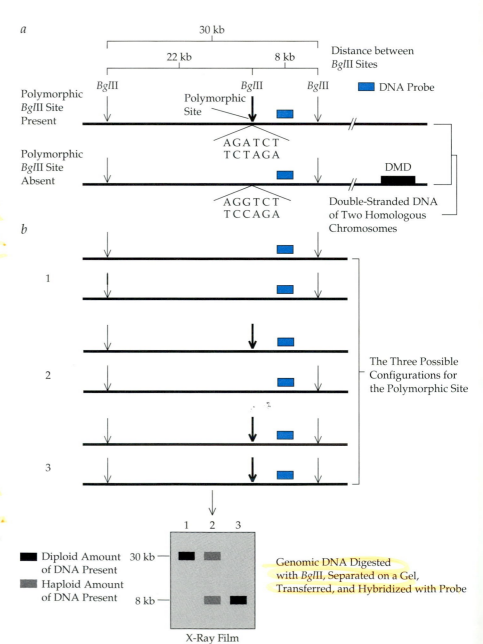

Figure 2 In this illustration of RFLPs, each continuous line represents the double-stranded DNA molecule of one of the two homologous chromosomes (a). In this example, there can be up to three BglII sites (that is, sites that the restriction enzyme BglII recognizes and cuts) in this region of DNA, and one of these BglII sites is polymorphic. The sites are closely linked with the DMD (Duchenne's muscular dystrophy) locus, which encodes dystrophin. The polymorphic site (b) may be absent from the DNA of both chromosomes (1), present on one and absent from the other (2), or present on both (3). In its absence, a single fragment 30 kb long is produced by cleavage with BglII, and when the polymorphic site is present, fragments of 22 kb and 8 kb are produced. A DNA probe that anneals to the DNA strands at the position indicated hybridizes to the 30 kb and 8 kb fragments when used to probe a Southern blot.

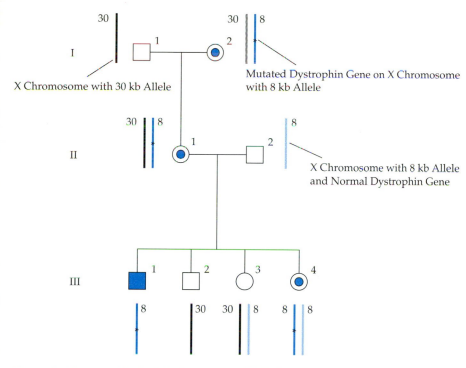

Figure 3 *Illustrated is the inheritance of an RFLP linked to the X chromosome mutation that gives rise to Duchenne's muscular dystrophy. The probe–restriction enzyme combination detects a polymorphism giving fragments of sizes of 30 and 8 kb [see Figure 2]. In this family, the mutation is carried on the chromosome with the 8 kb allele (that is, the allele with the restriction enzyme site that produces an 8 kb DNA fragment). The affected boy (III-1) carries the 8 kb allele on the chromosome that he inherited from his mother (II-1), who is a carrier (males inherit their X chromosome only from their mother). This chromosome had come from the grandmother (I-2). The unaffected boy (III-2) has inherited his mother's chromosome with the 30 kb polymorphism that had come from the grandfather (I-1), who was unaffected. Of the two daughters, III-3 has inherited her mother's normal X chromosome (carrying the 30 kb allele), while the other daughter (III-4) is also a carrier, having inherited the chromosome with the 8 kb allele and the mutant allele.*
Note that the RFLP is not the mutation itself. *This is shown clearly by II-2 and III-1, who both have the 8 kb fragment, but in II-2 this allele is linked with a normal dystrophin allele, whereas in III-1 it is linked with a mutated dystrophin gene.*

roughly 100 amino acids long and similar to one another; only four such segments are found in α-actinin. Because α-actinin exists as a short rodlike structure capped at both ends by globular domains that bind the cytoskeletal protein actin, it seems most likely that dystrophin assumes a long rodlike structure that may bind to cytoskeletal components at each end. Immunochemical and biochemical studies have shown that dystrophin is found at the inner surface of the muscle plasma membrane or sarcolemma, where it is closely associated with at least four membrane glycoproteins.[36,37] This observation suggests an organization similar to that of the erythrocyte membrane, in which the long cytoskeletal protein spectrin (which also contains α-actininlike repeats), in combination with the globular proteins ankyrin and band 4.1, stabilizes the integral membrane proteins band 3 and glycophorin C.

The analogy between erythrocyte and muscle cell membranes may apply to diseased as well as normal tissue. Absence of band 4.1 is the primary cause of the hematologic disorder of hereditary elliptocytosis, which is accompanied by very low levels of glycophorin C. Likewise, absence of dystrophin in Duchenne's muscular dystrophy seems to be associated with very low levels of one of the sarcolemmal glycoproteins normally associated with dystrophin. It remains to be determined, however, how this defect might lead to the abnormal regulation of Ca^{+2} channels, elevated levels of free Ca^{+2}, and eventual breakdown of muscle fiber and its fibrous replacement that characterize Duchenne's muscular dystrophy.[5]

In addition to being present in skeletal, smooth, and cardiac muscle, dystrophin is found in most tissues of the central nervous system.[38] Neuronal cells express the dystrophin gene with a different promoter and first exon from those involved in other tissues; that, along with alternative splicing, results in brain-specific dystrophin isoforms. Dystrophin appears rather early in neuronal development and appears to localize to the postsynaptic plasma membrane.[39,40] It has been difficult to correlate the presence of mental retardation in Duchenne's muscular dystrophy with specific dystrophin abnormalities, and the function of dystrophin in the central nervous system remains obscure.

The Natural History and Molecular Defect in Becker's Muscular Dystrophy

Becker's muscular dystrophy is similar to Duchenne's muscular dystrophy in the pattern of affected muscles, appearance on muscle biopsy, and X-linked recessive inheritance, but it exhibits a milder course. Onset generally occurs between midchildhood and early adult life, cardiac and central nervous system involvement occur much less frequently than in Duchenne's muscular dystrophy, and the mean lifespan is about 50 years.[41] Although some early genetic linkage studies suggested that Duchenne's and Becker's muscular dystrophy involved separate loci, it is now clear that the conditions are allelic, both resulting from dystrophin mutations.[17,42-45] At the protein level, the conditions can usually be distinguished on the basis of differences in the amount of dystrophin that is present: most patients with Duchenne's dystrophy have little or no dystrophin, whereas patients with Becker's dystrophy have reduced levels of dystrophin, dystrophins of abnormal size, or both. The mutational mechanisms underlying the two conditions are similar, however. Large intragenic deletions or duplications account for about two thirds of cases of Becker's and Duchenne's muscular dystrophy, and neither the size nor the precise location of the deletion or duplication seems to correlate with severity. The difference in the amounts of dystrophin seems instead to arise from the fact that nearly all the rearrangements observed in Becker's dystrophy maintain the normal translational reading frame [*see Figure 4*], giving rise to dystrophins that contain internal deletions or duplications. In rearrangements observed in Duchenne's dystrophy, however, the normal translational reading frame is lost and so translation terminates prematurely, giving rise to a shortened and unstable protein with an altered carboxyl terminus.

Animal Models and Potential Treatments for Duchenne's Dystrophy

Although prenatal diagnosis has become an effective means of preventing Duchenne's dystrophy, the high rate of new mutation in this disorder will maintain the need for effective treatments. The discovery that a previously identified classical mouse mutation, mdx, is caused by complete absence of dystrophin has provided a model in which to test potential treatments.[46] Although the mutant phenotype in the mouse is extremely mild and histological examination of mdx limb muscle shows few, if any, of the severe dystrophic changes that characterize Duchenne's dystrophy, diaphragm muscle from mdx mice is quite similar to that of affected humans.[47]

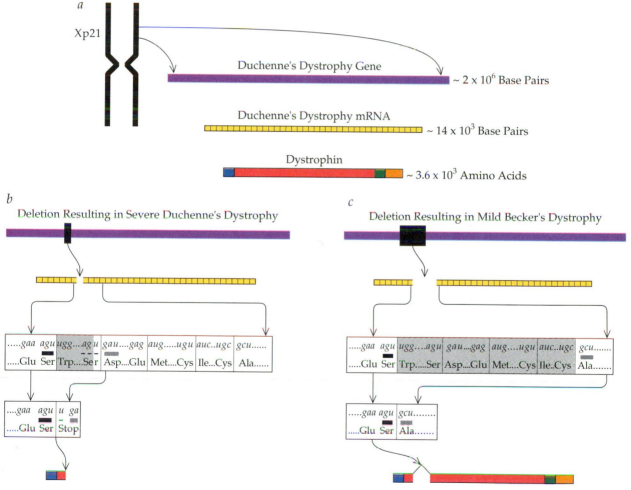

Figure 4 *The molecular basis for Duchenne's dystrophy and Becker's dystrophy phenotypes is shown here. (a) Indicated here are the Xp21 map position of the Duchenne's dystrophy gene and the approximate sizes of the gene, its transcription product (mRNA), and the dystrophin protein product. (b) A single-exon, out-of-frame deletion (shaded gray) is small, but it disrupts the translational reading frame, leading to a severely truncated dystrophin molecule that is rapidly degraded by the cell and, therefore, to severe Duchenne's dystrophy. (c) A relatively larger in-frame deletion (shaded gray) preserves the reading frame, resulting in an internally deleted protein. This protein is not degraded by the cell and is probably semifunctional, accounting for the milder Becker's dystrophy phenotype.*

Conventional medical and surgical treatment of the disease is generally limited to treating such complications as pulmonary infection, cardiac abnormalities, and contractures of the Achilles tendon. Aside from physical and occupational therapy programs directed at preserving joint mobility, attempts to alter the course of Duchenne's dystrophy have not proved effective. Two recent developments in developmental and molecular biology suggest new opportunities, however. First, specialized muscle cells known as satellite cells have the potential to migrate to, proliferate in, and eventually regenerate areas of muscle-fiber necrosis.[48] Second, direct injection of DNA vectors into mouse muscle results in stable expression of genes they encode.[49] Transplantation of nonmutant satellite cells into diseased muscle could result in muscle regeneration. A potential difficulty in overcoming histocompatibility barriers might be addressed either by autologous transplantation of mutant cells engineered to express normal dystrophin or by direct injection into Duchenne's dystrophy muscle of DNA vectors coding for human dystrophin (although more efficient methods for DNA delivery will be required if clinical improvement is to occur).[50,51] Even if such approaches should be successful, they will not address either the CNS problems seen in some patients with Duchenne's dystrophy or the cardiac problems likely to affect all patients with Duchenne's dystrophy if their skeletal muscle disease improves.

Cystic Fibrosis and the CFTR Gene

The name cystic fibrosis was formulated originally to describe the pathological abnormalities of the pancreas and the lungs in affected individuals.[52] Obstruction of exocrine ducts followed by cystic dilatation and fibrosis is accompanied by pancreatic insufficiency and an inability to clear pulmonary secretions, which lead to the clinical hallmarks of cystic fibrosis: recurrent respiratory infections and malabsorption.[53] Like Duchenne's dystrophy, cystic fibrosis is extremely common, but it is inherited in an autosomal recessive fashion. In Caucasian populations, approximately 1 in 20 individuals carries a mutant allele for this autosomal recessive disorder, accounting for a disease incidence of about 1 in 2,000.[54] Cystic fibrosis is usually diagnosed in early childhood and accounts for most pulmonary and pancreatic disease in the pediatric age group. The relatively high frequency of the cystic fibrosis gene has been difficult to understand because, unlike Duchenne's dystrophy, the rate of new mutations in cystic fibrosis is very low. The gene responsible for cystic fibrosis, the cystic fibrosis transmembrane conductance regulator (CFTR), was isolated in 1989,[55-57] two years after dystrophin was cloned. As in the case of Duchenne's disease, isolation of the gene has had a tremendous impact on diagnosis, and the major challenge in the next several years will be to understand how mutations in the CFTR gene lead to the abnormalities in chloride transport and exocrine insufficiency that characterize cystic fibrosis.

Natural History and Pathogenesis of Cystic Fibrosis

Most individuals affected with cystic fibrosis are diagnosed in the first several years of life when recurrent respiratory infection, growth retardation, steatorrhea, or a combination of these disorders prompts administration of a chloride sweat test. Under standardized conditions for collection of sweat after pilocarpine administration, more than 99 percent of individuals affected with cystic fibrosis have sweat chloride levels exceeding 60 mEq/L.[58,59] False positive tests are almost always the result of such salt-wasting states as adrenal insufficiency or nephrogenic diabetes insipidus, which are not easily confused with cystic fibrosis. About 10 percent of newly diagnosed cases of cystic fibrosis present in the newborn period with so-called meconium ileus, thought to be caused by pancreatic exocrine insufficiency in utero that leads to small bowel obstruction. Uncommon presentations include bowel obstruction later in life and atypical pulmonary disease, such as asthma or bronchiolitis; a few patients with cystic fibrosis are not diagnosed until their second or third decade.[53]

The primary abnormality in cystic fibrosis is aberrant regulation of chloride transport across epithelial cells in the pulmonary tree, the intestine, the exocrine pancreas, and apocrine sweat glands.[60,61] Electrophysiological studies have characterized the defect most fully in airway and sweat gland epithelia. In cells lining the tracheobronchial tree, transepithelial voltage and fluid secretion are determined by the balance between transport of sodium from the mucosa to the submucosa and transport of chloride from the submucosa to the mucosa.[62] Chloride transport is controlled directly by channels in the apical membrane (at the mucosal surface) that are normally activated by elevated levels of intracellular cyclic adenosine monophosphate (cAMP). In the airways of patients with cystic fibrosis, cAMP fails to activate these chloride channels, leading to decreased chloride transport and altered transepithelial voltage and ultimately to decreased fluid secretion and retention of mucus.[63,64]

A similar defect is found in apocrine sweat glands, in which salt and fluid concentrations are influenced normally by the balance between luminal chloride transport in the basal secretory coil and chloride reabsorption in the absorptive ducts that lie close to the skin surface.[65,66] In the sweat glands of patients with cystic fibrosis, the chloride channels in the absorptive duct are relatively impermeable, which accounts for the higher salt concentrations in sweat and forms the basis for the chloride sweat test. In addition, the elevated cAMP levels that normally activate luminal chloride transport in the secretory coil fail to do so in the sweat glands of patients with cystic fibrosis.[67]

Decreased fluid secretion is thought to be the initial step leading to thickening of pancreatic secretions, obstruction of the pulmonary tree with mucus, and dilatation of sweat glands.[53,61] Because pancreatic exocrine insufficiency begins in utero, complications secondary to abnormal digestion often are the earliest manifestation of cystic fibrosis. In addition to meconium ileus, distal intestinal obstruction, rectal prolapse, and fat malabsorption all may occur in early childhood.[68] About 40 percent of patients older than 10 years of age develop pancreatic endocrine insufficiency, manifested by abnormal glucose tolerance tests, and about 10 percent eventually require insulin therapy.[69] Islet cell destruction is usually not as severe as in type I diabetes mellitus; older patients with cystic fibrosis may develop microvascular disease as a complication of diabetes, but frank ketoacidosis is extremely rare. Other gastrointestinal complications include hepatobiliary cirrhosis, cholelithiasis, or both in about five to 10 percent of patients: such complications are thought to be caused by abnormalities in biliary secretion.[53]

The first pulmonary symptom of cystic fibrosis is usually intermittent coughing, which later becomes chronic and productive of sputum from which mucoid strains of *Pseudomonas aeruginosa* may be cultured. Colonization and recurrent pulmonary infection may be caused not only by an inability to clear mucus normally but also by altered posttranslational modification of mucus glycoproteins. Pulmonary function initially reflects obstructive disease, which progresses to a mixed restrictive and obstructive deficit as more lung tissue is destroyed.[53,70] Chronic hypoxemia leads to digital clubbing and about a 20 percent incidence of hypertrophic pulmonary osteoarthropathy.[71] Frequent infections develop in both the lower and upper airways: chronic rhinitis, leading to nasal polyps, occurs in about 20 percent of patients.[72] Hospitalization for intensive bronchodilator treatment, postural drainage, and intravenous antibiotic therapy for *Pseudomonas* infection becomes increasingly frequent as the disease progresses. Complications secondary to pulmonary infection or pulmonary hypertension with right heart failure are the most serious causes of morbidity in cystic fibrosis.[73] Median survival is 26 years of age, but the course is highly variable: 10 percent of affected individuals die before 10 years of age, and a small proportion survive to the fifth and sixth decades of life.[74]

The sweat chloride test is abnormal at birth in virtually all patients with cystic fibrosis, but clinical symptoms caused by sweat gland dysfunction are rare. Mainly, excessive loss of salt is responsible for a chronic state of hyperaldosteronism and a propensity to develop hypochloremic alkalosis after vomiting and diarrhea in early childhood.

More than 95 percent of male patients with cystic fibrosis are sterile.[75] Contributing factors may include defects in sperm maturation and anatomic abnormalities of Wolffian duct structures that lead to altered production and content of seminal secretions. The CFTR gene is expressed in postmeiotic spermatids, but its potential role in male gametogenesis has not been clarified.[76] Analogous abnormalities are not present in the female genitourinary system, although secondary amenorrhea or oligomenorrhea is a frequent complication of poor nutrition and chronic lung infection.

The CFTR Gene

Taking a systematic approach based on an RFLP map of the human genome, investigators mapped the mutation responsible for cystic fibrosis to chromosome 7q in 1985, very close to the previously isolated *met* oncogene.[77-79] By generating high-resolution physical and genetic maps of newly isolated molecular markers, they narrowed the region containing the cystic fibrosis gene to about 500 kb. Because it was difficult to predict sequence characteristics or a pattern of expression for the cystic fibrosis gene and because new mutations for this disease are difficult to identify, several potential candidate genes were considered at first.[80,81] In 1989, attention focused on one candidate gene when it was found to be mutated in a large number of cystic fibrosis chromosomes derived from different populations.[55-57] Because it was not clear whether this gene coded for a chloride channel defective in the cells of patients with cystic fibrosis or

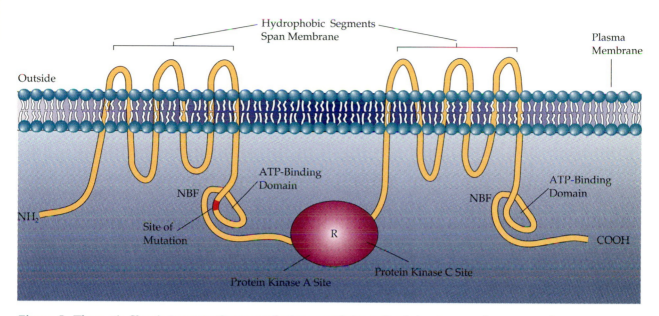

Figure 5 *The cystic fibrosis transmembrane conductance regulator molecule has two membrane-spanning regions, each made of six hydrophobic segments. On the carboxy-terminal side of each membrane domain is a consensus sequence for nucleotide-binding folds (NBF) that bind ATP. The central portion of the molecule (the R region) is characterized by the presence of a large number of charged residues. This R region contains sites that can be phosphorylated by protein kinases A and C. The site of the 3 bp deletion in the first ATP binding domain [see Figure 6] is indicated.*

for a protein that affected the conductance of a separate chloride channel, it was named the cystic fibrosis transmembrane conductance regulator (CFTR). Ultimate proof that this gene was responsible for cystic fibrosis came when the normal CFTR gene was expressed in airway cells derived from a patient with cystic fibrosis and was found to correct the defect in cAMP-dependent chloride permeability.[82]

The predicted amino acid sequence of the protein encoded by the CFTR gene is 1,480 residues long and is similar to the so-called TM6-NBD family of energy-dependent transport proteins.[55,83] Many of these proteins contain six membrane-spanning domains (i.e., TM6) and a cytoplasmic domain, the NBD, that can bind a nucleotide triphosphate such as ATP. In some members of this protein family (e.g., the multidrug-resistance P glycoprotein and the yeast STE6 gene product), hydrolysis of ATP is thought to provide energy to move small hydrophobic molecules from one side of the membrane to the other. The CFTR protein [*see Figure 5*] contains two TM6-NBD segments, each roughly 675 amino acids in length. These are separated by a cytoplasmic domain 128 amino acids in length—the regulatory, or R, region—that contains a large number of charged amino acids and potential sites for phosphorylation by protein kinase A.[78] Because the R region contains several sites that can be phosphorylated by cAMP-dependent protein kinase, it seems most likely that the CFTR gene product is itself a chloride channel whose activity depends on phosphorylation of particular residues within the R domain.

About 75 percent of cystic fibrosis mutations are accounted for by the delta F508 mutation, a 3 bp deletion that removes a phenylalanine residue within the first nucleotide-binding domain at position 508 [*see Figure 6*].[57,84] A large number of other CFTR alterations are accounted for by different mutations in the cystic fibrosis gene, although most of the mutations, like delta F508, affect the first nucleotide-binding domain, and a significant proportion of the remainder affect the second nucleotide-binding domain.[85-88] Precisely how any of these mutations alter CFTR activity is not yet clear; some mutations block intracellular processing and transport of the protein, whereas others seem to interact with the R domain to prevent cAMP-dependent activation.[89,90] A dearth of mutations in the cystic fibrosis gene that produce no CFTR protein at all suggests that complete loss of CFTR may be lethal in utero.

As decribed above, the course of cystic fibrosis is variable. Once it became clear that defects in CFTR accounted for all cases of cystic fibrosis, attention turned toward allelic heterogeneity as a source of variable expressivity. Attempts to correlate clinical findings with exact genotype for a large number of patients with cystic fibrosis demonstrated that the delta F508 mutation is associated with a more severe form of the disease (with regard to age at diagnosis and to the development of pancreatic insufficiency).[57,91] In the population of patients with cystic fibrosis who were under study, 52 percent were homozygous for delta F508, and nearly all of these patients exhibited pancreatic insufficiency. About 40 percent of the population carried one delta F508 allele (compound heterozygotes), and of these, 72 percent exhibited pancreatic insufficiency. Only eight percent of the population with cystic fibrosis lacked the delta F508 mutation, and

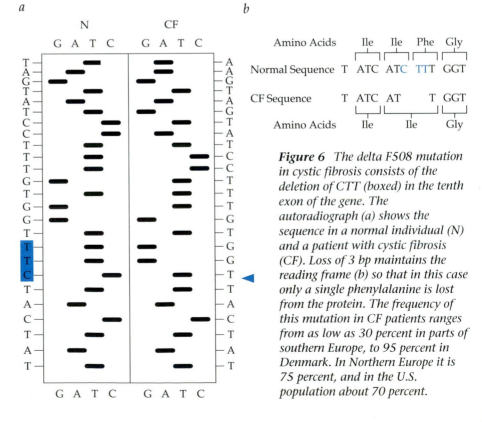

Figure 6   *The delta F508 mutation in cystic fibrosis consists of the deletion of CTT (boxed) in the tenth exon of the gene. The autoradiograph (a) shows the sequence in a normal individual (N) and a patient with cystic fibrosis (CF). Loss of 3 bp maintains the reading frame (b) so that in this case only a single phenylalanine is lost from the protein. The frequency of this mutation in CF patients ranges from as low as 30 percent in parts of southern Europe, to 95 percent in Denmark. In Northern Europe it is 75 percent, and in the U.S. population about 70 percent.*

only 36 percent of this group exhibited pancreatic insufficiency. The presence of delta F508 does not appear to predict increased severity of cystic fibrosis apart from its effect on pancreatic insufficiency, however; delta F508 has no separate effects on other aspects of phenotypic heterogeneity in cystic fibrosis. For example, homozygosity for delta F508 does not seem to influence the incidence of meconium ileus.

Direct testing for delta F508 and several other cystic fibrosis mutations by a polymerase chain reaction (PCR)-based assay is now offered by many clinical laboratories to determine if individuals with a positive family history are carriers.[88,92] Heterozygote testing is most informative when the affected individual and other family members are available, because direct analysis will fail to detect a small proportion of cystic fibrosis mutations. For the same reason, programs for heterozygote detection in the general population have not been instituted widely.[93,94] There has been a long-standing controversy as to whether the high incidence of cystic fibrosis in Caucasian populations is caused by some selective advantage for carriers of the cystic fibrosis gene or some form of genetic drift.[95] The structure and function of CFTR do not suggest any role that affects fertility or decreased disease susceptibility in carriers, and the equal transmission of mutant and nonmutant chromosomes does not support earlier suggestions of segregation distortion.[96]

The feasibility of newborn screening has been examined in several pilot studies in which elevated levels of immunoreactive trypsinogen in dried blood samples served to identify patients for subsequent sweat chloride analysis.[97,98] The incidence of false-positive and false-negative test results is significant, but there is some evidence that identification of cystic fibrosis patients at birth results in lower morbidity during early childhood. As improved methods of direct mutation analysis lead to population-based programs for heterozygote testing, the need for newborn screening programs should become less compelling.

Models and Treatment of Cystic Fibrosis

Although combined heart-lung transplantation has been performed in a few patients with cystic fibrosis who had end-stage respiratory disease and heart failure,[99] the mainstay of treatment is supportive care. After diagnosis, most patients are referred to specialized care centers that offer periodic pulmonary and nutritional screening, supportive care, and genetic counseling. Regular chest physical therapy, vitamin and pancreatic enzyme supplementation, and vigorous treatment of lung infections all have been demonstrated to reduce morbidity and mortality. The development of an aerosolized recombinant human DNAse that degrades thickened mucus and allows it to be cleared more easily appears promising; clinical testing has recently begun.[100] In addition, gelsolin, a protein that dismembers actin, may prove useful as a mucolytic agent.[101]

As in Duchenne's dystrophy, the lack of a suitable animal model has made it difficult to test therapeutic agents, but advances in experimental mouse embryology should soon make possible the development of mice with CFTR mutations. Unlike the defects in Duchenne's dystrophy, those in cystic fibrosis are qualitative rather than quantitative: attempts to increase the expression of mutant CFTR genes in cystic fibrosis cells are unlikely to affect abnormalities in chloride transport. On the other hand, cystic fibrosis is a recessive disease, and the presence of mutant CFTR protein in a heterozygous or homozygous mutant cell does not inhibit the ability of normal CFTR to correct abnormalities of chloride transport. This suggests a role for direct gene therapy in cystic fibrosis, that is, the introduction of the normal CFTR gene into mutant tissues.[102] Future efforts toward this goal are likely to focus on problems of expression and delivery, because current DNA vectors are not efficient enough to be delivered to more than a small fraction of epithelial cells.

Neurofibromatosis

Neurofibromatosis type 1, tuberous sclerosis, Sturge-Weber syndrome, and von Hippel–Lindau disease are associated with discrete lesions involving the skin, and so these conditions have been termed the phakomatoses, from *phakos*, the Greek word for spots. Neurofibromatosis type 1 is, however, genetically, developmentally, and pathologically distinct from the other conditions. Neurofibromatosis type 1 (also called von Recklinghausen's neurofibromatosis) is the most frequent autosomal dominant single-gene disorder affecting human populations. It is characterized by extremely variable expressivity, a high new mutation rate, and pleiotropic manifestations; diagnosis frequently requires input from several subspecialists.[103] The gene responsible for this disorder, termed NF-1, was isolated in 1990, but compared with dystrophin and the CFTR gene, little is known of its cellular function.[104-106] Because neurofibromatosis type 1, along with Gardner syndrome and Li-Fraumeni syndrome, is associated with an increased susceptibility to malignancy, studying the NF-1 gene ultimately may yield fundamental insights into the pathways controlling cellular proliferation.

Clinical, Genetic, and Diagnostic Aspects

Because the incidence of neurofibromatosis type 1 is 1 in 3,000 and roughly 50 percent of cases result from new mutations, nearly all primary care physicians encounter several affected individuals, some of whom have no family history.[103,107,108] Three of the hallmarks of this disorder, café au lait spots, neurofibromas, and Lisch nodules, are thought to represent, respectively, increased melanogenesis in epidermal melanocytes, disturbances of Schwann cell growth regulation, and melanocytic hamartomas of the iris.[109-112] Because these tissues are all derived from neural crest, neurofibromatosis type 1 has sometimes been called a neurocristopathy. Formal diagnostic criteria for this disorder, as established by an NIH consensus conference, require the presence of at least two of the following cardinal manifestations: (1) six or more café au lait spots greater than 15 mm in length in postpubertal individuals or greater than 5 mm in length in prepubertal individuals, (2) two or more neurofibromas of any type or one plexiform neurofibroma, (3) two or more Lisch nodules, (4) axillary or inguinal freckling, (5) characteristic bony lesions such as sphenoid dysplasia or a pseudoarthrosis, (6) optic gliomas, or (7) a first-degree relative previously diagnosed with neurofibromatosis type 1.[112-114] These criteria are specific but not tremendously sensitive, especially in very early childhood.

In the first year of life, usually the only signs of the disorder are the café au lait spots, which become more distinct and numerous later in childhood.[115] Axillary freckling, macrocephaly, and learning disability may also be present in later childhood, but neurofibromas usually do not develop until puberty. The prevalence of Lisch nodules in gene carriers is greater than 50 percent by midchildhood and close to 100 percent in adults.[116-119] Most adults with neurofibromatosis type 1 have multiple café au lait spots, Lisch nodules, and neurofibromas; areolar neurofibromas are especially common in affected females.[103] Although the penetrance of this disorder is thought to be complete (i.e., nearly all gene carriers manifest some aspect of the condition), a small proportion of gene carriers may have very mild findings.[120] In the 50 percent of cases that result from new mutations, there is no family history. In this situation, diagnosis may be difficult either in an adult with very mild expression of the mutation or in a young child with multiple café au lait spots.

Variable expressivity of neurofibromatosis type 1 has accounted, in part, for the confusion surrounding genetic heterogeneity in neurofibromatosis. There are at least two distinct genes that cause café au lait spots and brain tumors. In neurofibromatosis type 2, sometimes called central neurofibromatosis, there are few, if any, external neurofibromas, and there are always bilateral acoustic neuromas; this form of neurofibromatosis is caused by a mutation on chromosome 22.[121] In addition, there are rare clinical presentations of café au lait spots and neurofibromas that, for example, predominantly affect gastrointestinal organs or are associated with a particular set of dysmorphic features. It has not yet been determined whether these represent other genes, allelic heterogeneity of the NF-1 gene, or variable expression of one or a small group of alleles.[111,122]

The most worrisome complications of neurofibromatosis are developmental delay and malignancy. Although the incidence of significant mental retardation is probably less than five percent, as many as 30 percent of individuals with neurofibromatosis type 1 experience some learning disability.[108,123,124] Many individuals have macrocephaly and intracranial anatomic abnormalities detectable by a magnetic resonance imaging scan, but it is difficult to correlate a particular clinical feature with the likelihood of developmental delay.[112,125] Furthermore, unlike most conditions, the extent of intrafamilial variability in this disorder seems as great as interfamilial variability, and so it is difficult to predict an affected individual's course from the course of older first-degree relatives.

Malignancies of all types arise in about 10 percent of affected individuals. Neurofibrosarcomas, rhabdomyosarcomas, squamous cell and gastrointestinal carcinomas, pheochromocytomas, malignant schwannomas, and astrocytomas all occur with increased frequency in neurofibromatosis type 1. One of the most characteristic tumors, optic nerve gliomas, are seen often enough to warrant special screening studies.[125-128] Because the course of these tumors may be quite benign and they may not be detected without intracranial imaging procedures, some studies may have underestimated their true incidence.

Other complications of neurofibromatosis type 1 are mostly caused by neurofibromas that arise in confined places and exert pressure on vital structures. These can include aqueductal stenosis, diencephalic syndrome,

retroperitoneal or gastrointestinal bleeding, and renal artery stenosis.[103,112,129-132] Because expression of the disorder is so variable even within
a single family, it is often difficult to provide specific advice regarding the
natural history of the condition. A long-term study of 212 cases in
Denmark indicated that individuals in whom the disease was identified
after a hospitalization were more likely to experience serious complications than were their first-degree relatives who were also affected with
neurofibromatosis type 1.[133] This observation provides some foundation
for prognostication based on an individual's recent course.

The NF-1 Gene

The NF-1 gene was mapped to chromosome 17q by conventional RFLP
linkage studies in 1987.[134] It rapidly became clear that a single locus was
responsible for all cases of neurofibromatosis type 1 in which there was a
sufficient degree of pedigree information to allow linkage analysis.[135]
Increasingly refined mapping studies [*see Figure 7*] combined with molecular investigations of two patients who had developed the disorder as the
result of chromosomal rearrangements involving 17q11.2 ultimately led
to the isolation of the NF-1 gene in 1990.[106,136] Because several transcribed
sequences were present within this region, identification of the correct
gene depended on finding sequence alterations in individuals with disease
that, at the clinical level, was thought to represent a new mutation.
(Otherwise, sequence changes in affected members of a pedigree might be
the result of a neutral polymorphism closely linked to the actual NF-1
mutation.) The NF-1 gene covers at least 300 kb of genomic DNA and
contains, within one intron more than 40 kb long, three transcribed
sequences of unknown function whose orientation is opposite to that of
the NF-1 gene. Partial sequence characterization of the NF-1 cDNA, which
is about 13 kb long in total, has suggested that the product of this gene
plays a role in signal transduction pathways involving the *ras* proto-
oncogene.[104] Because mutations in *ras* are implicated in human tumors,
this finding has begun to indicate how mutations in NF-1 might lead to
the aberrant regulation of cell growth that is seen in neurofibromas.[105,137,138]

Within the sequenced portion of the NF-1 cDNA, there is a 2,485–amino
acid open reading frame that bears striking similarity (over a 1,500–amino
acid region) to two proteins in yeast, IRA1 and IRA2, that interact with the
yeast homologue of *ras*. In addition, an internal 360–amino acid segment
is similar to the GTPase activating protein for mammalian *ras* (*ras*GAP),
which interacts with the protein encoded by *ras*, p21^{ras}. Stimulation of cell
proliferation through the *ras* pathway involves binding of GTP by p21^{ras}.[139]
Hydrolysis of p21^{ras}-bound GTP is normally stimulated by GAP, the NF-1
gene product, or both and terminates the cycle of p21^{ras} activation.
Oncogenic mutations in *ras* prevent efficient GTP hydrolysis and result in
a persistent state of p21^{ras} activation. This has led to the suggestion that
reduced activity of the NF-1 gene product, which is sometimes referred to
as NF-1–GAP, may also block GTP hydrolysis and lead to persistent
activation of p21^{ras}.

This hypothesis implies that NF-1–GAP, and *ras*GAP are upstream
regulators of p21^{ras}, but it has also been suggested that these proteins lie
downstream of p21^{ras} in the signal-transduction pathway.[139,140] An analysis

of p21^{ras} activity in neurofibromas may help distinguish between these alternatives. Regardless, because many different molecular lesions can produce neurofibromatosis type 1, it seems most likely that these mutations inactivate the normal function of NF-1–GAP.[106,141,142] Furthermore, because the NF-1 gene is dominant and because neurofibromas do not exhibit a loss of heterozygosity for chromosome 17 markers (see below), it also seems likely that a 50 percent reduction of NF-1–GAP activity is sufficient to produce the altered regulation of melanogenesis manifested by café au lait spots and the disturbances in the regulation of Schwann cell growth manifested by neurofibromas.

Analysis of neurofibromas in individuals heterozygous for glucose-6-phosphate dehydrogenase (G6PD) isozymes suggests that multiple cells contribute to each neurofibroma.[143] By contrast, malignant tumors in patients with neurofibromatosis type 1 such as neurofibrosarcomas have a monoclonal origin, pointing to a pathogenetic process that requires

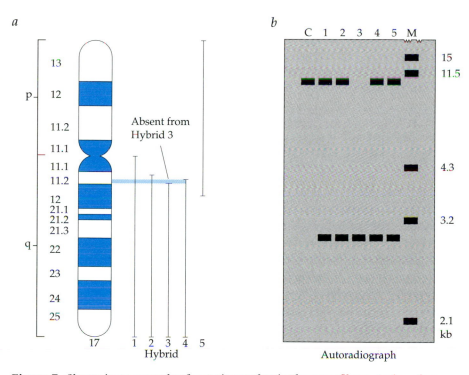

Figure 7 *Shown is an example of mapping probes in the neurofibromatosis region using somatic human-rodent cell hybrids. (a) Five cell hybrids (1–5), each containing a differing portion of the long arm (q) of chromosome 17, were used. The lengths of 17q included in each hybrid are shown by the lines. For example, hybrid 1 contains all of 17q, while hybrid 2 is missing segment 17q11.1 and a part of 11.2. (b) DNA was extracted from human cells (lane C in the blot) and from the five hybrids (lanes 1–5 in the blot), digested with a restriction enzyme, and Southern blotted with a probe from the gene EV12, a candidate for the neurofibromatosis gene. The probe hybridizes to human DNA present in all hybrids except hybrid 3. (The second set of bands at about 3.0 kb is the rodent gene that cross-hybridizes with the human probe.) Since the probe hybridizes to DNA from hybrid 4, the sequence must come from that portion of 17q present in hybrid 4 but absent from hybrid 3, that is, a small section of 17q11.2. The bands in lane M are fragments of known size, marked in kilobases.*

several genetic steps.[144-146] When tested for loss of heterozygosity, some malignant tumors in patients with neurofibromatosis type 1 appear to have lost one of their two chromosome 17 homologues. This suggests that, as in retinoblastoma, these tumors have developed after the loss of a recessive tumor suppressor gene, in which one copy is inactivated by a point mutation and the other copy by chromosomal loss. Because several potential tumor suppressor genes, including p53, are on chromosome 17, it is not yet possible to determine if NF-1 is indeed such a tumor suppressor gene and if the loss of both copies of the NF-1 gene affects a cell differently than the loss of just one copy.

New mutations in NF-1 are not strongly associated with advanced paternal age (unlike such single-gene disorders as achondroplasia and factor VIII deficiency[107]), even though more than 90 percent of new NF-1 mutations arise on the paternal chromosome[147] and so would be expected to show a paternal age effect. The paradox may be explained by mutations of a specific male germ cell that are not self-renewing. The reasons for the high mutation rate in NF-1, about 10^{-4} per generation per chromosome, are not yet clear. The NF-1 gene is large but is nonetheless about five times smaller than the dystrophin gene, which has a similar mutation rate. Both Duchenne's dystrophy and neurofibromatosis type 1 are caused by mutations that inactivate their respective gene products, and so perhaps a larger proportion of the NF-1–GAP protein than of dystrophin is susceptible to inactivating mutations, or perhaps local DNA sequence factors are responsible for a relatively higher frequency of deletions or other rearrangements per unit length on 17q than on Xp.

Management of NF-1

Routine management of neurofibromatosis type 1 is best accomplished with the consultation of a medical geneticist.[112] Appropriate screening examinations (including, for example, ophthalmologic, audiologic, and orthopedic examinations) can be coordinated on a regular basis, and genetic counseling and prenatal diagnosis can be provided for the individual and other family members.[108] The need for routine cranial imaging, either as an initial test or on a regular follow-up basis, is controversial, but as the availability and sensitivity of magnetic resonance imaging increases, it does seem likely that estimates of the incidence of intracranial lesions in this disorder will also increase. In general, surgery for benign neurofibromas in neurofibromatosis type 1 is not recommended. For lesions that cause functional complications or are especially disfiguring, however, dermabrasion and laser surgery have proved to be effective.[148,149] There is, as yet, no proven medical therapy that retards the progression of neurofibromatosis type 1 or prevents complications. As in cystic fibrosis, however, the development of animal models should aid these efforts.

Phenylketonuria and Hyperphenylalaninemia

Phenylketonuria, the urinary excretion of phenylacetate and phenylpyruvate, results from excess levels of circulating phenylalanine caused by a deficiency of the enzyme phenylalanine hydroxylase (PAH). A decade ago, the handling of phenylketonuria was often hailed as the pinnacle of success in applying biochemistry and molecular biology to societal problems that stem from inherited disease.[150-152] The condition was recognized in 1934, and public health programs for testing and treatment by phenylalanine restriction were instituted in the 1950s; they have had a tremendous impact on the course of phenylalanine hydroxylase deficiency.[153-155] Yet today the focus has shifted in several respects. For one thing, most adults who have been treated for phenylketonuria since birth show subtle neuropsychological defects, and issues surrounding alternative treatment strategies and mechanisms to improve compliance remain controversial.[156-158] Second, in a fraction of individuals detected by phenylketonuria screening programs, phenylalanine hydroxylase activity is normal and other treatment is required in addition to a low phenylalanine diet.[155] Identification and early treatment of these individuals remain problematic. Finally, in a generation of women with successfully treated phenylketonuria who are now of childbearing age, the phenomenon of maternal phenylketonuria has been recognized: in utero exposure to maternal hyperphenylalaninemia results in congenital abnormalities regardless of fetal genotype.[159-164] The number of pregnancies at risk has risen in proportion to the successful treatment of phenylketonuria, and their recurrence will challenge public health officials, physicians, and biochemical geneticists in the next decade.

Recognition and Diagnosis of Phenylketonuria

The phenotype of untreated phenylketonuria—characterized by postnatal growth retardation, moderate to severe mental retardation, recurrent seizures, hypopigmentation, and eczematous skin rashes—is rarely seen today because of the widespread implementation of newborn screening programs for hyperphenylalaninemia.[155,165] Affected patients are referred to specialized centers that provide dietary therapy and genetic counseling and monitor nutrition, growth, and development. In this situation, issues that commonly arise are whether problems with behavior or at school are related to the underlying condition, how best to monitor dietary therapy and distinguish inadequate therapy from noncompliance, and when therapy can be discontinued.[166] These issues are best addressed jointly by the primary care physician, genetic counselors, and dieticians who specialize in the care of phenylketonuria patients.

Administered by state or regional governments, most screening programs rely on a central laboratory to measure phenylalanine concentrations in dried blood samples obtained from the neonate between 24 and 72 hours of age. This initial screening reveals about a one percent incidence of positive or indeterminate test results, which are communicated to the primary physician and family so that more quantitative measurements of plasma phenylalanine can be made before the infant reaches two weeks of age. In neonates who undergo a second round of testing, the diagnosis of phenylketonuria is ultimately confirmed in about one percent, which indicates that the disease has a prevalence of one in 10,000. The false-negative rate of newborn screening programs for phenylketonuria is approximately one in 70; these individuals are usually not detected until early childhood, when developmental delay and seizures prompt a comprehensive evaluation for an inborn error of metabolism.[167-171]

Biochemistry of Hyperphenylalaninemia

Phenylalanine is an essential amino acid.[155] Its blood concentration is normally about 0.06 mmol/L and rarely rises above 0.1 mmol/L. Normally, most of the circulating phenylalanine is incorporated into protein and hydroxylated by phenylalanine hydroxylase to form tyrosine, and these processes persist even at the blood concentrations up to 1.0 mmol/L that may be seen in benign, or so-called nonphenylketonuria, hyperphenylalaninemia. At circulating phenylalanine concentrations higher than 1.2 mmol/L, however, phenylalanine is transaminated to form phenylpyruvate, which, along with its degradation product phenylacetate, is secreted in the urine, accounting for the name phenylketonuria. Damage to the CNS in partially treated phenylketonuria patients is more a function of phenylalanine itself than of its metabolites and is directly related to the degree of phenylalanine elevation.

The pathogenesis of CNS abnormalities in phenylketonuria seems to involve a combination of circumstances. Individuals with no phenylalanine hydroxylase activity at all require tyrosine as an essential amino acid, but tyrosine deficiency is not prevalent even among untreated phenylketonuria patients.[172-175] Elevated levels of phenylalanine can inhibit transport of other neutral amino acids across the blood-brain barrier, and this effect may lead to the deficiency of these amino acids specifically in the CSF.[176,177] Perhaps the most significant pathway is that resulting from the direct toxic effect of phenylalanine on the developing brain. Although the exact mechanism of toxicity is unclear, animal models indicate that high levels of phenylalanine (and, to a lesser extent, its metabolites) produce abnormalities in energy production, protein synthesis, and neurotransmitter homeostasis.[178,179] Pathological findings include abnormal areas of myelination, cell packing and density, and dendritic arborization.[180-183]

In about 90 percent of cases, hyperphenylalaninemia, regardless of the degree of elevation, is caused by a deficiency of phenylalanine hydroxylase. There is a stoichiometric requirement for the cofactor tetrahydrobiopterin in the hydroxylation reaction, which becomes converted to dihydrobiopterin and then may be regenerated to tetrahydrobiopterin by the enzyme dihydrobiopterin reductase. Defects in the synthetic pathway for tetrahydrobiopterin or in the enzyme dihydrobiopterin reductase account for about 10 percent of cases of hyperphenylalaninemia.[155,184,185] Because tetrahydrobiopterin is also a cofactor for the hydroxylation of tyrosine and tryptophan to produce catecholamines and serotonin, respectively, individuals with a defect in tetrahydrobiopterin metabolism suffer from abnormalities caused by a deficiency of neurotransmitters. Treatment of such individuals includes, in addition to restriction of dietary phenylalanine, supplementation with L-dopa and 5-hydroxytryptophan.

The pah Gene

Unlike the situation in Duchenne's dystrophy, cystic fibrosis, and neurofibromatosis type 1, much of the clinical biochemistry of phenylalanine metabolism and its disruption in hyperphenylalaninemia was already understood when a rat *pah* cDNA was isolated in 1982 with antibodies to previously purified phenylalanine hydroxylase protein.[186] The 13-exon human *pah* gene stretches over 90 kb and codes for a protein of 451 amino acids with a predicted molecular weight of 51 kd—in accord with previous biochemical analyses suggesting that the human enzyme was a 150 kd homotrimer.[187] Although *pah* was already implicated in the majority of hyperphenylalaninemias associated with phenylketonuria (i.e., those with phenylalanine concentrations persistently higher than 1.2 mmol/L), it rapidly became clear that allelic heterogeneity in *pah* mutations also accounts for the majority of benign hyperphenylalaninemias.[188,189]

DNA sequence analysis and the polymerase chain reaction have identified more than 40 *pah* mutations at the molecular level, helping to define structure-function relations for the phenylalanine hydroxylase protein.[190-194] Most of the mutations are single base-pair alterations that result in missense changes in the mature protein. One particularly common mutation (and also the first to be demonstrated) is, however, a single base-pair change at the splice acceptor site for intron 12, which results in the deletion of the preceding exon from the mature mRNA and therefore produces a truncated protein[195,196] [*see Figure 8*]. In addition, Southern blot analysis of eight polymorphic restriction sites in the *pah* gene has defined many different haplotypes, or unique combinations of RFLPs in linkage disequilibrium.[155,197] Consideration of the association of the various *pah* mutations with different haplotypes in particular populations has shed some light on the factors that account for the relatively high gene frequency of *pah* mutations.[190-194,198-200] In general, there are several mutant alleles within most populations, so that many affected individuals are actually compound heterozygotes at the molecular level. Furthermore, although most populations exhibit linkage disequilibrium between one or more pairs of *pah* mutant alleles and RFLP haplotypes, these relations do not, in general, extend between different ethnic groups.

For example, the initial analysis of Danish families demonstrated 12 different RFLP haplotypes (of the 1,152 that were theoretically possible), and four of these were associated with particular *pah* mutations.[155,197] The intron-12 *pah* mutation accounts for 25/66 of all *pah* mutations in this population and is associated almost exclusively with what has been

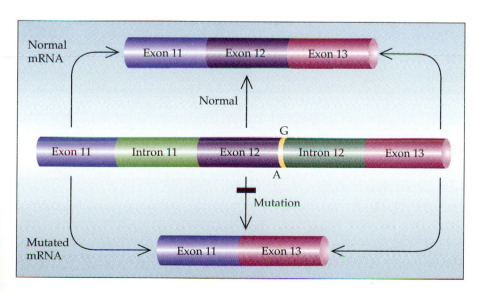

Figure 8 *A common* pah *mutation involves a single base pair change (G to A) at the splice acceptor site for intron 12. This causes exon 12 to be deleted from the mature mRNA and results in a truncated protein.*

designated haplotype 3. The next most frequent *pah* mutation, a base-pair change that causes an arginine-to-tryptophan substitution at position 408, accounts for 13/66 of all *pah* mutations and is associated with haplotype 2. Linkage disequilibrium is present for both mutations, as is indicated by the frequencies of haplotypes 2 and 3 in the general population: 3/66 and 2/66, respectively. Among individuals who have a phenylalanine hydroxylase deficiency, those who are homozygotes or compound heterozygotes for haplotypes 2 and 3 are more severely affected than those who carry haplotype 1 or 4. By contrast, in Chinese populations, 10 percent of *pah* mutations are caused by a nonsense substitution at position 111.[190,191] This mutation, which is not found in Caucasian populations, produces a severe phenotype and is associated with haplotype 4. It seems, therefore, that multiple *pah* mutations have occurred during the course of recent history and that multiple founder effects acting separately on individual mutations are responsible for linkage disequilibrium between particular mutations and RFLP haplotypes.

The incidence of hyperphenylalaninemia varies among different populations. In American blacks it is about one in 50,000, in Yemenite Jews it is about one in 50,000, and in most Northern European populations it is about one in 10,000.[155] The average mutant-gene frequency, about 10^{-2} per chromosome, is from 10 to 100 times higher than that in many other autosomal recessive conditions, and there is no evidence to suggest that the mutation rate is particularly high in this disorder. Because there are multiple *pah* mutant alleles, a selective advantage for phenylketonuria heterozygosity seems the most likely explanation for a high mutant-gene frequency, a suggestion in accord with the variation in phenylketonuria prevalence among different populations. One possible mechanism of selective advantage that has been suggested is that exposure to ochratoxin A, a mycotoxin and potential abortifacient that contaminates food stores in mild wet climates, is less damaging to fetuses of phenylketonuria heterozygotes than to fetuses of homozygous nonmutant individuals.[201,202]

Management of Phenylketonuria and Model Systems

The cornerstone of phenylketonuria management is dietary restriction of phenylalanine.[203] Each patient requires a diet tailored to his or her particular tolerance as determined by serial measurement of blood phenylalanine concentrations; most patients require between 250 and 500 mg of phenylalanine per day to avoid protein starvation. For infants, a program of semisynthetic formula can be combined with breast feeding; in early childhood, a low-protein diet supplemented with special protein hydrolysates or amino acid mixtures can provide sufficient restriction of phenylalanine without protein starvation.[204-206] Paradoxically, the complete phenylalanine restriction of general protein starvation can result in transient hyperphenylalaninemia stemming from a catabolic state and impaired protein synthesis. The goal of therapy is to maintain phenylalanine levels below 1.0 mmol/L, which is from five to 10 times the normal level but within the range of mild phenylalanine hydroxylase deficiency or benign hyperphenylalaninemia that has no phenotypic consequences.[155]

Although the outcome for phenylketonuria patients who are treated early is excellent compared with that for untreated patients, subtle neuropsychological abnormalities remain, which correlate with the degree of phenylalanine elevation over time.[156-158,207] Both treatment quality and patient compliance probably influence the outcome, and there is still a need for alternative treatment strategies. Because regulation of phenylalanine hydroxylase is complex, any attempt at gene therapy based on increasing the activity of this enzyme would probably require introduction of an expression vector into hepatocytes.[208,209] One alternative that has been suggested is based on bacterial phenylalanine-ammonia lyase, which converts phenylalanine into ammonia and *trans*-cinnamic acid, an inert metabolite.[210,211] Introduction of the bacterial enzyme into the gastrointestinal lumen in semipermeable microcapsules might allow phenylalanine to be converted into its metabolites without induction of immune rejection.

When centralized screening and treatment programs for phenylketonuria were first implemented, the dietary restriction of phenylalanine was discontinued at late childhood or adolescence in many clinics. It soon became clear that, even though the neonatal brain is indeed particularly susceptible to the damaging effects of hyperphenylalaninemia, early termination of treatment might be associated with a slow but progressive decline in cognitive function.[212] Although careful controlled trials have not yet been performed in individuals at all ages, most clinics currently recommend that treatment continue indefinitely.

Whereas mouse models for cystic fibrosis and neurofibromatosis type 1 will probably be developed by genetic engineering of embryonic stem cells, attempts to develop animal models for phenylketonuria have focused on chemical mutagenesis of the whole organism, followed by measurement of blood phenylalanine to screen for possible *pah* mutations. In 1987, a mouse mutation called *hph-1* (for hereditary persistence of hyperphenylalaninemia-1) was discovered; later it was shown to be a defect in the biosynthetic pathway for tetrahydrobiopterin.[213,214] In 1990, a true mutation in *pah* was discovered (*pahhph-5*) that appears to represent a partial loss of function.[215] Mice carrying these genes should be helpful for evaluating potential therapies for human phenylketonuria.

Maternal Phenylketonuria

As an increasing number of women who have been treated for phenylketonuria reach childbearing age, the problem, alluded to above, of fetal hyperphenylalaninemia resulting from intrauterine exposure will increase in magnitude.[159,160] In addition, pregnancies in women with benign hyperphenylalaninemia, who have not been treated and may only have been identified at birth through a screening program, may also be at increased risk for fetal hyperphenylalaninemia, because the concentration of phenylalanine is generally from two to three times as high in fetal blood as in maternal blood. Exposure to concentrations of phenylalanine higher than 1.2 mmol/L in utero produces mental retardation, microcephaly and growth retardation of prenatal onset, and congenital heart disease, regardless of the fetal genotype.[162] Rigorous control of maternal phenylalanine concentrations from before conception until birth may lower the incidence of fetal abnormalities in maternal phenylketonuria, but achieving practical results in large numbers of patients is problematic.[161,163] Future efforts will focus on identifying, tracking, and educating individuals at risk for these problems, either via central registries or by rescreening as adults.[164]

Beckwith-Wiedemann Syndrome

The combination of macroglossia (a large tongue), macrosomatia (somatic overgrowth), and umbilical abnormalities such as herniation, omphalocele, or both, are the cardinal features of Beckwith-Wiedemann syndrome: these characteristics account for the alternative designation, exomphalos-macroglossia-gigantism syndrome.[216,217] The condition is notable in several respects, and research into its causes illuminates many aspects of human genetics. First, Beckwith-Wiedemann syndrome exhibits a pattern of inheritance that can be explained only by extreme variability of expression or by an exception to mendelian principles. Second, Beckwith-Wiedemann syndrome can be caused either by a single locus inherited in an autosomal dominant fashion or (sporadically) by a partial duplication of chromosome 11p15 that involves the paternal homologue. In the latter case, association with a cytogenetic abnormality suggests that some of the phenotypic features of Beckwith-Wiedemann syndrome may be explainable as a contiguous-gene syndrome, in which altered expression of a group of linked genes contributes in an additive fashion to the syndromic phenotype. Finally, several lines of evidence have converged to suggest that development of Beckwith-Wiedemann syndrome involves parental imprinting, a recently discovered phenomenon wherein the expression of homologous genes depends on whether they were inherited from the mother or the father.

Phenotypic Features of Beckwith-Wiedemann Syndrome

The diagnosis of Beckwith-Wiedemann syndrome is usually made within the first few days of life when one or more suggestive physical features are recognized. The incidence has been estimated at one in 13,700.[218] In addition to omphalocele, macroglossia, and macrosomatia, the abnormalities frequently observed at birth include umbilical hernia; characteristic facial features; disproportionate overgrowth of one or more extremities (hemihypertrophy); hyperplasia or dysplasia of the kidneys, adrenal cortex, and pancreas; persistent hypoglycemia; and polycythemia.[216,219-222] The craniofacial abnormalities, which often become more apparent during the first year of life, include prominent eyes, capillary hemangiomas on the central forehead or eyelids, small pits on the posterior aspect of the external ear and unusual creases on the ear lobe, and a prominent mandible. Beckwith-Wiedemann syndrome patients also exhibit increased susceptibility to embryonal tumors including nephroblastoma, hepatoblastoma, gonadoblastoma, adrenocortical carcinoma, and rhabdomyosarcoma; occasionally, one of these tumors may be present at birth.[220,223,224]

There are no formal diagnostic criteria for Beckwith-Wiedemann syndrome, but the presence of several characteristic manifestations accompanied by a positive family history or partial duplication of 11p15 is usually considered confirmatory. Because many Beckwith-Wiedemann syndrome carriers manifest only subtle findings, a comprehensive family history that includes examination of first-degree relatives may be helpful.[217,225,226] Initial management of Beckwith-Wiedemann syndrome patients focuses on hypoglycemia and macroglossia.[227] Anticipation, careful monitoring, and (if necessary) treatment of hypoglycemia for the first few months of life may prevent subsequent neurologic complications. Pharyngeal obstruction by the large tongue can interfere with feeding and, in severe cases, with breathing, leading to positional or sleep-dependent oxygen desaturation.[228] These problems can be addressed by special nipples, careful positioning, and (if necessary) partial surgical resections of the tongue.[229] During early childhood, regular imaging studies of Beckwith-Wiedemann syndrome patients are indicated to detect embryonal tumors, which occur with a frequency of about 10 percent, Wilms' tumor being the most common.[220] Abdominal ultrasonography is recommended at three- to four-month intervals in early childhood and at six-month intervals in adolescence.[230]

In general, the natural history of Beckwith-Wiedemann syndrome is characterized by a decline in the excessive growth rate, and many childhood characteristics of the syndrome become less apparent with age.[231] Although there are some reports of mild to moderate developmental delay, this is not an invariable feature and may result, in part, from repeated hypoglycemia during the first few months of life.

Inheritance of Beckwith-Wiedemann Syndrome

The initial reports of Beckwith-Wiedemann syndrome in the 1960s noted several examples of familial occurrence. In several pedigrees, a Beckwith-Wiedemann syndrome gene has been mapped to chromosome 11p15, but the exact characteristics of inheritance are still controversial.[232,233] Pedigrees with affected members in multiple generations, a lack of evidence of sex-specific expression, and a mathematical analysis demonstrating that affected individuals transmit the condition to half of their offspring all suggest autosomal dominant inheritance.[234] However, there are many pedigrees in which obligate carriers from a single sibship manifest few if any signs of the condition, monozygotic twins are often discordant for the condition, and there is a peculiar lack of affected children born to male obligate carriers.[226,235] Several explanations have been proposed for these observations, including an unusual degree of variable expressivity, incomplete penetrance, or both; a role for parental-specific genomic imprinting (see below); or a two-step process in which nonpenetrant carriers transmit a so-called premutation that leads to full-blown Beckwith-Wiedemann syndrome only after a second event that is not yet understood.[226,234-236] (When the two-step process was proposed, there was no molecular basis in any human genetic condition for a premutation, but now it does appear that fragile X mental retardation may provide such a precedent (see below). Still, the epidemiologic data to support two-step mutation has always been much stronger in fragile X mental retardation than in Beckwith-Wiedemann syndrome, and so speculation regarding such a process in Beckwith-Wiedemann syndrome remains unjustified.)

A different line of research has led to the suggestion that Beckwith-Wiedemann syndrome may result from altered expression of several linked genes. In the 1980s it was recognized that partial duplication of chromosome 11p15 frequently accompanied sporadic cases of Beckwith-

Wiedemann syndrome, and that some familial cases that lacked the duplication exhibited linkage to 11p15 markers.[232,233,237,238] This chromosomal region contains the genes for insulin and insulinlike growth factor–2 (IGF-2) and the Ha-*ras*-1 and *int*-2 proto-oncogenes. Because each of these genes could logically be implicated in the pathogenesis of one or more aspects of Beckwith-Wiedemann syndrome, it has been suggested that increased expression of some or all of the genes in 11p15 contributes to the phenotype of Beckwith-Wiedemann syndrome and that patients who have no detectable chromosomal abnormality might have micro-duplications.[239] Subsequently, however, careful molecular studies of both the sporadic and familial forms of Beckwith-Wiedemann syndrome demonstrated that most patients with this syndrome do not carry more than the normal two copies of these genes.[240,241] Although it is not yet clear how Beckwith-Wiedemann syndrome might be caused in some cases by a single gene and in other cases by increased expression of several linked genes, this puzzle has been partially illuminated by the recent recognition of parental imprinting.

Elegant genetic studies in the mouse have revealed that for many genes the expression of each homologue depends on the parent from whom it was inherited.[242-245] In particular, the mouse gene for IGF-2 is expressed only on the chromosome inherited from the father, whereas the closely linked gene *H19* (whose function is not yet known) is expressed only on the chromosome inherited from the mother [*see Figure 9*].[246-248] This property is thought to be acquired during formation of the egg or sperm, when a gene is modified, or imprinted, in such a way that its state of expression during the life of the offspring remains constant. Although the molecular basis, persistence, and extent of this phenomenon have not yet been clarified, imprinting represents a fundamental aspect of mammalian development and is implicated in several human genetic diseases.[249]

The first suggestion that imprinting might play a pathogenetic role in Beckwith-Wiedemann syndrome came from the study of chromosomal abnormalities in Wilms' tumor, which can occur either in association with Beckwith-Wiedemann syndrome, as an isolated autosomal dominant condition, or as a sporadic event. Because studies of another childhood cancer, retinoblastoma, had revealed that tumor cells often lose one of the two homologues for the retinoblastoma gene, investigators made a systematic search for a similar loss of heterozygosity in Wilms' tumors from many patients.[140,250-254] The search first focused on chromosome 11p, because constitutional deletions (affecting every cell in the body) of 11p13 had already been implicated in a certain percentage of Wilms' tumors.[255] In some cases in which there was no cytogenetic abnormality, loss of heterozygosity for 11p13 was observed. This region was later found to contain a candidate gene for sporadic Wilms' tumor, WT-1.[256-258] Surprisingly, however, a large fraction of the tumors (some of them from Beckwith-Wiedemann syndrome patients) exhibited loss of heterozygosity for DNA markers on chromosome 11p15, distal to the WT-1 gene.[253,254] Furthermore, analysis of RFLPs of both parents showed that in most cases the maternal allele was lost and the paternal allele was retained.[252]

Substantive evidence of a role for genomic imprinting in the pathogenesis of Beckwith-Wiedemann syndrome came from a recent molecular

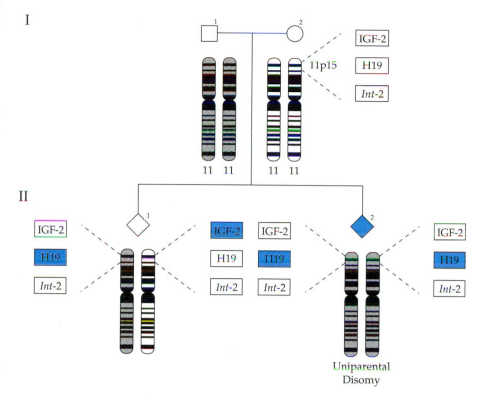

Figure 9   *The diagram illustrates parental-specific gene expression (genomic imprinting) and its potential consequences in the face of uniparental disomy. Normally, offspring inherit one homologue from each parent, as II-1 does. Epigenetic modifications during gametogenesis—so-called imprinting—may prevent a gene from being expressed in somatic cells of the zygote derived from that gamete (indicated by shading). In the mouse, for example, IGF-2 is not expressed from the maternally derived homologue, H19 is not expressed from the paternally derived homologue, and int-2 is expressed from both homologues. In some humans affected with Beckwith-Wiedemann syndrome, both copies of the region surrounding 11p15 originate from the paternal homologue. Consequent abnormalities in the overall level of gene expression for IGF-2, H19, and possibly other imprinted genes in the region may cause some of the features of the syndrome. (In II-2, both chromosome 11 homologues are of paternal origin in their entirety, but postzygotic events, including mitotic recombination, nondisjunction, and chromosomal reduplication, may also produce uniparental disomy for only part of the chromosome.)*

investigation of eight sporadic cases of the disease.[259] All patients were found to carry the normal two copies of chromosome 11p15 alleles, but pedigree analysis of RFLPs demonstrated that three patients had inherited both alleles from the father: so-called uniparental disomy [*see Figure 9*]. Although the origin and mechanism of uniparental disomy is unknown, because Beckwith-Wiedemann syndrome patients with partial trisomy for 11p15 usually carry an extra paternal rather than an extra maternal copy, it seems likely that, both in patients with uniparental disomy and in those with the trisomy, the condition develops via a common mechanism: overexpression of a gene or genes expressed only from the paternal homologue.[244,260]

As mentioned above, studies in mice also show that IGF-2 is expressed only from the paternal chromosome.[246-248] Overexpression of IGF-2 is an excellent candidate for some features of Beckwith-Wiedemann syndrome because in the mouse, the loss of IGF-2 leads to decreased fetal growth and low birthweight, and in the human, IGF-2 is often highly expressed in tumors from Beckwith-Wiedemann syndrome patients.[261,262]

In summary, there appear to be two distinct etiologies of Beckwith-Wiedemann syndrome. First, a single gene on 11p15 may be responsible in cases in which the condition is familial and there is no apparent cytogenetic abnormality. Second, altered expression of several linked genes, as in uniparental disomy and partial trisomy for 11p15, appears to cause some fraction of sporadic Beckwith-Wiedemann syndrome cases. It is intriguing to speculate that the familial form of the disorder represents a heritable mutation that affects the expression, or the susceptibility to imprinting, of closely linked genes. As with other human genetic diseases, answers to these questions are likely to come from mouse models that reproduce some or all components of the Beckwith-Wiedmann syndrome phenotype.

The Fragile X Mental Retardation Syndrome

Although it has long been appreciated that moderate to severe mental retardation affects about 25 percent more males than females, the association of male mental retardation with a cytogenetic abnormality of the X chromosome was not described until 1969.[263] In a variable fraction of an individual's cells, a region between bands Xq27 and Xq28 that fails to condense normally at metaphase appears as a thin constriction. This region, termed fraXq27.3, and similar ones elsewhere in the genome are designated fragile sites because normally condensed material distal to the constriction appears separated from the rest of the chromosome and because the constricted region is prone to breakage.[264,265] Males affected with the fragile X mental retardation syndrome exhibit several characteristic features involving several different systems; in fact, 26 years before its association with fraXq27.3, the clinical phenotype was recognized as a distinct mental retardation syndrome (by authors whose names account for the alternative designation for this disorder, Martin-Bell syndrome).[266] The unusual inheritance of the fragile X mental retardation syndrome and the molecular nature of the fragile site have intrigued and perplexed human geneticists over the past decade.[267,268] Even though the condition is X-linked, about a third of carrier females exhibit some degree of cognitive disability. More surprising, at least 20 percent of carrier males manifest no signs of the condition. Daughters of these nonpenetrant but transmitting males are themselves nonpenetrant but produce affected offspring, male and female, with frequencies close to mendelian expectations.[265] In general, nonpenetrant carriers of the condition do not exhibit the fragile X chromosome on cytogenetic testing, and so their diagnosis has depended on pedigree analysis. Among individuals in whom the fragile X mental retardation syndrome is considered because of suggestive clinical signs, diagnosis based on cytogenetic testing for the fragile site has been confounded by the special culture conditions required for fragile-site expression and the variable fraction of cells that express the fragile site.

A critical step was taken toward resolving these problems when the segment of DNA spanning the fragile site was isolated in 1991: it was found to include a highly repetitive region of DNA whose instability in length seemed to explain the unusual inheritance pattern.[269,270] Individuals with a slightly lengthened repetitive segment are clinically normal and are said to carry a premutation. Transformation to a full mutation comes when the slightly lengthened segment becomes even longer (in the course of transmission through the female germline) and produces the clinical features of fragile X mental retardation syndrome. Although the responsible mechanisms have yet to be clarified, these extraordinary findings are the basis for a fundamental new principle of human inheritance, the multistep mutation.

Phenotype and Incidence

The most consistent features of fragile X mental retardation syndrome in males are mental retardation and large testes.[271-274] About 90 percent of affected males have an IQ between 20 and 60 and a testicular volume greater than 30 ml (the normal range being from 10 to 20 ml). In early childhood, however, males usually come to clinical attention because of a delay in motor milestones or such behavioral problems as attention-deficit disorder, stereotypic hand movements, and rapid speech with stuttering or perseveration. Testes are usually not enlarged before puberty. In severely retarded fragile X mental retardation individuals, reduced speech and minimal social interactions may prompt an incorrect diagnosis of infantile autism. Characteristic craniofacial features (usually not apparent until later childhood) include mild coarsening of facial features, large ears, a prominent forehead and mandible, a long face, and relative macrocephaly (considered in relation to height).[274] Systemic features involving connective tissue are often present as well: hypotonia and small-joint hyperextensibility in infancy and early childhood and mitral-valve prolapse and bony deformities such as pes planus or pectus excavatum during adolescence. Females affected with the syndrome manifest most of the features seen in males but to a lesser degree. Most affected females have a nonverbal IQ below 85 and exhibit neuropsychological deficits in visuospatial abilities when compared to females who do not have this syndrome but have similar IQ scores.[275,276]

The incidence of fragile X mental retardation syndrome in males is about one in 1,500. It is the most common form of inherited mental retardation and ranks behind only trisomy 21, or Down syndrome, as a "genetic" cause of mental retardation.[277-280] The incidence in females is difficult to estimate precisely because many females with the condition are only mildly retarded. Given that there are no well-established cases of new mutations, for every affected male there are likely to be multiple female relatives who either are mildly retarded themselves or are at risk of producing affected male offspring.

Diagnosis

The fraXq27.3 site is one of 18 so-called rare fragile sites dispersed among 12 autosomes and the X chromosome. All the sites in this class are expressed in a small fraction of cells in a minority of individuals, but they are transmitted from one generation to the next as a single genetic locus. Only fraXq27.3 has been associated with a disease state. Initial attempts to use the presence of fraXq27.3 as the basis of a cytogenetic test for fragile X mental retardation syndrome were frustrated by the low fraction of cells that expressed the fragile site: no more than one or two percent of the lymphocytes from affected males, under normal culture conditions.[264] Eventually, several conditions that resulted in depletion of the intracellular pyrimidine deoxynucleotide triphosphates dTTP and dCTP (immediate precursors of DNA synthesis) were found to enhance fragile-site expression in lymphocytes. Under these conditions, from 10 to 50 percent of the cells in most affected males express the fragile site, making it possible to apply testing for the presence of fraXq27.3 widely and successfully in the diagnosis of the fragile X mental retardation syndrome in mentally retarded males.[265,281] Even under optimal culture conditions, however, most carrier females express the fragile site in only two to 10 percent of their cells. Because even individuals who are not carriers of fragile X mental retardation syndrome may exhibit fraXq27.3 in one or two percent of their cells, the detection of carrier females is complicated by diagnostic errors, both positive and negative.[281,282] Similarly, attempts to make the presence of fraXq27.3 in amniocytes the basis of prenatal diagnosis have been complicated by a generally lower level of fragile-site expression in such cells than in lymphocytes.[283] These and other problems with fragile-site analysis as a diagnostic test are likely to be resolved now that the DNA spanning the fragile site has been isolated (see below).

Inheritance Pattern

Even from the initial descriptions of Martin-Bell syndrome in 1943, in which two clinically normal brothers produced nine retarded grandsons, it was clear that this condition exhibited an unusual inheritance pattern.[266] Analysis of a large number of families has generated empirical risk figures that reflect a number of features of fragile X mental retardation syndrome inheritance[265,268] [see Figure 10]. First, for the offspring of affected carrier females, penetrance is 100 percent in sons and 56 percent in daughters, but for the offspring of unaffected carrier females, penetrance is 80 percent in sons and 32 percent in daughters. Simply stated (and counter to previously established genetic principles), the phenotype of an individual influences the likelihood that the offspring will be affected. Second, about 20 percent of carrier males manifest no signs of the condition and are diagnosed as carriers only by retrospective pedigree analysis. Daughters of these transmitting males are completely nonpenetrant, but maternal grandsons and granddaughters (children of a daughter) are 80 percent and 32 percent penetrant, respectively. This observation suggests that expression of the disease requires passage through the female germline. Third, transmitting males tend to occur in the same sibship with each other and with nonpenetrant carrier females. This is reflected in low penetrance figures for brothers and sisters of transmitting males—18 percent and 10 percent, respectively—compared with 80 percent and 32 percent for their maternal grandsons and granddaughters. (This last observation, occasionally referred to as the Sherman paradox, may be in part an artifact of ascertainment.)

Molecular Models

Various molecular models have been put forth to explain one or more aspects of the unusual inheritance pattern of fragile X mental retardation syndrome. Transposable elements whose expression depends on maternal transmission, an autosomal locus that modifies fragile X mental retardation syndrome expression, and explanations based on the cycle of X chromosome inactivation and reactivation have all been proposed, but with little experimental data or precedent.[284,285] In retrospect, a model that proposed several different states of mutability for the fragile X mental retardation syndrome locus now seems most consistent with current observations, although the factors that influence mutability are still unclear.[286] As originally envisioned, this two-step model suggested that the locus contained a pyrimidine-rich sequence that could exist as a normal allele, a premutation, and a full mutation, and that progression from one allele to the others involved DNA amplification of the pyrimidine-rich sequence during meiotic recombination. As described below, it now appears that progressive lengthening of an unstable DNA sequence accounts for the different steps in the development of the fragile X mental retardation syndrome. However, the sequence of this unstable region is not particularly pyrimidine-rich, and its amplification does not appear to be absolutely dependent on meiotic recombination.

Evidence for Molecular Basis of Disease

Molecular clones spanning fraXq27.3 were isolated by several groups in 1991. They used DNA markers that had been closely linked to the fragile X mental retardation syndrome in genetic analyses to isolate large frag-

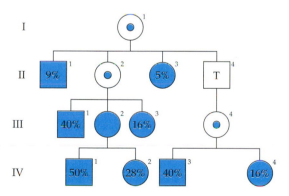

Figure 10 *Shown is an idealized pedigree of a fragile X family illustrating the risk of mental retardation in individual members (percentages). IV-1 and IV-2 are offspring of a penetrant female (III-2) and exhibit 100 percent and 56 percent penetrance, respectively. (Because carrier females may pass on either the mutant or the nonmutant X chromosome, the risk of mental retardation is equal to the penetrance divided by two.) IV-3 and IV-4 are offspring of a nonpenetrant female (III-4) and exhibit 80 percent and 32 percent penetrance, respectively. II-4 is a nonpenetrant (transmitting) male, recognized only because of his affected grandchildren. Penetrance in his offspring (III-4, an obligate carrier) is zero percent. Transmitting males (II-4) tend to occur in the same sibship with each other and with nonpenetrant females, as reflected by the lower risk of mental retardation in II-1 and II-3 than in IV-3 and IV-4. II-2 is an obligate carrier.*

ments of human genomic DNA in yeast artificial chromosome vectors.[354,355,379,380] The region of DNA that spanned the fragile site was rapidly localized to a 5.2 kb *Eco*RI restriction fragment, within which were found three remarkable clues to the molecular basis of the fragile X mental retardation syndrome.

METHYLATED CpG ISLAND

First, a short stretch of DNA subject to methylation was located in about the middle of the fragment.[270,287,288] Because methylation of cytosine to 5-methylcytosine occurs only when cytosine is followed by guanine (5′-CpG-3′) and because sites that are susceptible to methylation are often clustered together in eukaryotic genomes, these regions are referred to as CpG islands. Most CpG islands are unmethylated and are located close to housekeeping genes, which code for essential intracellular functions. In females, however, in whom nearly all the genes on one of the two X chromosomes are normally silenced by X chromosome inactivation, CpG islands on the inactive chromosome are methylated. The methylation status of the CpG island within the 5.2 kb *Eco*RI fragment has been determined (with restriction enzymes that distinguish between methylated and unmethylated DNA) in a large number of families affected by the fragile X mental retardation syndrome.[289] Surprisingly, the CpG island is methylated in affected males but unmethylated in nonpenetrant transmitting males. In females, the CpG island on the inactive X chromosome is always methylated, regardless of their fragile X mental retardation syndrome status; the CpG island on the active X chromosome is methylated in females affected with the fragile X mental retardation syndrome but unmethylated in nonpenetrant carrier females. That is to say, both for the single X chromosome in males and for the active X chromosome in females, methylation of the CpG island correlates almost precisely with expression of the fragile X mental retardation syndrome phenotype.

TRANSCRIBED SEQUENCE

A second clue to the molecular basis of the fragile X mental retardation syndrome became apparent when a transcribed region was found to lie within the 5.2 kb *Eco*RI fragment.[290] Molecular probes from this region detect a 4.8 kb mRNA that is expressed in fetal brain and lymphocytes but not in fetal liver, lung, or kidney. Partial sequence analysis of the cDNA, which has been termed the *fmr*-1 gene, has not indicated a particular function. A role in the fragile X mental retardation syndrome seems likely, however, because *fmr*-1 was not expressed in the lymphocytes of 16 out of 20 affected males.[291] Cells from the remaining four patients appeared to be a mixture of those that expressed *fmr*-1 and were not methylated at the nearby CpG island and those that did not express *fmr*-1 and were methylated at the nearby CpG island. In other words, the presence of methylation in just a fraction of cells seems sufficient to produce the fragile X mental retardation syndrome phenotype, even though the *fmr*-1 cDNA may still be expressed from the fraction of cells in which the CpG island is unmethylated.

UNSTABLE DNA SEGMENT

A final clue to the molecular basis of the fragile X mental retardation syndrome has come from the recognition that the *fmr*-1 coding region includes a segment of DNA that exhibits instability in length.[269,270,292] The unstable segment contains the sequence $(5'–CCG-3')_n$ and potentially codes for a polyarginine tract; n is equal to about 40 ± 25 in individuals who are neither affected with nor carriers of the fragile X mental retardation syndrome. In transmitting males and in unaffected carrier females, the length of the $(5'-CCG-3')_n$ tract is increased from 100 to 500 bp, which produces a corresponding increase in the 5.2 kb *Eco*RI fragment. In affected males and females, the length of the $(5'-CCG-3')_n$ tract is increased by more than 600 bp and is generally heterogeneous, suggesting that once this threshold is reached, additional amplification occurs frequently in somatic cells. Like the methylation of the CpG island, both cytogenetic expression of fraXq27.3 and the clinical fragile X mental retardation syndrome phenotype correlate almost precisely with increases in length greater than 600 bp. Most important, the 100 to 500 bp increases in length provide both a molecular explanation for the carrier state and a diagnostic tool for identifying unaffected carriers of the fragile X mental retardation syndrome premutation.

Restriction enzyme digests that examine both methylation of the CpG island and potential length increases of the 5.2 kb *Eco*RI fragment have now been performed on more than 500 individuals from 63 fragile X mental retardation syndrome families.[289] Together with the observations cited above, the results provide a unifying explanation for the inheritance and cytogenetics of the fragile X mental retardation syndrome. Although there is some polymorphism in the length of the $(5'-CCG-3')_n$ tract among normal individuals, amplification has not yet been observed if the number of repeats is less than 65. Larger numbers of repeats produce the premutation: the 100 to 500 bp increase in the size of the 5.2 kb *Eco*RI fragment. Individuals who carry the premutation are clinically and cytogenetically normal, but transmission of the premutation through the female germline is associated with a high probability (about 80 percent in this retrospective study) of further amplification to produce increases in length greater than 600 bp and the full mutation. In cells that carry the full mutation, the CpG island is methylated, and the *fmr*-1 gene is not expressed, and if the cells are exposed to appropriate culture conditions, the fraXq27.3 site can be visualized about 50 percent of the time. About 15 percent of the fragile X mental retardation syndrome patients who carry the full mutation also carry the premutation in some of their cells, but they are clinically indistinguishable from nonmosaic individuals with the fragile X mental retardation syndrome.

IMPLICATIONS OF FINDINGS

These findings will have a dramatic impact on the approach to inherited mental retardation. Because increases in length of the 5.2 kb *Eco*RI fragment can now be determined efficiently and precisely, female carriers of the full mutation can be identified unequivocally, and appropriate genetic counseling steps can be taken for related family members. Prenatal diagnosis of fragile X mental retardation syndrome can now be based on examination of amniocytes, so that pregnancies in which a premutation has progressed to a full mutation can be identified reliably. (It remains to be determined if somatic mosaicism for the full mutation can be diagnosed reliably from a sample of amniocytes or whether fetal blood sampling will be necessary to completely exclude false-negative diagnoses.) Finally, male and female carriers of the premutation can be identified prospectively to determine the mutation rate, the incidence, and the true likelihood of progression to the full mutation. A significant incidence of the premutation in the general population would have important societal and ethical implications.

Despite these dramatic advances, several questions remain. Daughters of transmitting males are always nonpenetrant, and it is not known why progression of the premutation to the full mutation requires passage through the female germline. Among individuals who carry the full mutation, it is not yet clear whether length amplification, CpG methylation, absence of *fmr*-1 expression, fraXq27.3 expression, or a combination of these events ultimately leads to the fragile X mental retardation syndrome phenotype. In particular, the relation of the *fmr*-1 gene product to the phenotype of the disease needs to be clarified. If the absence of an essential gene product encoded by *fmr*-1 leads to mental retardation, craniofacial abnormalities, and large testes, it remains to be explained why individuals mosaic for *fmr*-1 expression manifest phenotypic features indistinguishable from those of nonmosaic individuals, and why the alterations in the size of the *fmr*-1 gene product seen in the premutation are phenotypically silent. It is possible that there are additional nearby genes whose expression is affected by length amplification and CpG methylation in the 5.2 kb *Eco*RI fragment and that these genes have a role in the pathogenesis of the fragile X mental retardation syndrome. It is also possible that part of the disease phenotype results from a loss of distal X chromosomal material after the expression of fraXq27.3 in vivo and that cells of the CNS and gonads are more prone to conditions that perturb pyrimidine triphosphate levels. Regardless of the answers to these questions (which should come quite rapidly), the fragile X mental retardation syndrome has provided a new paradigm for understanding human heredity and disease.

The Future of Human Genetics

The tools of molecular biology have brought the field of human genetics into a new era. The isolation of genes responsible for specific inherited disorders not only has provided insight into their pathogenesis but also has made available new techniques for reliable diagnosis and informed genetic counseling and has illuminated new avenues to explore for treatment of genetic disease. Several ongoing areas of research are likely to have an additional impact on human genetics. Concerted attempts to map and to sequence the human genome will dramatically increase the rate at which new disease genes are identified and isolated. It is easy to foresee a time when most single-gene disorders can be diagnosed at or shortly after conception, providing opportunities for intervention and treatment at the earliest possible stage. Both conventional drugs and bioengineered agents as well as gene therapy are likely to have a role in the treatment of hereditary disorders, although the delivery of therapeutic agents to the proper tissues and at the appropriate time remains a considerable obstacle.

Attempts to understand the molecular basis of common diseases such as cancer and atherosclerosis have demonstrated that genetic susceptibility has an important role in their expression, even though these conditions are, for the most part, not inherited as mendelian characteristics. New techniques of analyzing populations that do not depend solely on mendelian relations will help define the number and relative importance of such genes. For example, it seems likely that alleles at several major loci that influence endothelial integrity, apolipoprotein metabolism, and vascular remodeling determine the probability that an individual will develop premature cardiovascular disease. These genes and their alleles may well be identified within the next decade, making it possible to distinguish susceptible individuals and to intervene appropriately before the onset of disease.

Finally, reproductive technologies that make possible the isolation and culture of gametes, in vitro fertilization, and limited preimplantation development will afford a number of dramatic opportunities for alleviating human disease. The potential consequences of such opportunities will need to be considered carefully. Most scientific and political bodies have agreed, for example, that even though germline alterations of vertebrate and invertebrate animals are permissible and worthwhile, manipulations that affect human eggs or sperm should not be entertained. The number of such decisions and their implications for individuals affected with hereditary disease will increase in the near future. As the opportunites for diagnosis and treatment of hereditary disease continue to increase, so will the responsibility of physicians and scientists to consider their societal and ethical implications.

References

1. Emery AEH: *Duchenne Muscular Dystrophy*. Oxford University Press, New York, 1987

2. Harper PS: The muscular dystrophies. *The Metabolic Basis of Inherited Disease*. Scriver CR, Beaudet AL, Sly WS, et al, Eds. McGraw-Hill, New York, 1989, p 2869

3. Duchenne GBA: Recherches sur la paralysie musculaire pseudohypertrophique ou paralysie myo-sclerosique. *Arch Gen Med* 11:5, 1868

4. Dubowitz V: Intellectual impairment in muscular dystrophy. *Arch Dis Child* 40:296, 1965

5. Turner PR, Westwood T, Regen CM, et al: Increased protein degradation results from elevated free calcium levels found in muscle from mdx mice. *Nature* 335:735, 1988

6. Boyd Y, Buckle VJ: Cytogenetic heterogeneity of translocations associated with Duchenne muscular dystrophy. *Clin Genet* 29:108, 1986

7. Boyd Y, Buckle V, Holt S, et al: Muscular dystrophy in girls with X;autosome translocations. *J Med Genet* 23:484, 1986

8. Francke U, Harper JF, Darras BT, et al: Congenital adrenal hypoplasia, myopathy, and glycerol kinase deficiency: molecular genetic evidence for deletions. *Am J Hum Genet* 40:212, 1987

9. Francke U, Ochs HD, De Martinville B, et al: Minor Xp21 chromosome deletion in a male associated with expression of Duchenne muscular dystrophy, chronic granulo-

matous disease, retinitis pigmentosa and McLeod syndrome. *Am J Hum Genet* 37:250, 1985

10. Kunkel LM, Monaco AP, Middlesworth W, et al: Specific cloning of DNA fragments absent from the DNA of a male patient with an X chromosome deletion. *Proc Natl Acad Sci USA* 82:4778, 1985

11. Monaco AP, Bertelson CJ, Middlesworth W, et al: Detection of deletions spanning the Duchenne muscular dystrophy locus using a tightly linked DNA segment. *Nature* 316:842, 1985

12. Worton RG, Duff C, Sylvester JE, et al: Duchenne muscular dystrophy involving translocation of the DMD gene next to ribosomal RNA genes. *Science* 224:1447, 1984

13. Ray PN, Belfall B, Duff C, et al: Cloning of the breakpoint of an X;21 translocation associated with Duchenne muscular dystrophy. *Nature* 318:672, 1985

14. Monaco AP, Neve RL, Colletti-Feener C, et al: Isolation of candidate cDNAs for portions of the Duchenne muscular dystrophy gene. *Nature* 323:646, 1986

15. Koenig M, Hoffman EP, Bertelson CJ, et al: Complete cloning of the Duchenne muscular dystrophy (DMD) cDNA and preliminary genomic organization of the DMD gene in normal and affected individuals. *Cell* 50:509, 1987

16. Kunkel LM: Analysis of deletions in DNA from patients with Becker and Duchenne muscular dystrophy. *Nature* 322:73, 1986

17. Gillard EF, Chamberlain JS, Murphy EG, et al: Molecular and phenotypic analysis of patients with deletions within the deletion-rich region of the Duchenne muscular dystrophy (DMD) gene. *Am J Hum Genet* 45:507, 1989

18. Den Dunnen JT, Grootscholten PM, Bakker E, et al: Topography of the Duchenne muscular dystrophy (DMD) gene: FIGE and cDNA analysis of 194 cases reveals 115 deletions and 13 duplications. *Am J Hum Genet* 45:835, 1989

19. Van Ommen GJ, Verkerk JM, Hofker MH, et al: A physical map of 4 million bp around the Duchenne muscular dystrophy gene on the human X-chromosome. *Cell* 47:499, 1986

20. Davie AM, Emery AE: Estimation of proportion of new mutants among cases of Duchenne muscular dystrophy. *J Med Genet* 15:339, 1978

21. Hoffman EP, Kunkel LM: Dystrophin abnormalities in Duchenne/Becker muscular dystrophy. *Neuron* 2:1019, 1989

22. Mulley JC, Haan EA, Sheffield LJ, et al: Recombination frequencies between Duchenne muscular dystrophy and intragenic markers in multigeneration families. *Hum Genet* 78:296, 1988

23. Abbs S, Roberts RG, Mathew CG, et al: Accurate assessment of intragenic recombination frequency within the Duchenne muscular dystrophy gene. *Genomics* 7:602, 1990

24. Chen JD, Hejtmancik JF, Romeo G, et al: A genetic linkage map of five marker loci in and around the Duchenne muscular dystrophy locus. *Genomics* 4:105, 1989

25. Wapenaar MC, Kievits T, Hart KA, et al: A deletion hot spot in the Duchenne muscular dystrophy gene. *Genomics* 2:101, 1988

26. Blonden LA, Grootscholten PM, den Dunnen JT, et al: 242 breakpoints in the 200-kb deletion-prone P20 region of the DMD gene are widely spread. *Genomics* 10:631, 1991

27. Beggs AH, Koenig M, Boyce FM, et al: Detection of 98% of DMD/BMD gene deletions by polymerase chain reaction. Hum Genet 86:45, 1990

28. Clemens PR, Fenwick RG, Chamberlain JS, et al: Carrier detection and prenatal diagnosis in Duchenne and Becker muscular dystrophy families, using dinucleotide repeat polymorphisms. *Am J Hum Genet* 49:951, 1991

29. Roberts RG, Barby TF, Manners E, et al: Direct detection of dystrophin gene rearrangements by analysis of dystrophin mRNA in peripheral blood lymphocytes. *Am J Hum Genet* 49:298, 1991

30. Murphy EA, Mutalik GS: The application of Bayesian methods in genetic counselling. *Hum Hered* 19:126, 1969

31. Haldane JBS: The rate of spontaneous mutation of a human gene. *J Genet* 31:317, 1935

32. Zatz M, Passos BM, Rapaport D, et al: Familial occurrence of Duchenne dystrophy through paternal lines in four families. *Am J Med Genet* 38:80, 1991

33. Hoffman EP, Brown RH, Kunkel LM: Dystrophin: the protein product of the Duchenne muscular dystrophy locus. *Cell* 51:919, 1987

34. Koenig M, Monaco AP, Kunkel LM: The complete sequence of dystrophin predicts a rod-shaped cytoskeletal protein. *Cell* 53:219, 1988

35. Mandel JL: Dystrophin. The gene and its product. *Nature* 339:584, 1989

36. Campbell KP, Kahl SD: Association of dystrophin and an integral membrane glycoprotein. *Nature* 338:259, 1989

37. Zubrzycka GE, Bulman DE, Karpati G, et al: The Duchenne muscular dystrophy gene product is localized in sarcolemma of human skeletal muscle. *Nature* 333:466, 1988

38. Jung D, Pons F, Leger JJ, et al: Dystrophin in central nervous system: a developmental, regional distribution and subcellular localization study. *Neurosci Lett* 124:87, 1991

39. Lidov HG, Byers TJ, Watkins SC, et al: Localization of dystrophin to postsynaptic regions of central nervous system cortical neurons. *Nature* 348:725, 1990

40. Chelly J, Hamard G, Koulakoff A, et al: Dystrophin gene transcribed from different promoters in neuronal and glial cells. *Nature* 344:64, 1990

41. Emery AE, Skinner R: Clinical studies in benign (Becker type) X-linked muscular dystrophy. *Clin Genet* 10:189, 1976

42. Beggs AH, Hoffman EP, Snyder JR, et al: Exploring the molecular basis for variability among patients with Becker muscular dystrophy: dystrophin gene and protein studies. *Am J Hum Genet* 49:54, 1991

43. Chelly J, Gilgenkrantz H, Lambert M, et al: Effect of dystrophin gene deletions on mRNA levels and processing in Duchenne and Becker muscular dystrophies. *Cell* 63:1239, 1990

44. England SB, Nicholson LV, Johnson MA, et al: Very mild muscular dystrophy associated with the deletion of 46% of dystrophin. *Nature* 343:180, 1990

45. Koenig M, Beggs AH, Moyer M, et al: The molecular basis for Duchenne versus Becker muscular dystrophy: correlation of severity with type of deletion. *Am J Hum Genet* 45:498, 1989

46. Sicinski P, Geng Y, Ryder CA, et al: The molecular basis of muscular dystrophy in the mdx mouse: a point mutation. *Science* 244:1578, 1989

47. Stedman HH, Sweeney HL, Shrager JB, et al: The mdx mouse diaphragm reproduces the degenerative changes of Duchenne muscular dystrophy. *Nature* 352:536, 1991

48. Hughes SM, Blau HM: Migration of myoblasts across basal lamina during skeletal muscle development. *Nature* 345:350, 1990

49. Acsadi G, Dickson G, Love DR, et al: Human dystrophin expression in mdx mice after intramuscular injection of DNA constructs. *Nature* 352:815, 1991

50. Partridge TA: Invited review: myoblast transfer: a possible therapy for inherited myopathies? *Muscle Nerve* 14:197, 1991

51. Partridge TA: Gene therapy. Muscle transfection made easy (news; comment). *Nature* 352:757, 1991

52. Anderson DH: Cystic fibrosis of the pancreas and its relation to celiac disease: a clinical and pathological study. *Am J Dis Child* 56:344, 1938

53. Boat TJ, Beaudet AL, Welsh M: Cystic fibrosis. *The Metabolic Basis of Inherited Disease.* Scriver CR, Beaudet AL, Sly WS, et al, Eds. McGraw-Hill, New York, 1989, p 2649

54. Brunecky Z: The incidence and genetics of cystic fibrosis. *J Med Genet* 9:33, 1972

55. Riordan JR, Rommens JM, Kerem B, et al: Identification of the cystic fibrosis gene: cloning and characterization of complementary DNA [published erratum appears in *Science* 245:1437, 1989]. *Science* 245:1066, 1989

56. Rommens JM, Iannuzzi MC, Kerem B, et al: Identification of the cystic fibrosis gene: chromosome walking and jumping. *Science* 245:1059, 1989

57. Kerem B, Rommens JM, Buchanan JA, et al: Identification of the cystic fibrosis gene: genetic analysis. *Science* 245:1073, 1989

58. Denning CR, Huang NN, Cuasay LR, et al: Cooperative study comparing three methods of performing sweat tests to diagnose cystic fibrosis. *Pediatrics* 66:752, 1980

59. Gibson LE, Cooke RE: A test for concentration of electrolytes in sweat in cystic fibrosis of the pancreas utilizing pilocarpine by iontophoresis. *Pediatrics* 23:545, 1959

60. Welsh MJ, Liedtke CM: Chloride and potassium channels in cystic fibrosis airway epithelia. *Nature* 322:467, 1986

61. Durie PR: The pathophysiology of the pancreatic defect in cystic fibrosis. *Acta Paediatr Scand Suppl* 363:41, 1989

62. Welsh MJ, Fick RB: Cystic fibrosis. *J Clin Invest* 80:1523, 1987

63. Frizzell RA, Rechkemmer G, Shoemaker RL: Altered regulation of airway epithelial cell chloride channels in cystic fibrosis. *Science* 233:558, 1986

64. Li M, McCann JD, Liedtke CM, et al: Cyclic AMP-dependent protein kinase opens chloride channels in normal but not cystic fibrosis airway epithelium. *Nature* 331:358, 1988

65. Bijman J, Fromter E: Direct demonstration of high transepithelial chloride-conductance in normal human sweat duct which is absent in cystic fibrosis. *Pflugers Arch* 407:S123, 1986

66. Bijman J, Quinton P: Permeability properties of cell membranes and tight junctions of normal and cystic fibrosis sweat ducts. *Pflugers Arch* 408:505, 1987

67. Sato K, Sato F: Defective beta-adrenergic response of cystic fibrosis sweat glands *in vivo* and *in vitro*. *J Clin Invest* 73:1763, 1984

68. Rosenstein BJ, Langbaum TS: Incidence of meconium abnormalities in newborn infants with cystic fibrosis. *Am J Dis Child* 134:72, 1980

69. Handwerger S, Roth J, Gorden P, et al: Glucose intolerance in cystic fibrosis. *N Engl J Med* 281:451, 1969

70. Fink RJ, Doershuk CF, Tucker AS, et al: Pulmonary function and morbidity in 40 adult patients with cystic fibrosis. *Chest* 74:643, 1978

71. Cohen AM, Yulish BS, Wasser KB, et al: Evaluation of pulmonary hypertrophic osteoarthropathy in cystic fibrosis: a comprehensive study. *Am J Dis Child* 140:74, 1986

72. Stern RC, Boat TF, Wood RE, et al: Treatment and prognosis of nasal polyps in cystic fibrosis. *Am J Dis Child* 136:1067, 1982

73. Stern RC, Borkat G, Hirschfield SS, et al: Heart failure in cystic fibrosis: treatment and prognosis of cor pulmonale with failure of the right side of the heart. Am J Dis Child 134:267, 1980

74. Knoke JD, Stern RC, Doershuk CF, et al: Cystic fibrosis: the prognosis for five-year survival. *Pediatr Res* 12:676, 1978

75. Kaplan E, Shwachman H, Perlmutter AD, et al: Reproductive failure in males with cystic fibrosis. *N Engl J Med* 279:65, 1968

76. Trezise AE, Buchwald M: In vivo cell-specific expression of the cystic fibrosis transmembrane conductance regulator. *Nature* 353:434, 1991

77. Wainwright BJ, Scambler PJ, Schmidtke J, et al: Localization of cystic fibrosis locus to human chromosome 7 cen-q22. *Nature* 318:384, 1985

78. White R, Woodward W, Leppert M, et al: A closely linked genetic marker for cystic fibrosis. *Nature* 318:382, 1985

79. Knowlton RG, Cohen-Haguenauer O, Van-Cong N, et al: A polymorphic DNA marker linked to cystic fibrosis is located on chromosome 7. *Nature* 318:380, 1985

80. Estivill X, Farrall M, Scambler PJ, et al: A candidate for the cystic fibrosis locus isolated by selection for methylation-free islands. *Nature* 326:840, 1987

81. Farrall MP, Stanier G, Feldman G, et al: Recombinations between IRP and cystic fibrosis. *Am J Hum Genet* 43:471, 1988

82. Rich DP, Anderson MP, Gregory RJ, et al: Expression of cystic fibrosis transmembrane conductance regulator corrects defective chloride channel regulation in cystic fibrosis airway epithelial cells. *Nature* 347:358, 1990

83. Hyde SC, Emsley P, Hartshorn MJ, et al: Structural model of ATP-binding proteins associated with cystic fibrosis, multidrug resistance and bacterial transport. *Nature* 346:362, 1990

84. Lemna WK, Feldman GL, Kerem B, et al: Mutation analysis for heterozygote detection and the prenatal diagnosis of cystic fibrosis. *N Engl J Med* 322:291, 1990

85. Dean M, White MB, Amos J, et al: Multiple mutations in highly conserved residues are found in mildly affected cystic fibrosis patients. *Cell* 61:863, 1990

86. Kerem BS, Zielenski J, Markiewicz D, et al: Identification of mutations in regions corresponding to the two putative nucleotide (ATP)-binding folds of the cystic fibrosis gene. *Proc Natl Acad Sci USA* 87:8447, 1990

87. Zielenski J, Bozon D, Kerem B, et al: Identification of mutations in exons 1 through 8 of the cystic fibrosis transmembrane conductance regulator (CFTR) gene. *Genomics* 10:229, 1991

88. Devoto M, Ronchetto P, Fanen P, et al: Screening for non-delta F508 mutations in five exons of the cystic fibrosis transmembrane conductance regulator (CFTR) gene in Italy. *Am J Hum Genet* 48:1127, 1991

89. Cheng SH, Gregory RJ, Marshall J, et al: Defective intracellular transport and processing of CFTR is the molecular basis of most cystic fibrosis. *Cell* 63:827, 1990

90. Gregory RJ, Rich DP, Cheng SH, et al: Maturation and function of cystic fibrosis transmembrane conductance regulator variants bearing mutations in putative nucleotide-binding domains 1 and 2. *Mol Cell Biol* 11:3886, 1991

91. Kerem E, Corey M, Kerem BS, et al: The relation between genotype and phenotype in cystic fibrosis—analysis of the most common mutation (delta F508). *N Engl J Med* 323:1517, 1990

92. Ng IS, Pace R, Richard MV, et al: Methods for analysis of multiple cystic fibrosis mutations. *Hum Genet* 87:613, 1991

93. Wilfond BS, Fost N: The cystic fibrosis gene: medical and social implications for heterozygote detection. *JAMA* 263:2777, 1990

94. Elias S, Annas GJ, Simpson JL: Carrier screening for cystic fibrosis: implications for obstetric and gynecologic practice. *Am J Obstet Gynecol* 164:1077, 1991

95. Knudsen AG Jr, Wayne L, Hallett WY: On selective advantage of cystic fibrosis heterozygotes. *Am J Hum Genet* 19:388, 1967

96. Kitzis A, Chomel JC, Kaplan JC, et al: Unusual segregation of cystic fibrosis allele to males. *Nature* 333:215, 1988

97. Waters DL, Dorney SF, Gaskin KJ, et al: Pancreatic function in infants identified as having cystic fibrosis in a neonatal screening program. *N Engl J Med* 322:303, 1990

98. Rock MJ, Mischler EH, Farrell PM, et al: Newborn screening for cystic fibrosis is complicated by age-related decline in immunoreactive trypsinogen levels. *Pediatrics* 85:1001, 1990

99. Yacoub MH, Banner NR, Khaghani A, et al: Heart-lung transplantation for cystic fibrosis and subsequent domino heart transplantation. *J Heart Transplant* 9:459, 1990

100. Aitken ML, Burke W, McDonald G, et al: Recombinant human DNase inhalation in normal subjects and patients with cystic fibrosis: a phase 1 study. *JAMA* 267:1947, 1992

101. Vasconcellos CA, Allen PG, Wohl ME, et al: Reduction in viscosity of cystic fibrosis sputum in vitro by gelsolin. *Science* 263:969, 1994

102. Stanley C, Rosenberg MB, Friedman T: Gene transfer into rat airway epithelial cells using retroviral vectors. *Somat Cell Mol Genet* 17:185, 1991

103. Riccardi VM: Von Recklinghausen neurofibromatosis. *N Engl J Med* 305:1617, 1981

104. Xu GF, O'Connell P, Viskochil D, et al: The neurofibromatosis type 1 gene encodes a protein related to GAP. *Cell* 62:599, 1990

105. Ballester R, Marchuk D, Boguski M, et al: The NF-1 locus encodes a protein functionally related to mammalian GAP and yeast IRA proteins. *Cell* 63:851, 1990

106. Wallace MR, Marchuk DA, Andersen LB, et al: Type 1 neurofibromatosis gene: identification of a large transcript disrupted in three NF-1 patients. *Science* 249:181, 1990

107. Huson SM, Compston DA, Clark P, et al: A genetic study of von Recklinghausen neurofibromatosis in south east Wales: I. Prevalence, fitness, mutation rate, and effect of parental transmission on severity. *J Med Genet* 26:704, 1989

108. Huson SM, Compston DA, Harper PS: A genetic study of von Recklinghausen neurofibromatosis in south east Wales: II. Guidelines for genetic counselling. *J Med Genet* 26:712, 1989

109. Williamson TH, Garner A, Moore AT: Structure of Lisch nodules in neurofibromatosis type 1. *Ophthalmic Paediatr Genet* 12:11, 1991

110. Kaufmann D, Wiandt S, Veser J, et al: Increased melanogenesis in cultured epidermal melanocytes from patients with neurofibromatosis 1 (NF 1). *Hum Genet* 87:144, 1991

111. Mulvihill JJ, Parry DM, Sherman JL, et al: NIH conference. Neurofibromatosis 1 (Recklinghausen disease) and neurofibromatosis 2 (bilateral acoustic neurofibromatosis): an update. *Ann Intern Med* 113:39, 1990

112. Riccardi VM: Neurofibromatosis. *Neurol Clin* 5:337, 1987

113. NIH NIoH: Consensus Development Conference on Neurofibromatosis Report 1988. *Neurofibromatosis* 1:172, 1988

114. DiSimone RE, Berman AT, Schwentker EP: The orthopedic manifestation of neurofibromatosis: a clinical experience and review of the literature. *Clin Orthop* May(230):277, 1988

115. Listernick R, Charrow J: Neurofibromatosis type 1 in childhood. *J Pediatr* 116:845, 1990

116. Huson S, Jones D, Beck L: Ophthalmic manifestations of neurofibromatosis. *Br J Oph-thalmol* 71:235, 1987

117. Ko W, Gorovoy K: Lisch nodules in neurofibromatosis. *J Ophthalmic Nurs Technol* 9:141, 1990

118. Lubs ML, Bauer MS, Formas ME, et al: Lisch nodules in neurofibromatosis type 1. *N Engl J Med* 324:1264, 1991

119. Toonstra J, Dandrieu MR, Ippel PF, et al: Are Lisch nodules an ocular marker of the neurofibromatosis gene in otherwise unaffected family members? *Dermatologica* 174:232, 1987

120. Riccardi VM, Lewis RA: Penetrance of von Recklinghausen neurofibromatosis: a distinction between predecessors and descendants. *Am J Hum Genet* 42:284, 1988

121. Wertelecki W, Rouleau GA, Superneau DW, et al: Neurofibromatosis 2: clinical and DNA linkage studies of a large kindred. *N Engl J Med* 319:278, 1988

122. Riccardi VM: Neurofibromatosis: past, present, and future. *N Engl J Med* 324:1283, 1991

123. Stine SB, Adams WV: Learning problems in neurofibromatosis patients. *Clin Orthop* 43, 1989

124. Wadsby M, Lindehammar H, Eeg OO: Neurofibromatosis in childhood: neuropsychological aspects. *Neurofibromatosis* 2:251, 1989

125. Hashimoto T, Tayama M, Miyazaki M, et al: Cranial MR imaging in patients with von Recklinghausen's disease (neurofibromatosis type I). *Neuropediatrics* 21:193, 1990

126. Alvord EJ Jr, Lofton S: Gliomas of the optic nerve or chiasm: outcome by patients' age, tumor site, and treatment. *J Neurosurg* 68:85, 1988

127. Duffner PK, Cohen ME: Isolated optic nerve gliomas in children with and without neurofibromatosis. *Neurofibromatosis* 1:201, 1988

128. Packer RJ, Bilaniuk LT, Cohen BH, et al: Intracranial visual pathway gliomas in children with neurofibromatosis. *Neurofibromatosis* 1:212, 1988

129. Finley JL, Dabbs DJ: Renal vascular smooth muscle proliferation in neurofibromatosis. *Hum Pathol* 19:107, 1988

130. Poston GJ, Grace PA, Venn G, et al: Recurrent near-fatal haemorrhage in von Recklinghausen's disease. *Br J Clin Pract* 44:755, 1990

131. Senveli E, Altinors N, Kars Z, et al: Association of von Recklinghausen's neurofibromatosis and aqueduct stenosis. *Neurosurgery* 24:99, 1989

132. Walsh MM, Brandspigel K: Gastrointestinal bleeding due to pancreatic schwannoma complicating von Recklinghausen's disease. *Gastroenterology* 97:1550, 1989

133. Sorenson SA, Mulvihill JJ, Nielsen A: Long-term follow-up of von Recklinghausen neurofibromatosis: survival and malignant neoplasms. *N Engl J Med* 314:1010, 1986

134. Barker D, Wright E, Nguyen K, et al: Gene for von Recklinghausen neurofibromatosis is in the pericentromeric region of chromosome 17. *Science* 236:1100, 1987

135. Clementi M, Murgia A, Anglani F, et al: Linkage analysis of neurofibromatosis type 1: study of a homogeneous North Italian population with five DNA markers of chromosome 17. *Hum Genet* 87:91, 1991

136. Fountain JW, Wallace MR, Bruce MA, et al: Physical mapping of a translocation breakpoint in neurofibromatosis. *Science* 244:1085, 1989

137. Xu GF, Lin B, Tanaka K, et al: The catalytic domain of the neurofibromatosis type 1 gene product stimulates ras GTPase and complements ira mutants of S. cerevisiae. *Cell* 63:835, 1990

138. Han JW, McCormick F, Macara IG: Regulation of Ras-GAP and the neurofibromatosis-1 gene product by eicosanoids. *Science* 252:576, 1991

139. Marshall CJ: How does p21ras transform cells? *Trends Genet* 7:91, 1991

140. Weinberg RA: Tumor suppressor genes. *Science* 254:1138, 1991

141. Upadhyaya M, Cheryson A, Broadhead W, et al: A 90 kb DNA deletion associated with neurofibromatosis type 1. *J Med Genet* 27:738, 1990

142. Wallace MR, Andersen LB, Saulino AM, et al: A de novo Alu insertion results in neurofibromatosis type 1. *Nature* 353:864, 1991

143. Fialkow PJ, Sagebiel RW, Gartler SM, et al: Multiple cell origin of hereditary neurofibromas. *N Engl J Med* 284:298, 1971

144. Menon AG, Anderson KM, Riccardi VM, et al: Chromosome 17p deletions and p53 gene mutations associated with the formation of malignant neurofibrosarcomas in von Recklinghausen neurofibromatosis. *Proc Natl Acad Sci USA* 87:5435, 1990

145. Skuse GR, Kosciolek BA, Rowley PT: The neurofibroma in von Recklinghausen neurofibromatosis has a unicellular origin. *Am J Hum Genet* 49:600, 1991

146. Glover TW, Stein CK, Legius E, et al: Molecular and cytogenetic analysis of tumors in von Recklinghausen neurofibromatosis. *Genes Chromosom Cancer* 3:62, 1991

147. Jadayel D, Fain P, Upadhyaya M, et al: Paternal origin of new mutations in von Recklinghausen neurofibromatosis. *Nature* 343:558, 1990

148. Roenigk RK, Ratz JL: CO2 laser treatment of cutaneous neurofibromas. *J Dermatol Surg Oncol* 13:187, 1987

149. Hanke CW, Conner AC, Reed JC: Treatment of multiple facial neurofibromas with dermabrasion. *J Dermatol Surg Oncol* 13:631, 1987

150. Scriver CR, Clow CL: Phenylketonuria: epitome of human biochemical genetics (pt 1 of 2). *N Engl J Med* 303:1336, 1980

151. Scriver CR, Clow CL: Phenylketonuria: epitome of human biochemical genetics. *N Engl J Med* 303:1394, 1980

152. Bickel H: Phenylketonuria: past, present, future. *J Inherited Metab Dis* 3:123, 1980

153. Fölling A: Über ausscheidung von phenylbrenztraubensaüre in den harn als stoffwechselanomalie in verbindung mit imbezillität. *Z Physiol Chem* 227:169, 1934

154. Nyhan WL: Asbjörn Fölling and phenylketonuria. *Trends Biochem Sci* 9:71, 1984

155. Scriver CR, Kaufman S, Woo SLC: The hyperphenylalaninemias. *The Metabolic Basis of Inherited Disease*. Scriver CR, Beaudet AL, Sly WS, et al, Eds. McGraw-Hill, New York, 1989, p 495

156. Michel U, Schmidt E, Batzler U: Results of psychological testing of patients aged 3–6 years. *Eur J Pediatr* 149(suppl):S34, 1990

157. Fishler K, Azen CG, Henderson R, et al: Psychoeducational findings among children treated for phenylketonuria. *Am J Ment Defic* 92:65, 1987

158. Krause W, Halminski M, McDonald L, et al: Biochemical and neuropsychological effects of elevated plasma phenylalanine in patients with treated phenylketonuria: a model for the study of phenylalanine and brain function in man. *J Clin Invest* 75:40, 1985

159. Lenke RR, Levy HL: Maternal phenylketonuria and hyperphenylalaninemia: an international survey of untreated and treated pregnancies. *N Engl J Med* 303:1202, 1980

160. Levy HL: Maternal PKU. *Prog Clin Biol Res* 177:109, 1985

161. Naughten E, Saul IP: Maternal phenylketonuria—the Irish experience. *J Inherit Metab Dis* 13:658, 1990

162. Luder AS, Greene CL: Maternal phenylketonuria and hyperphenylalaninemia: implications for medical practice in the United States. *Am J Obstet Gynecol* 161:1102, 1989

163. Guttler F, Lou H, Andersen J, et al: Cognitive development in offspring of untreated and preconceptionally treated maternal phenylketonuria. *J Inherit Metab Dis* 13:665, 1990

164. Waisbren SE, Doherty LB, Bailey IV, et al: The New England Maternal PKU Project: identification of at-risk women. *Am J Public Health* 78:789, 1988

165. Pitt DB, Danks DM: The natural history of untreated phenylketonuria over 20 years. *J Paediatr Child Health* 27:189, 1991

166. Schuett VE, Gurda RF, Brown ES: Diet discontinuation policies and practices of PKU clinics in the United States. *Am J Public Health* 70:498, 1980

167. AAP: American Academy of Pediatrics, Committee on Genetics: New issues in newborn screening for phenylketonuria and congenital hypothyroidism. *Pediatrics* 69:104, 1982

168. Jinks DC, Cuthrie R, Naylor EW: Simplified procedure for producing Bacillus subtilis spores for the Guthrie phenylketonuria and other microbiological screening tests. *J Clin Microbiol* 21:826, 1985

169. Kirkman HN, Carroll CL, Moore EG, et al: Fifteen-year experience with screening for phenylketonuria with an automated fluorometric method. *Am J Hum Genet* 34:743, 1982

170. McCabe ER, McCabe L, Mosher GA, et al: Newborn screening for phenylketonuria: predictive validity as a function of age. *Pediatrics* 72:390, 1983

171. Walker V, Clayton BE, Ersser RS, et al: Hyperphenylalaninemia of various types among three-quarters of a million neonates tested in a screening programme. *Arch Dis Child* 56:759, 1981

172. Thalhammer O, Pollak A, Lubec G, et al: Intracellular concentrations of phenylalanine, tyrosine and alpha-aminobytyric acid in 13 homozygotes and 19 heterozygotes for phenylketonuria (PKU) compared with 26 normals. *Hum Genet* 54:213, 1980

173. Thalhammer O, Lubec G, Konigshofer H, et al: Intracellular phenylalanine and tyrosine concentration in homozygotes and heterozygotes for phenylketonuria (PKU) and hyperphenylalaninemia compared with normals. *Hum Genet* 60:320, 1982

174. Koepp P, Held KR: Serum-tyrosine in patients with hyperphenylalaninaemia. *Lancet* 2:92, 1977

175. Batshaw ML, Valle D, Bessman SP: Unsuccessful treatment of phenylketonuria with tyrosine. *J Pediatr* 99:159, 1981

176. Choi TB, Pardridge WM: Phenylalanine transport at the human blood-brain barrier: studies with isolated human brain capillaries. *J Biol Chem* 261:6536, 1986

177. Christensen HN: Hypothesis: where the depleted plasma amino acids go in phenylketonuria, and why. *Perspect Biol Med* 30:186, 1987

178. Dwivedy AK, Shah SN: Effects of phenylalanine and its deaminated metabolites on Na$^+$, K$^+$-ATPase activity in synaptosomes from rat brain. *Neurochem Res* 7:717, 1982

179. Guttler F, Lou H: Dietary problems of phenylketonuria: effect on CNS transmitters and their possible role in behaviour and neuropsychological function. *J Inherit Metab Dis* 9:169, 1986

180. Heuther G, Kaus R, Neuhoff V: Brain development in experimental hyperphenylalaninaemia: myelination. *Neuropediatrics* 13:177, 1982

181. Bauman ML, Kemper TL: Morphologic and histoanatomic observations of the brain in untreated human phenylketonuria. *Acta Neuropathol* 58:55, 1982

182. Swaiman KF, Wu SR: Phenylalanine and phenylacetate adversely affect developing mammalian brain neurons. *Neurology* 34:1246, 1984

183. Pearsen KD, Gean-Marton A, Levy HL, et al: Phenylketonuria: MR imaging of the brain with clinical correlation. *Radiology* 177:437, 1990

184. Niederwieser A, Curtius H-CH: Tetrahydrobiopterin deficiencies in hyperphenylalaninemia. *Inherited Diseases of Amino Acid Metabolism: Recent Progress in Understanding, Recognition and Management.* Bickel H, Wachtel U, Eds. Georg Thieme Verlag, New York, 1985, p 104

185. Dhondt JL: Tetrahydrobiopterin deficiencies: preliminary analysis from an international survey. *J Pediatr* 104:501, 1984

186. Robson KJ, Chandra T, MacGillivray RT, et al: Polysome immunoprecipitation of phenylalanine hydroxylase mRNA from rat liver and cloning of its cDNA. *Proc Natl Acad Sci USA* 79:4701, 1982

187. DiLella AG, Kwok SCM, Ledley FD, et al: Molecular structure and polymorphic map of the human phenylalanine hydroxylase gene. *Biochemistry* 25:743, 1986

188. DiLella AG, Woo SLC: Molecular basis of phenylketonuria and its clinical applications. *Mol Biol Med* 4:183, 1987

189. Ledley FD, Levy HL, Woo SLC: Molecular analysis of the inheritance of phenylketonuria and mild hyperphenylalaninemia in families with both disorders. *N Engl J Med* 314:1276, 1986

190. Wang T, Okano Y, Eisensmith RC, et al: Missense mutations prevalent in Orientals with phenylketonuria: molecular characterization and clinical implications. *Genomics* 10:449, 1991

191. Wang T, Okano Y, Eisensmith RC, et al: Founder effect of a prevalent phenylketonuria mutation in the Oriental population. *Proc Natl Acad Sci USA* 88:2146, 1991

192. Hofman KJ, Steel G, Kazazian HH, et al: Phenylketonuria in U.S. blacks: molecular analysis of the phenylalanine hydroxylase gene. *Am J Hum Genet* 48:791, 1991

193. Kalaydjieva L, Dworniczak B, Kucinskas V, et al: Geographical distribution gradients of the major PKU mutations and the linked haplotypes. *Hum Genet* 86:411, 1991

194. DiLella AG, Marvit J, Brayton K, et al: An amino-acid substitution involved in phenylketonuria is in linkage disequilibrium with DNA haplotype 2. *Nature* 327:333, 1987

195. DiLella AG, Marvit J, Lidsky AS, et al: Tight linkage between a splicing mutation and a specific DNA haplotype in phenylketonuria. *Nature* 322:799, 1986

196. Marvit J, DiLella AG, Brayton K, et al: GT to AT transition at a splice donor site causes skipping of the preceding exon in phenylketonuria. *Nucleic Acids Res* 15:5613, 1987

197. Lidsky AS, Ledley FD, DiLella AG, et al: Extensive restriction site polymorphism at the human phenylalanine hydroxylase locus and application in prenatal diagnosis of phenylketonuria. *Am J Hum Genet* 37:619, 1985

198. Dianzani I, Devoto M, Camaschella C, et al: Haplotype distribution and molecular defects at the phenylalanine hydroxylase locus in Italy. *Hum Genet* 86:69, 1990

199. Zygulska M, Eigel A, Aulehla SC, et al: Molecular analysis of PKU haplotypes in the population of southern Poland. *Hum Genet* 86:292, 1991

200. Konecki DS, Lichter KU: The phenylketonuria locus: current knowledge about alleles and mutations of the phenylalanine hydroxylase gene in various populations. *Hum Genet* 87:377, 1991

201. Woolf LI: The heterozygote advantage of phenylketonuria. *Am J Hum Genet* 38:773, 1986

202. Woolf LI, McBea MS, Woolf FM, et al: Phenylketonuria as a balanced polymorphism: the nature of the heterozygote advantage. *Ann Hum Genet* 38:461, 1975

203. Woolf LI, Griffiths R, Moncrieff A: Treatment of phenylketonuria with a diet low in phenylalanine. *Br Med J* 1:57, 1955

204. Acosta PB, Trahms C, Wellman NS, et al: Phenylalanine intakes of 1- to 6-year-old children with phenylketonuria undergoing therapy. *Am J Clin Nutr* 38:694, 1983

205. Kindt E, Motzfeldt K, Halvorsen S, et al: Protein requirements in infants and children: a longitudinal study of children treated for phenylketonuria. *Am J Clin Nutr* 37:778, 1983

206. Link RM, Wachtel U: Clinical experiences with an amino acid preparation in children with phenylketonuria. *Rev Med Liege* 39:429, 1984

207. Holtzman NA, Kronmal RA, van Doorninck W, et al: Effect of age at loss of dietary control on intellectual performance and behavior of children with phenylketonuria. *N Engl J Med* 314:593, 1986

208. Ledley FD, Grenett HE, McGinnis-Shelnutt M, et al: Retroviral-mediated gene transfer of human phenylalanine hydroxylase into NIH 3T3 and hepatoma cells. *Proc Natl Acad Sci USA* 83:409, 1986

209. Ledley FD, Grenett HE, DiLella AG, et al: Gene transfer and expression of human phenylalanine hydroxylase. *Science* 228:77, 1985

210. Ambrus CM, Ambrus JL, Horvath C, et al: Phenylalanine depletion for the management of phenylketonuria: use of enzyme reactors with immobilized enzymes. *Science* 201:837, 1978

211. Ambrus CM, Anthone S, Horvath C, et al: Extracorporeal enzyme reactors for depletion of phenylalanine in phenylketonuria. *Ann Intern Med* 106:531, 1987

212. Smith I, Lobascher M, Stevenson J, et al: Effect of stopping the low phenylalanine diet on the intellectual progress of children with phenylketonuria. *Ann Clin Biochem* 14:134, 1977

213. Bode VC, McDonald JD, Guenet JL, et al: hph-1: a mouse mutant with hereditary hyperphenylalaninemia induced by ethylnitrosourea mutagenesis. *Genetics* 118:299, 1988

214. McDonald JD, Bode VC: Hyperphenylalaninemia in the hph-1 mouse mutant. *Pediatr Res* 23:63, 1988

215. McDonald JD, Bode VC, Dove WF, et al: Pahhph-5: a mouse mutant deficient in phenylalanine hydroxylase. *Proc Natl Acad Sci USA* 87:1965, 1990

216. Beckwith JB: Macroglossia, omphalocele, adrenal cytomegaly, gigantism and hyperplastic visceromegaly. *Birth Defects* 5:188, 1969

217. Engstrom W, Lindham S, Schofield P: Wiedemann-Beckwith syndrome. *Eur J Pediatr* 147:450, 1988

218. Higurashi M, Ijima K, Sugimoto Y, et al: The birth prevalence of malformation syndromes in Tokyo infants. *Am J Med Genet* 6:189, 1980

219. Filippi G, McKusick VA: The Beckwith-Wiedemann's syndrome. *Medicine* 49:279, 1970

220. Wiedemann HR: Tumor and hemihypertrophy associated with Wiedemann-Beckwith's syndrome. *Eur J Pediatr* 141:129, 1983

221. Sippell WG, Partsch CJ, Wiedemann HR: Growth, bone maturation and pubertal development in children with the EMG-syndrome. *Clin Genet* 35:20, 1989

222. Beckwith JB, Kiviat NB, Bonadio JF: Nephrogenic rests, nephroblastomatosis, and the pathogenesis of Wilms' tumor. *Pediatr Pathol* 10:1, 1990

223. Falik BT, Korenberg JR, Davos I, et al: Congenital gastric teratoma in Wiedemann-Beckwith syndrome. *Am J Med Genet* 38:52, 1991

224. Chitayat D, Friedman JM, Dimmick JE: Neuroblastoma in a child with Wiedemann-Beckwith syndrome. *Am J Med Genet* 35:433, 1990

225. Best LG: Familial posterior helical ear pits and Wiedemann-Beckwith syndrome. *Am J Med Genet* 40:188, 1991

226. Aleck KA, Hadro TA: Dominant inheritance of Wiedemann-Beckwith syndrome: further evidence for transmission of "unstable premutation" through carrier women. *Am J Med Genet* 33:155, 1989

227. Gerver WJ, Menheere PP, Schaap C, et al: The effects of a somatostatin analogue on the metabolism of an infant with Beckwith-Wiedemann syndrome and hyperinsulinaemic hypoglycaemia. *Eur J Pediatr* 150:634, 1991

228. Smith DF, Mihm FG, Flynn M: Chronic alveolar hypoventilation secondary to macroglossia in the Beckwith-Wiedemann's syndrome. *Pediatrics* 70:695, 1982

229. Kveim M, Fisher JC, Jones KC, et al: Early tongue resection for Beckwith-Wiedemann macroglossia. *Ann Plast Surg* 14:142, 1985

230. Azouz EM, Larson EJ, Patel J, et al: Beckwith-Wiedemann syndrome: development of nephroblastoma during the surveillance period. *Pediatr Radiol* 20:550, 1990

231. Friede H, Figueroa AA: The Beckwith-Wiedemann's syndrome: a longitudinal study of the macroglossia and dentofacial complex. *J Craniofac Genet Dev Biol* 1:179, 1985

232. Koufos A, Grundy P, Morgan K, et al: Familial Wiedemann-Beckwith syndrome and a second Wilms tumor locus both map to 11p15.5. *Am J Hum Genet* 44:711, 1989

233. Ping AJ, Reeve AE, Law DJ, et al: Genetic linkage of Beckwith-Wiedemann syndrome to 11p15. *Am J Hum Genet* 44:720, 1989

234. Niikawa N, Ishikariyama S, Takahashi S, et al: The Wiedemann-Beckwith syndrome: pedigree studies on 5 families with evidence for autosomal dominant inheritance with variable expressivity. *Am J Med Genet* 24:41, 1986

235. Olney AH, Buehler BA, Waziri M: Wiedemann-Beckwith syndrome in apparently discordant monozygotic twins. *Am J Med Genet* 29:491, 1988

236. Pettenati MJ, Haines JL, Higgins RR, et al: Wiedemann-Beckwith syndrome: presentation of clinical and cytogenetic data on 22 new cases and review of the literature. *Hum Genet* 74:143, 1986

237. Journel A, Lucas I, Allaire C, et al: Trisomy 11p15 and Beckwith-Wiedemann syndrome. *Ann Genet* 28:97, 1985

238. Waziri M, Patil SR, Hanson JW, et al: Abnormality of chromosome 11 in patients with features of BWS. *J Pediatr* 102:873, 1983

239. Henry I, Jeanpierre M, Couillin P, et al: Molecular definition of the 11p15.5 region involved in Beckwith-Wiedemann syndrome and probably in predisposition to adrenocortical carcinoma. *Hum Genet* 81:273, 1989

240. Spritz RA, Mager D, Pauli M, et al: Normal dosage of the insulin and IGF II genes in patients with Beckwith-Wiedemann syndrome. *Am J Hum Genet* 39:265, 1986

241. Schofield PN, Lindham S, Engstrom W: Analysis of gene dosage on chromosome 11 in children suffering from Beckwith-Wiedemann syndrome. *Eur J Pediatr* 148:320, 1989

242. Searle AG, Beechey CV: Genome imprinting phenomena on mouse chromosome 7. *Genet Res* 56:237, 1990

243. Engel E, DeLozier BC: Uniparental disomy, isodisomy, and imprinting: probable effects in man and strategies for their detection. *Am J Med Genet* 40:432, 1991

244. Little M, Van HV, Hastie N: Dads and disomy and disease [news; comment]. *Nature* 351:609, 1991

245. Surani MA, Kothary R, Allen ND, et al: Genome imprinting and development in the mouse. *Dev Suppl*, 1990, p 89

246. Bartolomei MS, Zemel S, Tilghman SM: Parental imprinting of the mouse H19 gene. *Nature* 351:153, 1991

247. DeChiara TM, Robertson EJ, Efstratiadis A: Parental imprinting of the mouse insulin-like growth factor II gene. *Cell* 64:849, 1991

248. Willison K: Opposite imprinting of the mouse Igf2 and Igf2r genes. *Trends Genet* 7:107, 1991

249. Hall JG: How imprinting is relevant to human disease. *Dev Suppl*, 1990, p 141

250. Devilee P, van den Broek, Mannens M, et al: Differences in patterns of allelic loss between two common types of adult cancer, breast and colon carcinoma, and Wilms' tumor of childhood. *Int J Cancer* 47:817, 1991

251. Mannens M, Devilee P, Bliek J, et al: Loss of heterozygosity in Wilms' tumors, studied for six putative tumor suppressor regions, is limited to chromosome 11. *Cancer Res* 50:3279, 1990

252. Pal N, Wadey RB, Buckle B, et al: Preferential loss of maternal alleles in sporadic Wilms' tumour. *Oncogene* 5:1665, 1990

253. Henry I, Grandjouan S, Couillin P, et al: Tumor-specific loss of 11p15.5 alleles in del11p13 Wilms tumor and in familial adrenocortical carcinoma. *Proc Natl Acad Sci USA* 86:3247, 1989

254. Reeve AE, Sih SA, Raizis AM, et al: Loss of allelic heterozygosity at a second locus on chromosome 11 in sporadic Wilms' tumor cells. *Mol Cell Biol* 9:1799, 1989

255. Francke U, Holmes LB, Atkins L, et al: Aniridia-Wilms' tumor association: evidence for specific deletion of 11p13. *Cytogenet Cell Genet* 24:185, 1979

256. Francke U: A gene for Wilms tumour? *Nature* 343:692, 1990

257. Gessler M, Poustka A, Cavenee W, et al: Homozygous deletion in Wilms tumours of a zinc-finger gene identified by chromosome jumping. *Nature* 343:774, 1990

258. Call KM, Glaser T, Ito CY, et al: Isolation and characterization of a zinc finger polypeptide gene at the human chromosome 11 Wilms' tumor locus. *Cell* 60:509, 1990

259. Henry I, Bonaiti PC, Chehensse V, et al: Uniparental paternal disomy in a genetic cancer-predisposing syndrome. *Nature* 351:665, 1991

260. Turleau C, de Grouchy J, Chavin-Colin F, et al: Trisomy 11p15 and Beckwith-Wiedemann syndrome: a report of two cases. *Hum Genet* 67:219, 1984

261. Scott I, Cowell J, Robertson M, et al: IFG II gene expression in Wilms' tumour and embryonic tissues. *Nature* 317:260, 1985

262. Ferguson SA, Cattanach BM, Barton SC, et al: Embryological and molecular investigations of parental imprinting on mouse chromosome 7. *Nature* 351:667, 1991

263. Lubs HA: A marker X chromosome. *Am J Hum Genet* 21:231, 1969

264. Sutherland GR: Fragile sites on human chromosomes: demonstration of their dependence on the type of tissue culture medium. *Science* 197:265, 1977

265. Nussbaum RL, Ledbetter DH: The fragile X syndrome. *The Metabolic Basis of Inherited Disease*. Scriver CR, Beaudet AL, Sly WS, et al, Eds. McGraw-Hill, New York, 1989, p 327

266. Martin JP, Bell J: A pedigree of mental defect showing sex-linkage. *J Neurol Neurosurg Psychiatry* 6:154, 1943

267. Sherman SL, Morton NE, Jacobs PA, et al: The marker (X) syndrome: a cytogenetic and genetic analysis. *Am J Hum Genet* 48:21, 1984

268. Sherman SL, Jacobs PA, Morton NE, et al: Further segregation analysis of the fragile X syndrome with special reference to transmitting males. *Hum Genet* 69:289, 1985

269. Kremer EJ, Pritchard M, Lynch M, et al: Mapping of DNA instability at the fragile X to a trinucleotide repeat sequence p(CCG)n. *Science* 252:1711, 1991

270. Oberle I, Rousseau F, Heitz D, et al: Instability of a 550-base pair DNA segment and abnormal methylation in fragile X syndrome. *Science* 252:1097, 1991

271. Turner G, Daniel A, Frost M: X-linked mental retardation, macroorchidism, and the Xq27 fragile site. *J Pediatr* 96:837, 1980

272. Chudley AE, Hagerman RJ: Fragile X syndrome. *J Pediatr* 110:821, 1987

273. Hagerman RJ, Smith ACM, Mariner R: Clinical features of the fragile X syndrome. *The Fragile X Syndrome: Diagnosis, Biochemistry, and Intervention*. Hagerman RJ, McBogg PM, Eds. Spectra Publishing, Dillon, CO, 1983

274. Butler MG, Allen GA, Haynes JL, et al: Anthropometric comparison of mentally retarded males with and without the fragile X syndrome. *Am J Med Genet* 38:260, 1991

275. Cianchetti C, Sannio FG, Fratta AL, et al: Neuropsychological, psychiatric, and physical manifestations in 149 members from 18 fragile X families. *Am J Med Genet* 40:234, 1991

276. Brainard SS, Schreiner RA, Hagerman RJ: Cognitive profiles of the carrier fragile X woman. *Am J Med Genet* 38:505, 1991

277. Jacobs PA, Mayer M, Abruzzo MA: Studies of the fragile (X) syndrome in populations of mentally retarded individuals in Hawaii. *Am J Med Genet* 23:567, 1986

278. Gustavson K-H, Blomquist HK, Son HB, et al: Prevalence of the fragile-X syndrome in mentally retarded boys in a Swedish county. *Am J Med Genet* 23:581, 1986

279. Webb TP, Bundey SE, Thake AI, et al: Population incidence and segregation ratios in the Martin-Bell syndrome. *Am J Med Genet* 23:573, 1986

280. Sanfilippo S, Ragusa RM, Musumeci S, et al: Fragile X mental retardation: prevalence in a group of institutionalized patients in Italy and description of a novel EEG pattern. *Am J Med Genet* 23:589, 1986

281. Sutherland GR, Hecht F: *Fragile Sites on Human Chromosomes.* Oxford University Press, New York, 1985, p 80

282. Jenkins ED, Brown WT, Brooks J, et al: Low frequencies of apparently fragile X chromosomes in normal control cultures: a possible explanation. *Exp Cell Biol* 54:40, 1986

283. Jenkins EC, Brown WT, Wilson MG, et al: The prenatal detection of the fragile X chromosome: review of recent experience. *Am J Med Genet* 23:297, 1986

284. Nussbaum RL, Ledbetter DH: Fragile X syndrome: a unique mutation in man. *Annu Rev Genet* 20:109, 1986

285. Laird CD: Proposed mechanism of inheritance and expression of the human fragile-X syndrome of mental retardation. *Genetics* 117:587, 1987

286. Pembrey ME, Winter RM, Davies KE: A premutation that generates a defect at crossing over explains the inheritance of fragile X mental retardation. *Am J Med Genet* 21:709, 1985

287. Heitz D, Rousseau F, Devys D, et al: Isolation of sequences that span the fragile X and identification of a fragile X-related CpG island. *Science* 251:1236, 1991

288. Bell MV, Hirst MC, Nakahori Y, et al: Physical mapping across the fragile X: hypermethylation and clinical expression of the fragile X syndrome. *Cell* 64:861, 1991

289. Rousseau F, Heitz D, Biancalana V, et al: Direct diagnosis by DNA analysis of the fragile X syndrome of mental retardation. *N Engl J Med* 325:1673, 1991

290. Verkerk AJ, Pieretti M, Sutcliffe JS, et al: Identification of a gene (FMR-1) containing a CGG repeat coincident with a breakpoint cluster region exhibiting length variation in fragile X syndrome. *Cell* 65:905, 1991

291. Pieretti M, Zhang FP, Fu YH, et al: Absence of expression of the FMR-1 gene in fragile X syndrome. *Cell* 66:817, 1991

292. Yu S, Pritchard M, Kremer E, et al: Fragile X genotype characterized by an unstable region of DNA. *Science* 252:1179, 1991

Acknowledgments

Figure 1   Adapted by Talar Agasyan from "The Morbid Anatomy of the Human Genome: A Review of Gene Mapping in Clinical Medicine," part 3 of 4, by V. A. McKusick, in *Medicine* 66:237, 1987.

Figures 2, 3, 5 through 7   Adapted from *Recombinant DNA*, 2nd ed., by J. D. Watson, J. Witkowski, M. Gilman, et al. Scientific American Books, New York, 1992. © 1992 James D. Watson, Jan Witkowski, Michael Gilman, Mark Zoller. Used with permission.

Figure 4   Tom Moore. Adapted from "Diseases of Muscle and the Neuromuscular Junction," by R. W. P. Cutler, in SCIENTIFIC AMERICAN *Medicine*, edited by E. Rubenstein and D. D. Federman, Section 11, Subsection I. Scientific American, Inc., New York, 1994. All rights reserved.

Figure 5   Adapted by Talar Agasyan.

Figure 8   Dimitry Schidlovsky and Talar Agasyan.

Figure 9   Talar Agasyan.

Figure 10   Adapted by Talar Agasyan from *The Metabolic Basis of Inherited Disease*, 6th ed., edited by C. R. Scriver, A. L. Beaudet, W. S. Sly, et al. McGraw-Hill, New York, 1989.

CHAPTER 10

Molecular Mechanisms of Carcinogenesis

Robert A. Weinberg, Ph.D.

Genes may be involved in carcinogenesis in at least two ways. A number of genes acquired at conception as normal or aberrant alleles may strongly affect the probability of cancer onset during an individual's lifetime. These cancer susceptibility genes may function at a variety of levels to affect the metabolism of potentially carcinogenic compounds, the ability to recognize and to repair genetic damage, the growth regulation of specific cell types, or the ability of the immune system to recognize and eradicate incipient tumors.

A second class of genes can become involved in cancer as a consequence of somatic mutational mechanisms that damage genes present in the cells of a target organ. After mutations occur, these somatically altered genes may confer advantageous growth properties on the cells, enabling mutant cells to proliferate more rapidly than their genetically normal counterparts, to acquire vascularization, or to metastasize.

Data from a variety of sources strongly reinforce the theory that genetic aberrations acquired by tumor cell genomes play an important role in cancer formation. For one thing, the carcinogenic potency of many chemicals is correlated with their ability to induce mutations in target cells.[1] Furthermore, analyses of tumor cell karyotypes have repeatedly revealed chromosomal abnormalities, many of which are characteristically associated with specific malignant disorders.[2] Although these and other findings indicated that inborn and somatic mutations play an important role in triggering cancer, they did not identify the specific genes that cause cells to exhibit malignant phenotypes. Over the past 10 years, gene-cloning techniques have allowed researchers to identify, isolate, and study in detail a series of oncogenes that, in mutant form, impart malignant traits to cells. Other, more recent work indicates that another class of genes—termed tumor suppressor genes, antioncogenes, or growth-suppressing genes—plays an equally important role in human cancer pathogenesis.

Oncogenes

Initial insight into the existence and workings of oncogenes was provided by studies of tumor viruses that can infect normal cells and transform them into tumor cells. These virus-transformed cells deviated from their normal counterparts in a number of ways, including abnormalities of morphology, intermediary metabolism, dependence on growth factor stimulation, and many other aspects of cell behavior. The complexity of these cellular responses contrasted strongly with the relatively small amount of genetic information used by these viruses to induce transformation. The virus-associated transforming genes, or oncogenes, were found to carry only several thousand nucleotides of genetic information, in contrast to the cell genome, which has a million times more DNA. This work established the principle that the small amount of genetic information embodied in an oncogene can act pleiotropically to induce multiple, complex alterations in cell phenotype.

The oncogenes carried by tumorigenic retroviruses, notably Rous sarcoma virus, commanded special attention. Detailed studies of the virus-associated oncogene, termed *src*, demonstrated that it was not a true viral gene. Instead, these studies showed, the *src* oncogene had originated in the chromosomal sequences of a normal chicken cell. A nontransforming ancestor of the Rous virus had captured this cellular gene, converted it into a potent oncogene, and exploited it to transform subsequently infected cells.[3]

This discovery had several important ramifications. It pointed to the existence of a preexisting cellular gene with a latent oncogenic potential that could be activated by a virus. This cellular antecedent, the *src* proto-oncogene, was found to be present in a wide variety of animal cell genomes, indicating that the normal *src* gene plays an essential role in normal cell or organism physiology. This discovery also suggested that oncogenes associated with other transforming retroviruses might derive, by analogous processes, from other cellular proto-oncogenes. Indeed, in the past 15 years, a cohort of as many as 20 cellular proto-oncogenes has been identified through the discovery of a cognate oncogene for each oncogene carried by a retrovirus genome.[3]

Oncogenes in Human Tumors

Although the study of transforming retroviruses constituted a powerful experimental approach, this line of research did not appear to address the genetic processes that trigger human cancers. With the exception of hepatocellular carcinomas, cervical carcinomas, adult T cell leukemias, and Burkitt's lymphomas, human tumors are rarely associated with viral infections. Therefore, nonviral genetic mechanisms have been sought as causal elements in human tumorigenesis. One strategy to uncover these mechanisms involves a functional test designed to screen for the presence of oncogenes in the DNA of chemically induced rodent tumors and spontaneously arising human tumors. This functional test depends on gene transfer, also known as transfection: a procedure in which DNA and associated genes from one cell type are extracted and introduced into a second, recipient cell. In these experiments, DNA is prepared from a variety of tumor cells and introduced into more normal, nontumorigenic recipient cells. Indeed, some of these recipient cells begin to grow in culture in a manner similar to transformed cells and, when introduced into host animals, proliferate into rapidly growing tumor masses [*see Figure 1*].[4]

This type of experiment indicated that the information orchestrating the cancer phenotype is carried in the DNA of cancer cells that have no exposure to transforming viruses. Moreover, the transforming genes found in chemically induced animal tumors were seen to be very similar to those detected in human tumors. This finding indicated that the animal and human tumors arise through similar molecular processes.

Several of the oncogenes detected through transfection were subsequently isolated by means of molecular cloning, which made it possible to ascertain their origin. Characterization of a human bladder carcinoma oncogene showed that its molecular structure was very similar to that of a gene present in the DNA of normal cells. Thus, as suspected, this oncogene was found to derive from a preexisting normal cellular gene, ostensibly via a somatic mutation that occurred during tumor pathogenesis.

Cloned copies of the normal gene were inactive in transfection-transformation assays, which demonstrated that the normal gene encodes a biologic activity distinct from that of its oncogenic derivative. This finding focused attention on the precise nature of the mutation that conferred oncogenic activity on the tumor-associated gene. The essential difference between the two genes, each 5,000 DNA bases in length, was traced to a single base change (termed a point mutation).[5] This subtle change in gene structure suffices to convert a normal cellular proto-oncogene into a virulent oncogene. Accordingly, the activation of oncogenes can be traced to specific mutations of the cell genome that arise during the process of tumor formation. The relation between human tumor oncogenes and the retrovirus-activated oncogenes was clarified when it was found that the two types arise from a common repertoire of cellular proto-oncogenes. In animals, proto-oncogenes may occasionally become activated by the intervention of retroviruses [*see Figure 2*]; in humans, the same proto-oncogenes can be activated by nonviral somatic mutations, such as the point mutation that gives rise to the bladder carcinoma oncogene. Indeed, many of the oncogenes that were discovered through their association with animal retroviruses were found in altered, activated form in human

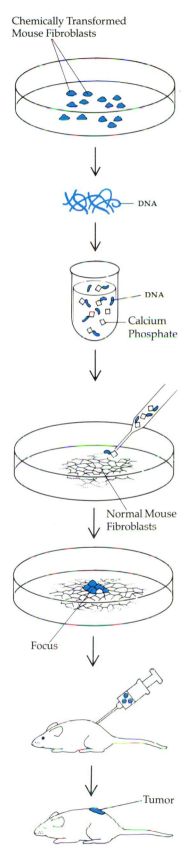

Chemically Transformed Mouse Fibroblasts

DNA

DNA

Calcium Phosphate

Normal Mouse Fibroblasts

Focus

Tumor

Figure 1 *Transfection experiments showed that tumor cell DNA can encode cancer traits. DNA was extracted from mouse cells that had been transformed by 3-methylcholanthrene, a carcinogen. The DNA was then coprecipitated with calcium phosphate to facilitate its entry into normal mouse cells. Transfected normal cells gave rise to foci of transformed cells, which produced a tumor when injected into mice.*

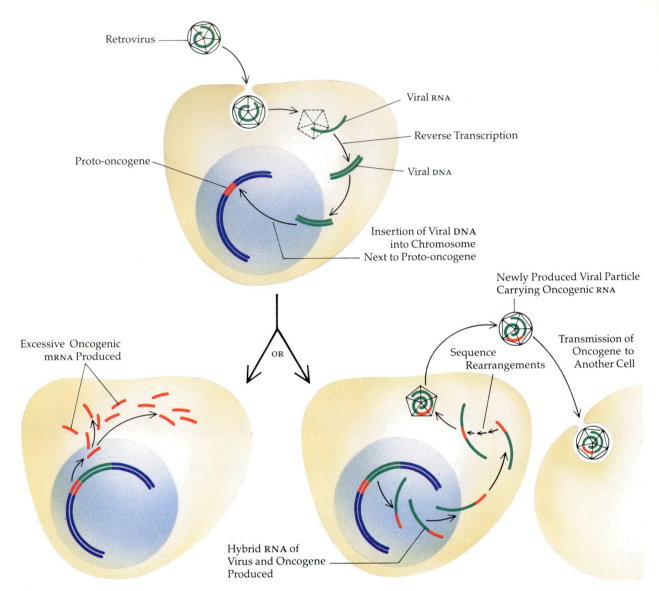

Figure 2 *Retroviruses, which cause cancer in many animals, can activate oncogenes when they infect a cell. Viral RNA is transcribed in reverse by reverse transcriptase into DNA that can be incorporated into the cellular chromosome (top). A virus may activate a cellular proto-oncogene such as* myc *by inserting its genome next to the proto-oncogene, thereby deregulating the expression of the cellular gene (lower left). Alternatively, a virus may pick up a cellular proto-oncogene in the course of an infection and activate it by incorporating it into the viral genome (lower right). In rare circumstances, sequential rearrangements occur that allow the viral progeny to leave the cell with a copy of the oncogenic RNA embedded in the viral genome; such new viral particles may then introduce the activated oncogene into another cell. The Rous sarcoma virus acquired its* src *oncogene from a cell in this way.*

tumors [*see Table 1*]. For example, many of the oncogenes detected by transfection are closely related to the *ras* oncogenes initially found in the genomes of rat sarcoma viruses; the *myc* oncogene, which was first detected in avian myelocytomatosis virus, has been shown to be activated in Burkitt's lymphoma; and the *abl* oncogene of Abelson murine leukemia virus has been found to be altered in virtually all chronic myelogenous leukemias.[6,7]

The proto-oncogenes appear to play important roles in the life of a normal cell, which explains their conservation in similar form in disparate organisms. It appears that they cannot be discarded or substantially changed by the processes that remodel most genes over extended evolutionary periods. The normal roles of many of these genes have now been elucidated (see below).

Like virtually all other genes, each proto-oncogene is composed of a regulatory region and a structural region. The regulatory region modulates the expression of the gene in response to various developmental or physiologic stimuli, whereas the structural region encodes the amino acid sequence of a protein. In principle, changes in either the regulatory or the structural portion of a proto-oncogene can create an active oncogene.

Table 1   Oncogenes in Human Tumors

Name of Oncogene	Tumor Associations	Mechanism of Activation	Properties of Gene Product
neu/erb-B2	Mammary, ovarian, and stomach carcinomas	Amplification	Cell surface growth factor receptor
erb-B	Mammary carcinoma, glioblastoma	Amplification	Growth factor receptor
ret	Papillary thyroid carcinomas	Rearrangement	Cell surface receptor
trk	Papillary thyroid carcinomas	Rearrangement	Growth factor receptor
raf	Stomach carcinoma	Rearrangement	Cytoplasmic serine/threonine kinase
Ha-ras	Bladder carcinoma	Point mutation	GDP/GTP binding
Ki-ras	Lung and colon carcinomas	Point mutation	Signal transducer
N-ras	Leukemias	Point mutation	Signal transducer
myc	Lymphomas, carcinomas	Amplification, chromosomal translocation	Nuclear transcription factor
N-myc	Neuroblastoma	Amplification	Nuclear transcription factor
L-myc	Small cell lung carcinoma	Amplification	Nuclear transcription factor
bcl-2	Follicular and undifferentiated lymphomas	Chromosomal translocation	Cytoplasmic membrane protein
gsp	Pituitary tumors	Point mutation	Cytoplasmic GDP/GTP signal transducer
hst	Stomach carcinoma	Rearrangement	Growth factor

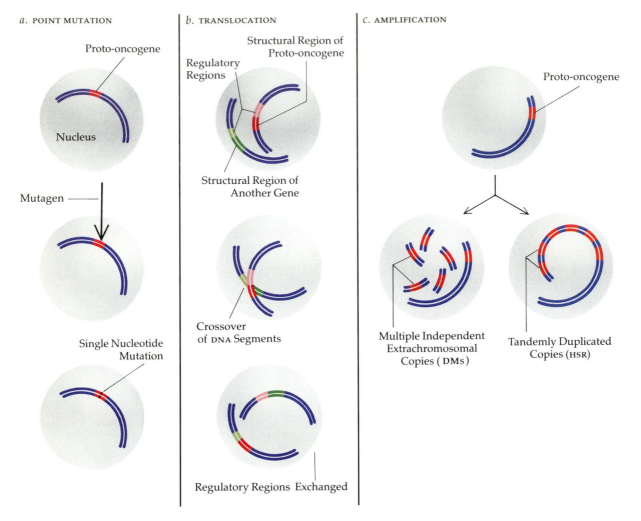

a. POINT MUTATION

Proto-oncogene

Nucleus

Mutagen

Single Nucleotide
Mutation

b. TRANSLOCATION

Structural Region of
Proto-oncogene

Regulatory
Regions

Structural Region of
Another Gene

Crossover
of DNA Segments

Regulatory Regions Exchanged

c. AMPLIFICATION

Proto-oncogene

Multiple Independent
Extrachromosomal
Copies (DMs)

Tandemly Duplicated
Copies (HSR)

Figure 3 *Activation of a proto-oncogene in the absence of retroviruses occurs either by means of mutations that affect the structure of the encoded protein or via genetic changes that alter the expression of this gene (regulatory alterations). A common source of structural alteration—the favored route of activation for* ras *oncogenes—is a point mutation (a); a single nucleotide in the gene is altered by exposure to radiation or to a chemical carcinogen, which results in a change of one amino acid in the encoded protein. In contrast, regulatory changes are often produced by translocation (b) or by amplification (c) of a large chromosomal segment carrying a proto-oncogene. In Burkitt's lymphoma, for example, translocation of DNA (b) juxtaposes the* myc *proto-oncogene and an unrelated immunoglobulin-encoding gene, leading to exchange of regulatory regions. Amplification (c) leads to deregulated replication of a proto-oncogene; multiple copies of the gene appear either as tandemly duplicated segments within the chromosome (homogeneously staining regions, or HSRs) or as extrachromosomal particles (double minutes, or DMs).*

Regulatory changes may lead to inappropriate levels of a growth-inducing protein, whereas structural mutations may lead to synthesis of a protein that has aberrant structure and function [*see Figure 3*]. Examples of both types of alterations have been found.

STRUCTURAL CHANGES

The point mutations that activate *ras* oncogenes are the simplest alterations that a DNA sequence can undergo. More dramatic alterations of

DNA sequence, such as deletions or inversions of large blocks of a gene, have not been observed among activated *ras* oncogenes.

The point mutations that activate *ras* oncogenes have been found at a limited number of sites within the structure-encoding portion of the gene.[8] Some *ras* oncogenes carry point mutations that affect amino acid residue 12 of the *ras* protein, whereas other independent mutations affect residue 13 or 61.[8,9] The normal *ras* protein acts in the cell as a signal-transducing device operating in a complex signaling cascade within the cell's cytoplasm: it acquires growth-stimulatory signals, often released by mitogen receptors at the cell surface, and passes them along a pathway to a downstream target that stimulates cell proliferation. Once it has received a growth-stimulatory signal, the normal *ras* protein binds the nucleotide guanosine triphosphate (GTP) and enters into an active, signal-emitting mode. The *ras* protein normally remains in its active conformation only briefly; having released a pulse of growth-stimulatory signals, it rapidly returns to a resting state by hydrolyzing its bound GTP into guanosine diphosphate (GDP). It is precisely this step that is defective in the oncogenic *ras* proteins found in human tumors. As a consequence, the *ras* protein becomes trapped in its excited, signal-emitting mode and thus floods the cell unrelentingly with growth-stimulatory signals.

Determination of the three-dimensional structure of a *ras* protein has revealed that the amino acid residues that are affected by oncogenic mutations are directly involved in the binding and hydrolysis of GTP.[9] Alterations in these residues compromise the ability of the *ras*-encoded protein to hydrolyze GTP to GDP. Consequently, the physiologic effects of the *ras* oncogene mutations can now be understood in terms of precisely defined changes in protein structure.

Study of the *abl* gene in cells from patients with chronic myelogenous leukemia (CML) has uncovered another example of an altered proto-oncogene protein. The chromosomal translocation that creates the Philadelphia (Ph[1]) chromosome found in CML cells also causes the *abl* proto-oncogene to become fused with a second, previously unlinked gene (*bcr*). The resulting hybrid gene specifies a hybrid *bcr-abl* protein, which functions differently from the normal *abl* protein.[10] The normal *abl* protein is a tightly regulated tyrosine kinase, which acts like the *src* protein to stimulate growth through its ability to phosphorylate specific target proteins; the *bcr-abl* fusion protein is constitutively active, and its kinase activity is no longer regulated physiologically. Once again, cell growth is driven by a steady, uncontrolled release of growth-stimulatory signals.

REGULATORY CHANGES

Whereas the oncogenes *ras* and *abl* are created by mutations that alter protein structure, oncogenes such as *myc* are created by mutations that affect the amount of encoded proteins. A variety of genetic changes can increase the level of *myc* expression. Perhaps the most dramatic change is the chromosomal translocation seen in Burkitt's lymphoma, in which the gene segment normally regulating levels of *myc* proto-oncogene expression is broken away and replaced by a regulatory sequence derived from an immunoglobulin gene [*see Figure 3*].[11] This translocation, like the one that occurs in CML cells, depends on reciprocal exchanges of chromosomal segments between two nonhomologous chromosomes. In the *myc* translocation, however, the restructured gene specifies a normal protein, but the amount of this protein is no longer regulated by physiologic stimuli, such as growth factor stimulation of a cell. Uncoupled from its normal physiologic regulators, *myc* is expressed continuously.

A second, quite distinct alteration can affect *myc* regulation. In certain tumor cells, the *myc* gene is present in multiple copies. Instead of the two copies characteristic of other genes on autosomal chromosomes, 50 to 100 copies of the *myc* gene may be present.[12] Such gene amplification results in a proportional increase in the level of the *myc*-encoded protein.

In both of these instances, deregulation of the level of *myc*-specified protein ensues from activation of the *myc* gene. Amplification of a related gene, termed N-*myc*, has frequently been found in childhood neuroblastomas, where it serves as a harbinger of aggressive tumor growth.[13] Small cell carcinomas often carry amplified copies of N-*myc* or a related gene, L-*myc*.

Cells from advanced breast and ovarian carcinomas often have amplified copies of the *neu*/*erb*-B2 (also termed HER-2/*neu*) gene, which specifies a cell surface mitogen receptor. Its overexpression leads to deregulated release of growth-stimulatory signals into these cells.[14]

Congenital Susceptibility to Cancer

The various genetic changes that activate oncogenes, including the point mutations and large-scale chromosomal rearrangements, are detectable in the genomes of tumor cells but not in the genomes of cells from adjacent normal tissue. It is apparent that these genetic lesions arose in a cell within the target tissue; that cell became the ancestor of the entire tumor cell population. Such somatic mutations have no effect on the germ cells and are not transmitted genetically to the progeny of an affected organism. Because activated oncogenes are not transmitted in the germ line, they cannot account for the well-known hereditary factors that influence susceptibility to various types of cancer. Inborn determinants affecting predisposition to specific types of cancer have been clearly documented, but they seem to involve genetic sequences distinct from the known oncogenes. As mentioned earlier, these susceptibility genes appear to act at various levels: some influence the rate at which carcinogens undergo metabolic activation in specific target organs[15]; others influence the ability of cells to repair DNA damage that either occurs spontaneously or is actively induced by carcinogens.[16,17] Inborn defects in recognizing and repairing DNA damage underlie the rare cancer syndromes xeroderma pigmentosum and ataxia telangiectasia. Still other alleles may affect the ability of the immune system to recognize and destroy incipient tumors, but the mechanism of action of these genes is poorly understood.[18,19]

Tumor Suppressor Genes

A new class of cancer susceptibility genes, termed tumor suppressor genes, has come into view, largely through successes in genetic mapping and gene cloning [*see Table 2*].[20-23] In contrast to proto-oncogenes, which induce cancer when they are converted into the deregulated, hyperactive alleles that are termed oncogenes, these tumor suppressor genes trigger cancer as inactive or null alleles. This finding suggests that suppressor genes act in normal cells to constrain or suppress proliferation; accordingly, cells deprived of the services of a suppressor gene exhibit the unconstrained growth that leads to malignancy. The best studied tumor suppressor gene is the retinoblastoma (Rb) gene. Both copies of this gene are invariably found to be inactivated in retinoblastoma tumor cells (i.e., the nullizygous state). This total loss of genetic function can occur in several ways [*see Figure 4*]. Children afflicted with familial retinoblastoma

Table 2 Tumor Suppressor Genes in Human Tumors

Chromosomal Localization	Name of Locus	Tumor Involvement	Nature of Gene Product
1p	—	Melanoma, multiple endocrine neoplasia type 2, neuroblastoma, pheochromocytoma, ductal cell carcinoma	—
3p	—	Small cell carcinoma and adeno-carcinoma of lung, cervical carcinoma, renal cell carcinoma, von Hippel-Lindau disease	—
5p	APC	Familial adenomatous polyposis, colorectal carcinoma	Cytoplasmic protein
9p13	MLM	Familial melanoma	—
9q	—	Bladder carcinoma	—
10q	—	Astrocytoma, multiple endocrine neoplasia type 2	—
11p	WT-1	Wilms' tumor, rhabdomyo-sarcoma, breast carcinoma, hepatoblastoma, transitional cell bladder carcinoma, lung carcinoma	DNA-binding protein, perhaps regulator of transcription
11q	—	Multiple endocrine neoplasia type 1	—
13q	Rb-1	Retinoblastoma, osteosarcoma, ductal breast carcinoma, bladder carcinoma	DNA-binding protein, perhaps regulator of transcription
17p	p53	Small cell lung carcinoma, colo-rectal carcinoma, breast carcin-oma, osteosarcoma, squamous cell lung carcinoma, and others	DNA-binding protein
17q	NF-1	Neurofibromatosis type 1 (von Recklinghausen NF)	Interacts with *ras* pro-tein, induces GTP hydrolysis
18q	DCC	Colorectal carcinoma	Cell surface receptor
22q	—	Neurofibromatosis type 2, acoustic neuroma, pheochromocytoma	—

carry one intact and one defective copy of the Rb gene in all their cells, having acquired a defective allele from sperm or egg at conception. Tumor cell growth is triggered when a random somatic mutation inactivates the surviving, intact allele in one of their retinal cells. In nonfamilial (so-called sporadic) cases of retinoblastoma, both copies of this gene are inactivated somatically in one retinal cell, which then proliferates into a tumor cell population.

The mechanism discovered for the Rb gene applies to other members of this class of genes: when defective alleles are passed through the germ line, they confer inborn cancer susceptibility and lead to associated familial cancer syndromes; when these same genes are inactivated solely through somatic mutations, they trigger sporadic forms of the same tumors.[24-29] For example, the gene coding for adenomatous polyposis coli (the APC gene) is an inactivated form of a tumor suppressor gene that causes familial

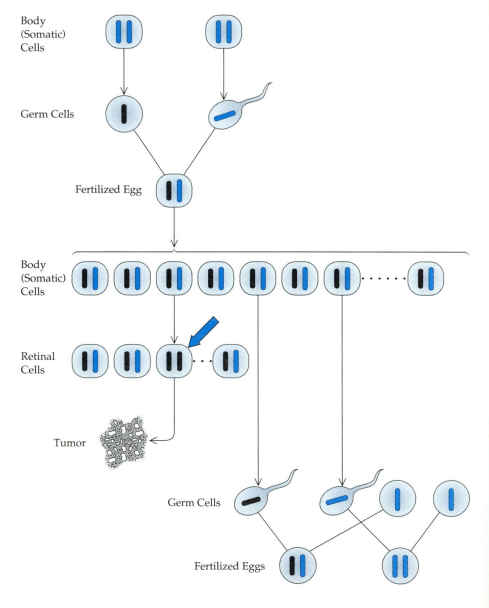

Figure 4 *Hypothetical case of familial retinoblastoma is traced at the cellular level. As the result of a genetic accident in the first generation, the region carrying Rb, the retinoblastoma gene, is deleted from the single chromosome 13 in an ovum. The chromosome (black) carrying the deletion is inherited by a son and is present in all his body cells, including retinal cells. A somatic mutation in infancy or early childhood inactivates the second copy of the gene in one retinal cell (red arrow), and so a tumor develops. The tumor is excised and about half of his sperm cells carry the deleted form of chromosome 13, and so about half of his children inherit the predisposition to retinoblastoma.*

polyposis when it is passed through the germ line; it may also become inactivated somatically, as seems to occur in most cases of sporadic, nonfamilial colon carcinoma.[25] Again, the p53 gene may be passed in mutant form through the germ line, as it is in families that suffer the rare, multitumor Li-Fraumeni syndrome; this same gene is altered by somatic mutation during the genesis of more than half of the human tumor types examined to date.[28,29]

Both normal alleles of a tumor suppressor gene must usually be defective for cell growth to become deregulated. The first allele may be altered through either a germ line mutation or a somatic mutation. The second, surviving allele is then altered somatically. Often, the surviving allele is simply discarded and replaced by a replicate of the mutant allele. As a consequence, the suppressor gene locus carries two identical (albeit mutant) alleles of the gene. This process, termed either a loss of heterozygosity or a reduction to homozygosity, often involves a large chromosomal domain flanking the tumor suppressor gene, which also loses heterozygosity during this process. By studying the behavior of genetic markers located within these flanking domains, investigators can trace the behavior of linked suppressor genes.[24]

A powerful strategy for discovering new suppressor genes in human tumors has emerged. By tracing genetic markers scattered throughout the genome, researchers have found specific markers that are repeatedly reduced to homozygosity in many tumors of a given type. This marker homozygosity suggests the presence of a closely linked suppressor gene whose second gene copy has been eliminated from the evolving tumor cell by this process. For example, advanced colon carcinoma cells often show a loss of heterozygosity of markers mapping to the long arm of chromosome 18. This result suggests the presence of a suppressor gene on this chromosomal arm whose loss often accompanies (and perhaps causes) the conversion of benign growths to more malignant colonic growths. On the basis of this indirect evidence, researchers proceeded to identify and isolate the responsible gene, now termed DCC (for "deleted in colon carcinoma").[30]

Similar strategies have led to the isolation of the WT-1 gene, homozygous inactivation of which triggers the childhood kidney neoplasm known as Wilms' tumor.[26] Other work led to the cloning of the NF-1 gene, whose inactivation triggers neurofibromatosis type 1.[27]

The inactivation of genes like NF-1 and WT-1 appears to lead to a narrow range of tumors. Unexpectedly, the inactivation of the Rb gene, initially uncovered through its association with a rare eye tumor, plays a role in the genesis of a large range of tumors, including many sarcomas, small cell lung carcinomas, and bladder and breast carcinomas.

Alteration of the p53 suppressor gene, which maps to the short arm of chromosome 17, appears to be involved in a very wide range of tumors[28,29] (see above). The somatic mutations that alter p53 genes are almost always point mutations. Indeed, p53 may be the most frequently mutated gene in human cancer.

The genetics of p53 involvement in tumorigenesis distinguish the p53 gene from most other tumor suppressor genes. In the case of the Rb gene, a single mutant allele is phenotypically silent (or recessive); in contrast, mutant p53 alleles often affect cell phenotype even in the presence of a coexpressed, wild-type allele.[21,22,29] This effect is attributable to the biochemistry of the p53 protein, which assembles as a tetramer. Cells that carry both mutant and wild-type p53 alleles form mixed tetramers, whose functioning is compromised by the defective subunits encoded by the mutant p53 allele; the mutant allele inhibits its wild-type counterpart. This inhibition is not complete, however, and most tumor cells gain further growth advantage by eventually discarding the surviving wild-type allele.

Two theories are currently being examined to explain how a tumor suppressor gene functions in the normal cell. The first theory is based on the fact that a normal cell receives various growth-inhibitory signals that cause it to cease proliferating. Such a cell must maintain an elaborate machinery that allows it to brake its growth in response to these negative signals. This theory proposes that when both copies of a gene encoding a component of this response machinery are deleted, the cell loses its ability to receive and process these exogenous growth-inhibitory signals properly. As a consequence, the cell may continue to grow under conditions where such growth would be inappropriate. Tumor suppressor genes could encode proteins that form part of this response apparatus.

The second theory proposes, as does the first, that tumor suppressor genes encode growth-inhibitory proteins but proposes that the signals that activate these suppressor proteins originate within the cell. Much evidence has accumulated indicating that normal cell lines are allocated a limited number of cell divisions before they die out. The allocation of cell divisions may be determined by the cell's internal generational clock. Cells that survive senescence and become immortalized often carry mutant p53 genes. This finding suggests that although these cells have reached the number of generations allocated by their generational clock, they are unable to shut down growth because they lack functioning p53 proteins.

Furthermore, p53 mutant cells show another peculiarity. Unlike normal cells, p53 mutant cells replicate their genomes after DNA-damaging doses of x-rays. In contrast, normal cells tarry, repair the x-ray–induced damage, and only then replicate their DNA. The p53 gene, then, may respond to an internal signal generated by the cell apparatus that monitors the intactness of the genome and may thus shut down growth if extensive damage has been detected.[31]

The roles of the p53 and Rb suppressor genes in normal organism function have been demonstrated dramatically by the changes observed in genetically altered mice that lack both copies of either the p53 or the Rb genes. The p53-negative mice develop normally but succumb to cancer in high numbers beginning at two months of age.[32-34] The Rb-negative mice die between day 13 and day 15 of gestation because their red blood cell precursors cannot mature properly. These findings provide the first clues to the normal roles of these genes. The Rb gene seems to play an important role in enabling red blood cell precursors in the murine embryonic liver to enter end-stage differentiation.

Chromosomal Alterations in Cancer

The mutational processes that activate oncogenes or inactivate tumor suppressor genes may or may not have manifestations at the karyotypic level (i.e., may or may not grossly alter chromosome structure).[35] Point mutations that activate *ras* oncogenes or inactivate the Rb gene represent such minor perturbations that they have little effect on overall gene structure and no effect on the chromatin associated with the gene. In contrast, many of the mutational processes that lead to *myc* activation depend on massive reorganization of DNA segments and often produce observable karyotypic abnormalities.

The association of the *myc* proto-oncogene with immunoglobulin segments is achieved only by a major reshuffling of chromosomal arms—a reciprocal translocation that is readily observable in banded metaphase chromosomes. A similar translocation creates the *bcr-abl* fusion gene seen in CML.

These two translocations provide models for other translocations that have been studied at the molecular level. In several leukemias, specific genes (often encoding transcription factors) are joined to the regulatory sequences of immunoglobulin or T cell receptor genes in a situation analogous to that seen with *myc* [*see Table 3*]. Such translocations appear to occur because the machinery that normally rearranges immunoglobulin and T cell receptor genes malfunctions.

Alternatively, the fusion genes resulting from a translocation may follow the pattern of *bcr-abl*, creating a hybrid protein that has novel functions. One of these fusion genes arises from the 15;17 chromosomal translocations that occur in acute promyelocytic leukemias (PMLs). A novel protein arises from the fusion of a product of the PML gene with the retinoic acid receptor–α protein. The connection between this fusion product and the often observed dramatic response of PMLs to retinoic acid treatment is not clearly understood.

Gene amplification also often leads to karyotypic abnormalities that are visible under the light microscope. Usually, both the oncogene and the flanking DNA sequences are amplified. If the amplified DNA segments remain associated with a chromosome, they are often found in a large tandem array that manifests itself, at the karyotypic level, as a homogeneously staining region (HSR). When the amplified DNA segments break loose from the chromosome, they may replicate as extrachromosomal particles known as double minutes (DMs) [*see Figures 3 and 5*]. DMs are characteristic of certain types of tumors. For example, advanced childhood neuroblastomas often carry several hundred DMs per cell. Each of these DMs carries a copy of the N-*myc* gene.[13,35] The overexpression of certain growth-regulating genes, however, often occurs without any clearly karyotypic alterations of the chromosomes that carry them.

Other chromosomal aberrations involve tumor suppressor genes, which may be deleted or inactivated during tumorigenesis. Usually, these genetic changes create relatively minor alterations in gene structure, which are not apparent microscopically at the karyotypic level. Occasionally, however, a large stretch of chromosomal DNA that includes the tumor suppressor gene may be lost; such a loss is seen as an interstitial deletion that involves one or more chromosomal bands. These deletions first alerted cytologists to the presence of the retinoblastoma gene on chromosome 13 and of the WT-1 gene on chromosome 11.

Although many karyotypic abnormalities have been associated with certain types of tumors, only a few are well understood at the molecular level. It is likely that many of these changes reflect the activation of cellular genes that promote tumor cell growth or the inactivation of genes that restrict growth. In most cases, however, the nature of these genes is not known.

Multistep Tumorigenesis

Tumor cells must acquire a number of distinct aberrant traits to proliferate. Reflecting this requirement is the fact that the genomes of certain well-studied tumors carry several different independently altered genes, including activated oncogenes and inactivated tumor suppressor genes. Each of these genetic changes appears to be responsible for imparting some of the traits that, in aggregate, represent the full neoplastic phenotype.[36-38] For example, *ras* oncogenes appear to exert strong effects on cell shape and on the ability to grow in the absence of attachment to normal substrate; they can induce cells to secrete a number of growth-stimulating factors. The *myc* oncogene seems to specialize in affecting other cellular traits. Cells in which this oncogene is activated are readily immortalized and thus are able to divide an unlimited number of times in culture. This behavior contrasts dramatically with that of most normal cells, whose replicative potential in vitro and in vivo is limited. Cells carrying the *myc* oncogene are also more responsive to growth factors that may be present in the surrounding medium. Mutations of the p53 tumor suppressor gene enable

Table 3 Human Tumor–Associated Chromosomal Translocations

Chromosomal Sites	Name	Tumor Association	Nature of Active Effector
9;22	*bcr-abl*	Chronic and acute myeloid leukemias	Tyrosine kinase
14;11	*bcl*-1	B cell lymphomas and multiple myelomas	Cyclin D1
14;22	*bcl*-2	Chronic B cell leukemias	Cytoplasmic protein
14;19	*bcl*-3	B cell chronic lymphocytic leukemias	Transcription factor
8;2, 14, 22	*myc*	Burkitt's lymphoma	Helix-loop-helix transcription factor
7;19	*lyl*-1	T cell leukemias	Helix-loop-helix transcription factor
1;14	*tal/scl/tcl*-5	T cell leukemias	Helix-loop-helix transcription factor
10;14	*tcl*-3/*hox*-11	T cell leukemias	Homeodomain and helix-loop-helix transcription factors
1;19	E2a-*pbx*1	Childhood acute pre-B cell leukemia	Homeodomain transcription factor
	ttg/rhom-1	T cell leukemias	Zinc finger transcription factor
	rhom-2	T cell leukemias	Zinc finger transcription factor
15;17	*PML-RARa*	Acute promyelocytic leukemia	Zinc finger transcription factor
			Retinoic acid receptor
6;9	*dek-can*	Acute myeloid leukemia	Unknown

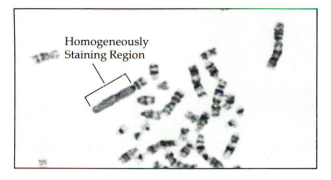
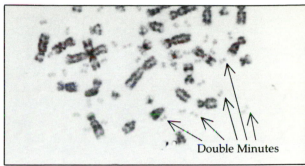

Figure 5 *Amplified oncogenes can produce karyotypic abnormalities that are visible under a light microscope. A homogeneously staining region (HSR) occurs when a large tandem array of amplified genes remains associated with a chromosome (left). Double minutes (DMs) appear when copies of amplified genes are not integrated into the chromosome (right).*

a cell line to become immortalized (see above). This immortalization appears to be important for an expanding clone of tumor cells that need to replicate without limitation.

Tumor cells may also gain growth advantage by escaping programmed cell death, or apoptosis, the process used by many normal tissues to limit cell population size. This process may be disrupted during the pathogenesis of a variety of tumor cell types, yielding a large population of premalignant cells that may then develop further into frankly neoplastic cell types. Overexpression of the *bcl-2* gene and the resulting abnormally high levels of its gene product block apoptosis in a variety of cell types. This gene was initially discovered at the breakpoint region of a chromosomal translocation found in follicular and diffuse B cell lymphomas, but its overexpression is now thought to play a role in the pathogenesis of other tumors as well, including non–small cell carcinomas, in which high levels of *bcl-2* expression are correlated with poor long-term survival.

This model of multiple collaborating genetic changes can be verified experimentally by transferring various oncogenes into normal embryo fibroblasts. When either a *ras* or a *myc* oncogene is introduced into an embryo fibroblast, it is unable to impart tumorigenicity to this cell. When *ras* and *myc* oncogenes are introduced concomitantly, however, the previously normal cells can form actively growing tumors in appropriate hosts.[36-38] Such data suggest that cancer should be seen as a long progression of genetic alterations, each of which imparts some changes that together succeed in transforming a normal cell into a cancer cell.

A dramatic example of this multistep transformation has been documented in the case of colon carcinoma, which is thought to evolve through a series of histopathologic forms, beginning with dysplastic areas of the colonic epithelium, passing through a stage of adenomatous polyps, and ultimately progressing to frank carcinoma.

Many early adenomas carry lesions that inactivate their APC gene, the tumor suppressor gene that in mutant form leads to familial polyposis. More than half of the more advanced adenomas also carry activated *ras* oncogenes that presumably contribute to their premalignant growth traits. The carcinomas that arise from these adenomas carry still more genetic abnormalities, on chromosomes 17 and 18.[39,40] The gene affected on chromosome 17 is the previously described p53 suppressor gene; in vitro tissue culture studies have shown that the p53 gene can collaborate with *ras* oncogenes in the full transformation of cells. Inactivation of the chromosome 18 target gene, the DCC tumor suppressor gene, also aids in progression to a fully malignant state. It appears that the critical steps of colon carcinogenesis will soon be defined in terms of a succession of precisely characterized lesions in well-studied genes. This represents a model for similar multistep tumor progression occurring in other organ systems.

Other Molecular Mechanisms of Tumor Development

Over the past 10 years, most research on the molecular mechanisms of carcinogenesis has focused on growth-deregulating mechanisms and their underlying genetic changes. However, it is clear that cancer cells require more than the growth impetus supplied by these genetic changes. Early in tumor progression, cancer cells must successfully evade the host immune surveillance system, which is designed to seek out and rapidly destroy tumor cells as they arise throughout the body. Once cancer cells form a tumor mass of substantial size, they must acquire vasculature to supply nourishment and remove metabolic waste. Cancer cells also often display biochemical changes that enable them to invade adjacent tissue and ultimately to metastasize to distant sites.

The biochemical basis for immune system recognition of tumor cells is still unclear. The tumorigenicity of cells may increase when their display of class I histocompatibility antigens is reduced[41] and may decrease when these antigens are redisplayed.[18,42] These class I antigens, displayed in conjunction with tumor-specific antigens, are essential for recognition of tumor cells by cytolytic thymus-dependent lymphocytes (CTLs).

One experimental approach has shown some success in revealing the molecular nature of human tumor-specific antigens. Researchers have developed lines of CTLs that originate in a tumor-bearing patient and that are toxic to that patient's tumor cells in vitro. These CTLs can be used to identify the genes encoding the tumor cell antigens that CTLs recognize. This approach has yielded a group of cloned genes encoding antigens that are displayed by human melanoma cells but not by normal cells from various tissues. Tumor cells that have lost one of these genes escape being killed by the corresponding reactive CTLs.[19] This work paves the way for defining the molecular immunology of human tumor cells in terms of specific genes and gene products.

Of great importance to a growing tumor is its ability to receive nourishment and remove metabolic waste. Early, small tumors depend on passive diffusion to exchange molecules with the surrounding tissue, but once a tumor reaches a diameter greater than 1 mm, it requires intimate contact with the circulatory system. For this reason, more advanced tumors release angiogenic factors, which encourage the growth of blood vessels from the surrounding tissue into the tumor mass.[43,44] Among the angiogenic factors that provoke neovascularization are several well-known mitogens, such as the fibroblast growth factor (FGF) and the endothelial cell growth factor

(ECGF). These angiogenic factors are presumably used during wound healing and by developing tissue to create well-vascularized tissue; also, they are elaborated as part of the physiologic response of normal tissue to hypoxia. The mechanisms enabling tumor cells to secrete angiogenic factors are poorly understood.

Neovascularization may be an essential precursor to metastasis for two reasons. It is required for the large increase in tumor cell number, which in turn allows the appearance of rare metastatic variants. Moreover, it provides a direct portal of entry into the circulatory system for metastasizing cells.

Products of Oncogenes and Tumor Suppressor Genes

Although the effects of oncogenes on cellular phenotype have been studied extensively, a thorough understanding of oncogene function will ultimately derive from detailed biochemical characterization of the proteins that they encode. Such characterization should eventually provide answers to a pressing question: how can a single protein species induce the multiple physiologic changes in the cell that are associated with the cancer state? Indeed, complex regulatory pathways appear to control cellular growth. The oncogenic proteins can intervene at key points in these regulatory pathways and disrupt their normal functioning.[45,46]

The primary structures (i.e., amino acid sequences) of virtually all the oncogene-encoded proteins are now known. This information has been obtained by decoding the nucleotide sequences of the oncogene clones. However, such structural details afford little insight into the function of proteins. Instead, knowledge of oncogene function has come from enzymological analyses of these proteins. Such analyses have been pursued most extensively in the characterization of the tyrosine kinase oncoproteins, including those specified by the *src*, *abl*, and *neu*/*erb*-B2 oncogenes. These kinases all transfer phosphate groups from adenosine triphosphate (ATP) to the tyrosine residues of a number of target proteins. By covalently modifying a target protein, a kinase is often able to change the functional state of this target. Because a single type of kinase may act on many distinct target proteins, it may perturb a number of regulatory pathways or enzymatic functions. This capacity is most important for an oncogenic protein, which must act pleiotropically to elicit multiple changes in the cellular phenotype.

Many growth factor receptors, which are used by the cell to detect the presence of growth factors in the extracellular space, also possess a tyrosine kinase catalytic domain in their cytoplasmic portions. This finding indicates that phosphorylation of tyrosine residues on cytoplasmic proteins represents a generalized growth-promoting signal within the cell. These growth factor receptors all appear to act similarly. Among them are the receptors for platelet-derived growth factor (PDGF), epidermal growth factor (EGF), and the recently identified *neu*/*erb*-B2 ligand. The last two receptors are frequently overexpressed in breast and ovarian carcinomas.[14] After the extracellular domains of these receptors bind ligands, their cytoplasmic tyrosine kinases become activated, and specific tyrosine residues of the receptors become autophosphorylated. The phosphotyrosines then attract a series of cytoplasmic proteins, each on its own an important signal transducer, including phospholipase C; the GTPase-activating protein, or GAP (a partner of the *ras* protein; see below); and several others. These proteins now become phosphorylated and, in turn, appear to activate several downstream signaling cascades. For example, phospholipase C can degrade a form of phosphatidylinositol (PI) found in the plasma membrane. Two breakdown products of PI, diacylglycerol and inositol trisphosphate, act in turn as potent growth agonists.[46,47]

As described, the normal *ras* p21 proteins cycle between an active state and an inactive state; oncogenic forms of p21 are trapped in the active state. This relatively small protein would seem to act as a regulator, switching on and off yet another protein that can release growth-stimulatory signals in the cell. The identity of the second protein and the nature of its emitted signals remain unclear. Candidates include GAP and the product of the NF-1 (neurofibromatosis) gene.[27,48,49]

In contrast to these oncogene proteins, which act in the cell cytoplasm, a number of other proteins act in the cell nucleus, where they may serve as transcription factors regulating the expression of other genes. The protein product of the *myc* gene (and, by extension, products of the related N-*myc* and L-*myc* genes) has been found to be capable of binding to specific DNA sequences that appear to be part of a control sequence present in several responder genes controlled by the *myc* gene.[50] Expression of the *myc* gene favors cell growth, because the *myc* protein apparently activates a bank of responder genes whose expression in turn is essential to the proliferation program of the cell.

The protein products of tumor suppressor genes have quite different functions. For example, the receptorlike protein encoded by the DCC gene is displayed on the surface of many epithelial cell types.[30] This protein appears to enable these cells to detect an inhibitory signal, either a diffusible factor or a component of the extracellular matrix. The NF-1 protein, which is found in the cytoplasm, is either absent or present in reduced amounts in the tumor cells of individuals having a susceptibility to neurofibromatosis. The NF-1 protein interacts with the growth-promoting *ras* protein of the cell; it may limit cell growth either by inactivating GTP-activated *ras* protein or by promoting postmitotic differentiation.[49]

Several proteins encoded by tumor suppressor genes are found in the cell's nucleus. The best known of these are the products of the p53 and Rb genes. Both appear to curb cell proliferation by stopping the cell late in the G_1 period of its growth cycle. The Rb protein appears to curb cell growth by reversibly sequestering a series of cellular growth-promoting proteins, among them possibly the *myc* protein.[51] The p53 protein is itself a transcription factor that binds to a specific DNA sequence and activates the transcription of a nearby gene; however, the identities of the genes controlled by the p53 protein are still unknown. The WT-1 protein, which is absent in Wilms' tumor cells, also functions as a transcription factor that regulates a bank of responder genes.[26] Initial work suggests that it represses rather than induces gene function.

Oncogenes and Growth Factors

Cancer represents a breakdown in the communication between tumor cells and their normal neighbors. Both growth-stimulatory and growth-inhibitory signals are exchanged between cells within a tissue. Most normal cells do not divide unless they are stimulated to do so by exogenous growth factors. These factors are generally secreted at specific sites in response to developmental, homeostatic, or wound-healing requirements. The neoplastic state is characterized by the ability of a cell to grow in the absence of some or all of these normally required exogenous growth-stimulating factors.

Oncogenes might intervene in a variety of ways to provide autonomy from exogenous growth factors.[52] The simplest mechanism involves deregulation of cellular genes that specify secreted growth factors. The expression of such genes is usually tightly controlled and limited to specific cell types. Activation of an oncogene may result in the deregulation of a growth factor gene and the secretion of large amounts of a growth factor; once secreted, the factor may then stimulate growth of the cell that has just produced it. The oncogene may encode the growth factor itself, or it may encode a protein that can stimulate expression of the growth factor gene. In either case, an autostimulatory, or autocrine, mechanism ensues: growth factor independence is achieved because cell division is driven by the cell's own secreted factors [*see Figure 6*]. One example of this mechanism involves the *sis* oncogene, which arose from alterations of the normal cellular gene encoding PDGF.[53] Cells that carry this oncogene are presumed to have escaped from their dependence on exogenous PDGF. A less direct autocrine process is connected with *src* oncogenes: expression of a *src* oncogene indirectly activates other cellular genes that control growth factor secretion.[54] A variety of human tumor cells have been shown to secrete growth factors that are presumed to play an important role in driving tumor cell growth.

Another mechanism that confers growth factor autonomy stems from changes in the receptors that are displayed on the cell surface and used by the cell to recognize the presence of growth factors in its surroundings. For example, the EGF receptor normally transmits growth-stimulatory signals to the interior of the cell only when it binds an EGF molecule. Mutation of the EGF-receptor gene may alter the structure of the receptor molecule so that it sends growth-stimulatory signals into the cell in the absence of bound growth factor.[55] The *erb*-B oncogene is an altered version of an EGF-receptor gene. The mutant receptor specified by the *erb*-B oncogene can emit mitogenic signals in the absence of EGF [*see Figure 6*]. Another oncogene, *fms*, has been found to encode an altered form of the mononuclear phagocyte receptor that detects macrophage colony-stimulating factor (also known as colony-stimulating factor–1).[56] Deregulated growth is also driven by the overexpression of receptor proteins, which appears to trigger receptor firing that is independent of ligand (i.e., growth factor) binding. One such example is the *neu/erb*-B2 receptor (see above).[57]

Most proto-oncogenes and the related oncogenes encode proteins that reside deep within the cell, seemingly far removed from the activity at the cell surface. It is likely that many of these proteins are involved in a complex signaling pathway that normally relays signals from the growth factor receptors to critical sites within the cell. For example, it is now apparent that *ras* proteins relay growth-stimulatory signals from cell surface receptors to physiologically important intracellular targets, such

AUTOCRINE MECHANISM

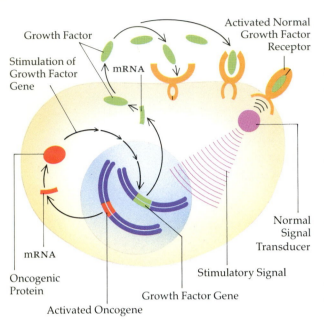

Growth Factor

Stimulation of Growth Factor Gene

mRNA

Activated Normal Growth Factor Receptor

mRNA

Oncogenic Protein

Activated Oncogene

Growth Factor Gene

Stimulatory Signal

Normal Signal Transducer

Figure 6 Oncogenes may provide independence from growth factors in at least four ways. The autocrine mechanism (top) is characterized by excessive secretion of growth factors that act on the tumor cell itself; an oncogene may indirectly stimulate expression of a growth factor gene (as shown), or it may encode the growth factor and directly cause excessive secretion of the factor. A second mechanism (bottom, left) involves production of altered growth factor receptors; the oncogene may encode faulty receptors that transmit stimulatory signals to the cell even in the absence of extracellular growth factors. A third mechanism (bottom, right) is characterized by interference with the signaling pathway that normally carries the stimulatory message from growth factor receptors to other sites in the cell. A normal gene may encode a protein that transduces signals from the receptor; the oncogenic version of this gene may produce a protein that sends out stimulatory signals even in the absence of signaling by the growth factor receptor. A fourth mechanism of growth factor independence (not shown here) involves downstream elements that respond to these signaling pathways.

RECEPTOR ALTERATION

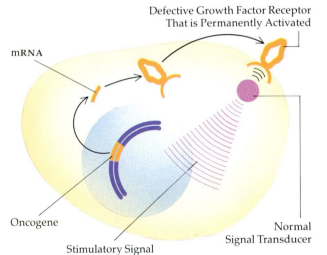

mRNA

Defective Growth Factor Receptor That is Permanently Activated

Oncogene

Stimulatory Signal

Normal Signal Transducer

TRANSDUCER ALTERATION

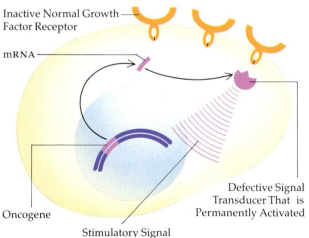

Inactive Normal Growth Factor Receptor

mRNA

Oncogene

Stimulatory Signal

Defective Signal Transducer That is Permanently Activated

as GAP and the NF-1 protein. The oncogenic versions of the *ras* proteins are able to release signals to their downstream targets even in the absence of stimulation from an activated growth factor receptor [*see Figure 6*][46]; thus a signaling pathway that is normally mitogen dependent is activated without the presence of mitogen (see above).

A fourth mechanism of growth factor independence involves elements farther downstream in these signaling cascades; these elements respond by activating gene expression in the cell nucleus.[58] The proto-oncogene forms of genes such as *myc, fos,* and *jun* encode nuclear proteins that are normally produced in large amounts in direct response to growth factor stimulation and in turn elicit growth response from the cell. The oncogenic versions of these genes specify these proteins constitutively, resulting in another form of growth factor independence. Hence, at least four physiologic mechanisms serve to confer oncogene-induced growth factor independence. The individual steps in these complex signaling cascades are rapidly being uncovered.

Diagnostic and Therapeutic Implications

Advances in molecular and cellular biology have made it possible to pinpoint some of the molecular lesions that play central causative roles in neoplastic transformation. Although these findings have important implications for basic biology, their immediate impact on clinical medicine is less apparent.

The use of monoclonal antibodies and nucleic acid sequence probes should make it possible to detect a variety of activated oncogenes in tumor biopsy specimens. In several cases, these reagents either have been developed or are expected to be developed soon. The resulting data may have great diagnostic utility. For example, a probe for the N-*myc* oncogene can be used for staging childhood neuroblastoma; this oncogene is characteristically amplified in advanced, but not in early, stages of the disease.[59] Other probes, including those using the *neu/erb*-B2 and *abl* oncogenes, may also be useful as diagnostic or prognostic assays. Amplification of the *neu/erb*-B2 oncogene in mammary carcinomas appears to be correlated with invasive disease.[57] Structural analysis of the *abl* oncogene provides an accurate diagnosis of chronic myelogenous leukemia at the molecular level. An *abl* oncogene assay may also prove useful in the diagnosis of a virulent subtype of acute lymphocytic leukemia.[60] Measures of neovascularization may also have great diagnostic utility: immunofluorescent staining for factor VIII, a component of newly formed capillaries, should detect new capillaries infiltrating primary tumors and help predict future metastatic behavior of breast carcinoma cells.[61]

The *ras* proto-oncogene may undergo a number of different types of activating point mutations, each of which leads to the substitution of a distinct amino acid. The transforming potencies of the resulting oncogenic alleles differ greatly: some alleles have virulent effects on cell behavior, whereas others seem quite benign. A diagnostic test could therefore be developed on the basis of analysis of the *ras* oncogene.[62] The development of the polymerase chain reaction (PCR) gene amplification procedure has made it possible to detect mutations, such as those that activate the *ras* oncogene, in DNA extracted from minute amounts of colon tumor tissue present in stool.[63,64] Detection of mutant alleles of the Rb and WT-1 suppressor genes is already being used for genetic diagnosis of familial disease. It is still unclear, however, whether oncogenes and tumor suppressor genes will be effective for diagnosing and assessing the prognosis of all types of cancer.

It is evident that the most attractive aspect of oncogene and suppressor gene research originates from the insights it may yield into new therapeutic modalities. A widely recognized limitation of current therapy is its lack of specificity; adverse effects on normal tissue limit the dosages that can be administered. Characterization of some oncogenes and suppressor genes provides the possibility of absolute specificity: certain tumor-associated proteins are qualitatively distinct from comparable proteins that are found elsewhere in the body. For example, the structures of the oncogenic *bcr-abl* and *ras* proteins differ from the structures of their counterparts in normal cells. These altered structures should provide unique targets for therapeutic agents that may be developed in the coming decades. Rapidly evolving knowledge of the molecular mechanisms of cancer is likely soon to provide other totally new insights into cancer management, many of which cannot yet be anticipated.

References

1. McCann J, Ames BN: Detection of carcinogens as mutagens in the *Salmonella*/microsome test: assay of 300 chemicals: discussion. *Proc Natl Acad Sci USA* 73:950, 1976

2. Yunis JJ: The chromosomal basis of human neoplasia. *Science* 221:227, 1983

3. Bishop JM: Cellular oncogenes and retroviruses. *Annu Rev Biochem* 52:301, 1983

4. Shih C, Shilo BZ, Goldfarb MP, et al: Passage of phenotypes of chemically transformed cells via transfection of DNA and chromatin. *Proc Natl Acad Sci USA* 76:5714, 1979

5. Tabin CJ, Bradley SM, Bargmann CI, et al: Mechanism of activation of a human oncogene. *Nature* 300:143, 1982

6. Bishop JM: The molecular genetics of cancer. *Science* 235:305, 1987

7. Bishop JM: Molecular themes in oncogenesis. *Cell* 64:235, 1991

8. Barbacid M: *ras* genes. *Annu Rev Biochem* 56:779, 1987

9. Krengel U, Schlichting L, Scherer A, et al: Three-dimensional structures of H-ras p21 mutants: molecular basis for their inability to function as signal switch molecules. *Cell* 62:539, 1990

10. Sawyers CL, Denny CT, Witte ON: Leukemia and the disruption of normal hematopoiesis. *Cell* 64:337, 1991

11. Leder P, Battey J, Lenoir G, et al: Translocations among antibody genes in human cancer. *Science* 222:765, 1983

12. Collins S, Groudine M: Amplification of endogenous *myc*-related DNA sequences in a human myeloid leukemia cell line. *Nature* 298:679, 1982

13. Brodeur GM, Seeger RC, Schwab M, et al: Amplification of N-*myc* in untreated human neuroblastomas correlates with advanced disease stage. *Science* 224:1121, 1984

14. Slamon DJ, Godolphin W, Jones LA, et al: Studies of the HER-2/neu proto-oncogene in human breast and ovarian cancer. *Science* 244:707,1989

15. Guengerich FP, Shimada T, Distlerath LM, et al: Human cytochrome P-450 isozymes: polymorphism and potential relevance in chemical carcinogenesis. *Biochemical and Molecular Epidemiology of Cancer*. Harris CR, Ed. Alan R Liss, Inc, New York, 1986, p 205

16. Friedberg EC: *DNA Repair*. WH Freeman and Co, New York, 1985

17. Willis AE, Lindahl T: DNA ligase I deficiency in Bloom's syndrome. *Nature* 325:355, 1987

18. Wallich R, Balbuc N, Hammerling GJ, et al: Abrogation of metastatic properties of tumour cells by *de novo* expression of H-2k antigens following H-2 gene transfection. *Nature* 315:301, 1986

19. Van der Bruggen P, Traversari C, Chomez P, et al: A gene encoding an antigen recognized by cytolytic T lymphocytes on a human melanoma. *Science* 254:1643, 1991

20. Klein G: The approaching era of the tumor suppressor genes. *Science* 238:1539, 1987

21. Weinberg RA: Tumor suppressor genes. *Science* 254:1138, 1991

22. Marshall CJ: Tumor suppressor genes. *Cell* 64:313, 1991

23. Ponder BAJ: Inherited predisposition to cancer. *Trends Genet* 6:213, 1991

24. Hansen MF, Cavenee WK: Genetics of cancer predisposition. *Cancer Res* 47:5518, 1987

25. Groden J, Thliveris A, Samowitz W, et al: Identification and characterization of the familial adenomatous polyposis coli gene. *Cell* 66:589, 1991

26. Call KM, Glaser T, Ito CY, et al: Isolation and characterization of a zinc finger polypeptide gene at the human chromsome 11 Wilms' tumor locus. *Cell* 60:509, 1990

27. Cawthon RM, Weiss R, Xu GF, et al: A major segment of the neurofibromatosis type 1 gene: cDNA sequence, genomic structure, and point mutations. *Cell* 62:193, 1990

28. Malkin D, Li FP, Strong LC, et al: Germ line p53 mutations in a familial syndrome of breast cancer, sarcomas, and other neoplasms. *Science* 250:1233, 1990

29. Michalovitz D, Halevy O, Oren M: p53 mutations: gains or losses. *J Cell Biochem* 45:22, 1991

30. Fearon ER, Cho KR, Nigro JM, et al: Identification of a chromosome 18q gene that is altered in colorectal cancers. *Science* 247:49, 1990

31. Kuerbitz SJ, Plunkett BS, Walsh WV, et al: Wild-type p53 is a cell cycle checkpoint determinant following irradiation. *Proc Natl Acad Sci USA* 89:7491, 1992

32. Donehower LA, Harvey M, Slagle BL, et al: Mice deficient for p53 are developmentally normal but susceptible to spontaneous tumours. *Nature* 356:215, 1992

33. Lee EY, Chang C-Y, Hu N, et al: Mice deficient for Rb are nonviable and show defects in neurogenesis and haematopoiesis. *Nature* 359:288, 1992

34. Jacks T, Fazeli A, Schmitt EM, et al: Effects of an *Rb* mutation in the mouse. *Nature* 359:295, 1992

35. Rowley JD: Human oncogene locations and chromosome aberrations. *Nature* 301:290, 1983

36. Land H, Parada LF, Weinberg RA: Cellular oncogenes and multistep carcinogenesis. *Science* 222:771, 1983

37. Ruley HE: Adenovirus early region 1A enables viral and cellular transforming genes to transform primary cells in culture. *Nature* 304:602, 1983

38. Hunter T: Cooperation between oncogenes. *Cell* 64:249, 1991

39. Bos JL, Fearon ER, Hamilton SR, et al: Prevalence of *ras* gene mutations in human colorectal cancers. *Nature* 327:293, 1987

40. Vogelstein B, Fearon ER, Hamilton SR, et al: Genetic alterations during colorectal-tumor development. *N Engl J Med* 319:525, 1988

41. Schrier PI, Bernards R, Vaessen RTMJ, et al: Expression of class I major histocompatibility antigens switched off by highly oncogenic adenovirus 12 in transformed rat cells. *Nature* 305:771, 1983

42. Tanaka K, Isselbacher KJ, Khoury G, et al: Reversal of oncogenesis by the expression of a major histocompatibility complex class I gene. *Science* 228:26, 1985

43. Folkman J, Klagsburn M: Angiogenic factors. *Science* 235:442, 1987

44. Liotta LA, Steeg PS, Stetler-Stevenson WG: Cancer metastasis and angiogenesis: an imbalance of positive and negative regulation. *Cell* 64:327, 1991

45. Hunter T: The proteins of oncogenes. *Sci Am* 251(2):70, 1984

46. Cantley LC, Auger KR, Carpenter C, et al: Oncogenes and signal transduction. *Cell* 64:281, 1991

47. Morrison DK, Kaplan DR, Rhee SG, et al: Platelet-derived growth factor (PDGF)–dependent association of phospholipase C-γ with PDGF receptor signaling complex. *Mol Cell Biol* 10:2359, 1990

48. Trahey M, McCormick F: A cytoplasmic protein stimulates normal N-ras p21 GTPase, but does not affect oncogenic mutants. *Science* 238:542, 1987

49. Xu GF, O'Connell P, Viskochil D, et al: The neurofibromatosis type 1 gene encodes a protein related to GAP. *Cell* 62:599, 1990

50. Blackwell TK, Kretzner L, Blackwood EM, et al: Sequence-specific DNA binding by the c-myc protein. *Science* 250:1149, 1990

51. Rustgi AK, Dyson N, Bernards R: Amino-terminal domains of c-*myc* and N-*myc* proteins mediate binding to the retinoblastoma gene product. *Nature* 352:541, 1991

52. Cross M, Dexter TM: Growth factors in development, transformation, and tumorigenesis. *Cell* 64:271, 1991

53. Waterfield MD, Scrace GT, Whittle N, et al: Platelet-derived growth factor is structurally related to the putative transforming protein p28[sis] of simian sarcoma virus. *Nature* 304:35, 1983

54. Sporn MB, Todaro GJ: Autocrine secretion and malignant transformation of cells. *N Engl J Med* 303:878, 1980

55. Downward J, Yarden Y, Mayes E, et al: Close similarity of epidermal growth factor receptor and v-*erb-B* oncogene protein sequences. *Nature* 307:521, 1984

56. Sherr CJ, Rettenmier CW, Sacca R, et al: The c-*fms* proto-oncogene product is related to the receptor for the mononuclear phagocyte growth factor CSF-1. *Cell* 41:665, 1985

57. Slamon DJ, Clark GM, Wong SG, et al: Human breast cancer: correlation of relapse and survival with amplification of the Her-2/*neu* oncogene. *Science* 235:177, 1987

58. Lewin B: Oncogenic conversion by regulatory changes in transcription factors. *Cell* 64:303, 1991

59. Seeger RC, Brodeur GM, Sather H, et al: Association of multiple copies of the N-*myc* oncogene with rapid progression of neuroblastomas. *N Engl J Med* 313:1111, 1985

60. Clark SS, McLaughlin J, Crist WN, et al: Unique forms of the *abl* tyrosine kinase distinguish Ph[1]-positive CML from Ph[1]-positive ALL. *Science* 235:85, 1987

61. Weidner N, Semple JP, Welch WR, et al: Tumor angiogenesis and metastasis—correlation in invasive breast carcinoma. *N Engl J Med* 324:1, 1991

62. Forrester K, Almoguera C, Han K, et al: Detection of high incidence of K-*ras* oncogenes during human colon tumorigenesis. *Nature* 327:298, 1987

63. Sidransky D, Tokino T, Hamilton SR, et al: Identification of ras oncogene mutations in the stool of patients with curable colorectal tumors. *Science* 256:102, 1992

64. Saiki RK, Gelfand DH, Stoffel S, et al: Primer-directed enzymatic amplification of DNA with a thermostable DNA polymerase. *Science* 239:487, 1988

Acknowledgments

This article has been adapted from "Molecular Mechanisms of Carcinogenesis," by R. A. Weinberg, in SCIENTIFIC AMERICAN *Medicine*, edited by E. Rubenstein and D. D. Federman, Section 12, Subsection II. Scientific American, Inc., New York, 1994. All rights reserved.

Figure 1 Bunji Tagawa. Reprinted from "A Molecular Basis of Cancer," by R. A. Weinberg, in *Scientific American* 249(5):126, 1983. © 1983 Scientific American, Inc. All rights reserved.

Figures 2, 3, 6 Dana Burns.

Figure 4 Tom Moore. Adapted from "Finding the Anti-Oncogene," by R. A. Weinberg, in *Scientific American* 259(3):44, 1988. © 1988 Scientific American, Inc. All rights reserved.

Figure 5 Courtesy of Dr. June L. Biedler, Sloan-Kettering Institute for Cancer Research, Rye, New York.

Table 1 Adapted from "The Proteins of Oncogenes," by T. Hunter, in *Scientific American* 251(2):70, 1984. © 1984 Scientific American, Inc. All rights reserved.

CHAPTER 11

Bioengineered Agents in Clinical Medicine

Curtis L. Scribner, M.D., Charles Durfor, Ph.D., Dennis Klinman, M.D., Robert Kozak, Ph.D.

The rapid advances of the past few decades in understanding life at the molecular level have changed the practice of medicine in many ways, as has been demonstrated in the preceding chapters. Molecular biology has also given birth to a new industry that is making novel diagnostic and therapeutic agents available to the clinician. Biotechnology is only some 10 years old, but its potential impact on medicine and health care seems almost limitless.

The immensity of that potential could be glimpsed when the first genes were cloned, inserted in foreign cells, and expressed. Today, the Food and Drug, Administration's definition of biotechnology encompasses a number of processes and manipulations: recombinant DNA or RNA technology, hybridoma or other cell fusion technology, molecular modification of cellular receptors, and applications of cells, tissues, or their components whose potential biologic activity has been modified with these techniques. In particular, the identification of human DNA sequences and their transfer to long-lived cell lines has made possible the production of gram and kilogram quantities of very pure material that is almost identical to normal human proteins—and in some cases an improved version of such proteins—for investigation and for clinical application. This chapter will concentrate on the two major classes of biotechnology products: monoclonal antibodies (antibodies directed against a single epitope of a particular antigen) and cytokines (small proteins or glycoproteins that mediate cell-to-cell interactions by way of specific cell-surface receptors).

The journey from molecular biologic research and discovery to manufacture and clinical application is not an easy one. Difficult scientific, clinical, and production problems can slow or even halt development; indeed, fewer than 20 percent of the products that enter clinical trials are ever approved for general use. For some products, the clinical effect is not nearly as great as laboratory or preclinical studies predicted. For many more, significant and serious side effects outweigh the potential clinical benefit. And even with the most promising drugs, the basic problem of scaling up production from milligrams to tons can be staggering.

Still, a number of products of biotechnology, including erythropoietin, human insulin [*see Figure 1*], and tissue plasminogen activator (t-PA), have made it to market [*see Table 1*]. Many, many more—notably monoclonal antibodies and cytokines—are under clinical investigation. As advances in understanding of normal physiology and disease are made at the molecular level, new therapeutic agents are being developed, and then often modified, by biotechnology to prevent disease or to treat it more specific-

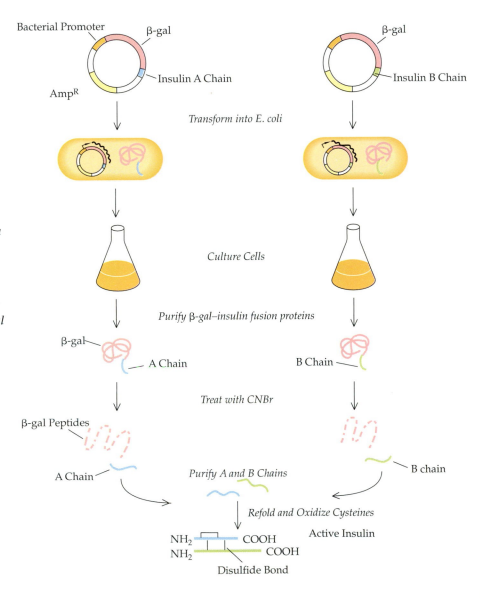

Figure 1 Diagram depicts the expression of human insulin in Escherichia coli. *Recombinant insulin is first made by expressing the A and B chains of insulin separately and then refolding them into a mature insulin molecule. The expression vectors are transformed into E. coli, and the β-galactosidase (β-gal)–insulin fusion proteins accumulate inside the bacterial cells. The cells are harvested, and each β-gal–insulin fusion protein is purified. Treatment of the fusion protein with the chemical cyanogen bromide (CNBr) results in cleavage of peptide bonds after all methionine amino acids. In this way, the natural insulin peptides are obtained. The insulin chains are cleaved further because they do not contain internal methionines. The A and B chains are purified and then mixed together to form active recombinant insulin.*

Table 1 Approved Biotechnology Products

Agent	Indication
Erythropoietin	Anemia of chronic renal disease Anemia related to human immunodeficiency virus (HIV) infection
Granulocyte colony-stimulating factor (G-CSF)	Chemotherapy-induced granulocytopenia
Granulocyte-macrophage colony-stimulating factor (GM-CSF)	Granulocytopenia after bone-marrow transplantation
Hepatitis B vaccine	Vaccination against hepatitis B
Interferon alfa-2a	Hairy cell leukemia HIV-related Kaposi's sarcoma
Interferon alfa-2b	Hairy cell leukemia Genital warts HIV-related Kaposi's sarcoma Non-A, non-B hepatitis
Interferon alfa-n3*	Genital warts
Interferon beta	Multiple sclerosis
Interferon gamma-1b	Chronic granulomatous disease
Interleukin-2	Renal cell carcinoma
OKT3	Treatment of acute renal allograft rejection
Human growth hormone	Growth hormone deficiency
Human insulin	Treatment of diabetes
Tissue plasminogen activator (t-PA)	Treatment of acute myocardial infarction
Factor VIII	Hemophilia A
Indium-labeled murine monoclonal antibody (anti–colon carcinoma)	Detection of colon cancer

Note: table includes agents approved by the U.S. Food and Drug Administration as of October 1993.

* Interferon alfa-n3 is derived from induced pooled leukocytes.

ally in a rational approach. Many products will be discussed in this chapter, but we shall begin with an example that shows the true power of biotechnology-derived products to influence the course of human disease dramatically.

Success Story: Recombinant Human Erythropoietin

The treatment of chronic renal failure has been altered radically by innovative technology not once but twice in the past 40 years. The first advance was the development and widespread use of renal dialysis to correct life-threatening fluid and electrolyte imbalances. The dialysis patient's chances for long-term survival improved markedly. Many patients with chronic renal failure nevertheless remained moderately to severely limited in activity because of chronic and severe anemia.[1]

The major cause of the anemia is the loss of endogenous erythropoietin, a 30 kilodalton (kd) glycoprotein made in the peritubular interstitial cells of the outer renal cortex.[2] Erythropoietin normally is secreted into the blood in response to changes in tissue oxygenation and is the maturation signal for the terminal steps in red blood cell development.[3,4] When the kidneys are destroyed or removed, the small amount of erythropoietin made in the liver usually is not enough to sustain red cell development[5] and the hematocrit rapidly falls to a steady state that may not meet the body's oxygen demand. It is here that the second significant technological advance was made in the treatment of patients with chronic renal failure: the introduction of recombinant erythropoietin.

The existence of a protein in the plasma of anemic animals that could cause an elevation in red blood cells had been known for many years. Jacobson demonstrated in 1957 that the primary source of erythropoietin was the kidney,[6] and Miyake and Goldwasser showed that erythropoietin could be isolated from urine.[7] Unfortunately, the quantities of erythropoietin in urine were so low that the commercial fractionation of erythropoietin from large quantities of urine proved not to be economical.

The erythropoietin gene was isolated from a human liver cell complementary DNA (cDNA) library in 1985 and cloned and characterized.[8,9] Its subsequent expression in cells from a Chinese hamster ovary line quickly led to the production of relatively large quantities of pure erythropoietin for human studies.

The results of the first clinical administration of erythropoietin were almost miraculous. Patients who had been incapacitated because of anemia and chronic angina were suddenly able to move about with comfort, take interest in outside activities, and resume a more normal life. Changes were noted over time in the onset and severity of the neuropathy of renal failure. In fact, patients who would have been started on dialysis on the basis of conventional biochemical markers felt so well that they declined to be dialyzed; the rate of pregnancy in women on dialysis began to rise, presenting difficult (but welcome) problems to both the patient and the nephrologist.

Since recombinant erythropoietin's clinical introduction in 1985, this bioengineered product has not only allowed many patients to live more normal lives but also revolutionized thinking about disease causation in chronic renal failure. As new receptors, cytokines, activation pathways, and inhibitory routes are discovered, the clinical application of bioengineered products to the prevention, diagnosis, and treatment of human disease will undoubtedly have even more startling results.

Advantages of Biotechnology

This battery of new technologies offers many opportunities to change or modify the initial gene product as needed to engineer a specific protein for a specific use. For example, a human DNA sequence can be transferred into bacterial, yeast, insect, or mammalian cells for expression depending on the specifications of the desired product. In each expression system the product is often physically slightly different from the human material because of subtle variations in the amount and type of posttranslational changes that occur in given cells. In some cases, as in posttranslational glycosylation, changes in the carbohydrate constituents of the cell (or even, as in the case of material produced in *Escherichia coli*, the complete lack of glycosylation) have little or no effect on product activity or plasma half-life; in the case of erythropoietin, however, although glycosylation is not necessary for in vitro activity, it is critical for in vivo activity. Such significant changes in biologic activity, immunogenicity, or pharmacokinetics can occur unexpectedly after seemingly minor changes in secondary, tertiary, or quaternary protein structure.

Other advantages of DNA manipulation and transfer include the ability to change the final product to alter its specificity, to eliminate unwanted activity, or to increase its production. For example, PIXY 321 is an end-to-end fusion of two very important hematopoietic cytokines: interleukin-3 and granulocyte-macrophage colony-stimulating factor.[10] Each alone will stimulate the growth of hematopoietic progenitor cells, but the new fusion protein has been specifically engineered to markedly increase cell growth by optimally stimulating the receptors for both cytokines at once.

Drawbacks of Biotechnology

There are disadvantages to these technologies as well. It is still very difficult to produce human monoclonal antibodies [*see* Monoclonal Antibodies, *below*]: it is difficult to find human B cells secreting immunoglobulins of interest, to fuse them to a long-lived human plasmacytoma, and to get the resulting hybridomas to grow and synthesize human monoclonal antibodies in large quantities. Most monoclonal antibodies currently in development are murine in origin because murine antibodies are relatively easy to elicit against specific antigens and they can regularly be produced in large quantities.

Even murine antibodies—and indeed many other biotechnology-derived products—have three potential drawbacks. First, as nonhuman proteins they can rapidly induce an antibody response in humans.[11] The human anti-murine antibodies (HAMA) can be directed both to the antigen-binding site (anti-idiotype) and to the rest of the antibody. Anti-idiotype antibodies can rapidly block the specific activity of any subsequently administered murine monoclonal antibody. HAMA against the rest of the antibody can not only bind to the original antibody but also cross-react with many other murine monoclonal antibodies, resulting in rapid clearance of the antibody from the blood. The development of both forms of HAMA may mean that many murine antibodies can only be administered once. Similarly, the immunogenicity of all new bioengineered products must be addressed. In fusion proteins, unexpected and potentially immunogenic changes may be introduced in the tertiary or quaternary structure of either individual protein. Additionally, administration of recombinant copies of normally cell-bound receptors may expose previously hidden intracytoplasmic or intramembrane regions to the immune system.

A second concern is the ease with which monoclonal antibodies—and, again, all bioengineered products—can be contaminated with infectious agents. Producing a sterile product for injection into humans is problematic with any manufacturing technology; in the case of bioengineered products, the very cells that make the product can be infected with mycoplasmas or viruses that are not easy to detect and that can find their way into the final product. For example, essentially every cell of murine origin has retrovirus DNA in its genome. Many murine B cell–derived hybridomas regularly secrete large quantities of retroviruses into the cell media that can copurify with the product. Although the degree of specific risk to humans associated with these viruses is still hypothetical, special care must be taken to insure that the final product is free of any potentially infectious agent.

Finally, as mentioned above, relatively minor changes in the manufacture of these products can result in major changes in the activity or immunogenicity of the product. Indeed, even changes in the materials added to the production process can cause subtle but potentially significant changes in the product. As a result, both the manufacture and the final release of these products must be tightly controlled.

Many bioengineered products have already been approved by the Food and Drug Administration [*see Table 1*], and many more are under active clinical development. The next several sections deal in more detail with specific bioengineered molecules, including various monoclonal antibodies and the cytokines.

Monoclonal Antibodies

Animal polyclonal immunoglobulins have figured in clinical practice for many years. Many animal-derived products have high titers against specific antigens and remain effective for immunosuppression and for passive immunotherapy. There are at least three drawbacks to their use, however. First, even though the titer of antibody against specific antigens is high in comparison with standard intravenous immunoglobulin products, only a very small absolute quantity of highly specific antibody is infused. Second, subtle changes in the immunizing antigen's structure, the immunization regimen, or the humoral response of the species that was immunized can make it hard to achieve consistent potency in successive batches of polyclonal immunoglobulins. Third, nonhuman immunoglobulin proteins, especially from the horse, are extremely immunogenic, so that rechallenge of a sensitized human with an antiserum from the same source can bring on a catastrophic clinical reaction.

To overcome some of these problems, a major research goal was to produce large quantities of a single immunoglobulin against a specific epitope on a defined antigen. This became possible when Kohler and Milstein prepared the first hybridoma cell line. Their procedure,[12] for which they were awarded the 1984 Nobel Prize in Physiology or Medicine, involves the fusion (with polyethylene glycol) of an immortalized myeloma (B cell tumor) line with short-lived normal antibody-producing B cells from an animal immunized against the desired antigen [*see Figure 2*]. To facilitate selection of fused cells, murine myeloma cells lacking hypoxanthine-guanosine phosphoribosyl transferase (HGPRT) activity are used: only cells containing genetic information from both parent cell lines (i.e., hybridomas) survive in a hypoxanthine-aminopterin-thymine (HAT) growth medium. Individual antibody-secreting cells are then isolated to insure that each new cell line will be derived from one and only one cell. The monoclonal antibodies they secrete can subsequently be selected for further development on the basis of specific antigen binding or a variety of other screening methods (e.g, inhibition of virus replication, cell function, or enzyme activity).

From 80 to 90 percent of all monoclonal antibodies currently in clinical trials are of mouse origin because of the ease with which murine antibodies can be made. However, as noted above, there are at least two major drawbacks to the use of murine antibodies in humans. First, because the murine monoclonal antibodies are xenogeneic proteins, they are cleared

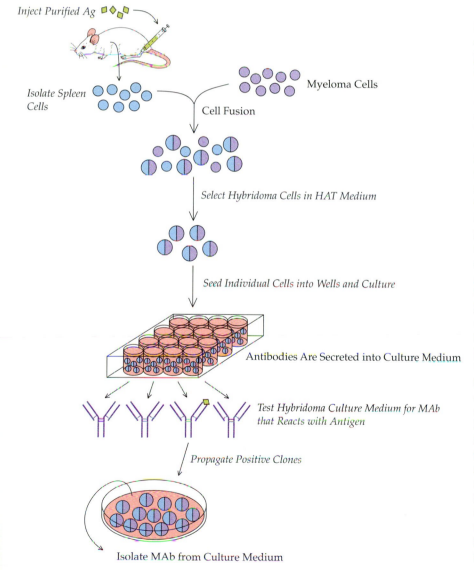

Inject Purified Ag

Isolate Spleen Cells

Myeloma Cells

Cell Fusion

Select Hybridoma Cells in HAT Medium

Seed Individual Cells into Wells and Culture

Antibodies Are Secreted into Culture Medium

Test Hybridoma Culture Medium for MAb that Reacts with Antigen

Propagate Positive Clones

Isolate MAb from Culture Medium

Figure 2 *Diagram presents series of steps involved in the production of a monoclonal antibody (MAb). A mouse is inoculated with an antigen (Ag) of interest. This step stimulates the proliferation of lymphocytes expressing antibodies against the antigen. Lymphocytes are taken from the spleen and fused to myeloma cells by treatment with polyethylene glycol. Hybrid cells are selected by growth in a medium containing hypoxanthine, aminopterin, and thymidine (HAT). The myeloma cells lack the enzyme hypoxanthine phosphoribosyltransferase (HPRT) and thus die in this medium unless they become fused with a lymphocyte, which expresses the missing enzyme. Unfused lymphocytes soon die as well, because they do not grow for long in culture. Individual hybrid cells are transferred to the well of a microtiter dish and cultured for several days. Aliquots of the culture fluids are removed and tested for the presence of antibody (Ab) that binds the antigen. Cells that test positive are cultured for monoclonal antibody production.*

from the human body much more rapidly than human antibodies. Second, and more important, patients who receive murine monoclonal antibodies often develop human anti-murine antibodies.[11]

The HAMA Problem

Unlike the human immune response to horse sera, the incidence of immune-complex disease or anaphylactic or anaphylactoid reactions related to the reinfusion of murine antibody into a HAMA-positive patient appears to be rare. HAMA can, however, further decrease the already short plasma half-life of murine antibodies, thereby reducing the likelihood that the immunoglobulin will reach the target tissue and making repeated infusions of mouse antibody of very limited clinical benefit. In addition, HAMA may also seriously confound the clinical laboratory's diagnosis of disease: human anti-murine antibodies can cross-react with the murine monoclonal antibody reagents relied on for in vitro diagnostic tests, such as those for detecting carcinoembryonic antigen (CEA) or cancer antigen-125 (CA-125) levels, giving erroneous results.[12]

Several approaches have been taken in an effort to prevent the development of or to eliminate HAMA. One approach has been to digest the antibody by papain and pepsin proteolysis to yield Fab and F(ab')2 fragments; removal of the immunoglobulin constant region (Fc) can reduce immunogenicity, prevent Fc receptor–mediated hepatic clearance, and increase renal excretion to give a shortened plasma half-life ($t_{1/2} \approx 1$ to 12 hours)—all without substantial loss of antigen-binding affinity or selectivity.

A second approach to reducing the development of HAMA is to graft a murine antigen-binding site to human immunoglobulin constant regions to make a mouse-human chimeric antibody [*see Figure 3*]. This approach combines the murine system's effective derivation of antigen-specific antibodies with the more natural or nonforeign human antibody framework. The immune response against these so-called chimeric antibodies—that is, the development of human anti-chimeric antibodies (HACA)—is sometimes significantly reduced, the plasma clearance of the chimeric antibodies is generally from eight to 10 times longer than that of the corresponding murine antibody, and the human constant regions are more effective in activating human complement or mediating antibody-

MOUSE ANTIBODY

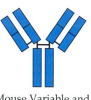

Mouse Variable and
Constant Regions
Mouse CDRs

CHIMERIC ANTIBODY

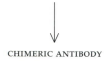
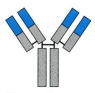

Human Constant
Regions
Mouse Variable
Regions, including CDRs

HUMANIZED ANTIBODY

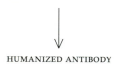
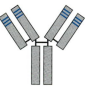

Human Variable
Framework and
Constant Regions
Mouse CDRs only

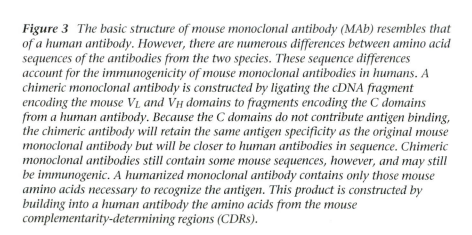

Figure 3   *The basic structure of mouse monoclonal antibody (MAb) resembles that of a human antibody. However, there are numerous differences between amino acid sequences of the antibodies from the two species. These sequence differences account for the immunogenicity of mouse monoclonal antibodies in humans. A chimeric monoclonal antibody is constructed by ligating the cDNA fragment encoding the mouse V_L and V_H domains to fragments encoding the C domains from a human antibody. Because the C domains do not contribute antigen binding, the chimeric antibody will retain the same antigen specificity as the original mouse monoclonal antibody but will be closer to human antibodies in sequence. Chimeric monoclonal antibodies still contain some mouse sequences, however, and may still be immunogenic. A humanized monoclonal antibody contains only those mouse amino acids necessary to recognize the antigen. This product is constructed by building into a human antibody the amino acids from the mouse complementarity-determining regions (CDRs).*

dependent cellular cytotoxicity. Chimeric antibodies have the potential to be far more effective than the murine monoclonal antibodies from which they were derived. They may, however, still not be optimal for repetitive and long-term treatment because the anti-chimeric antibodies can still arise unless exquisitely detailed bioengineering techniques are used to prepare and analyze the chimeric protein so as to eliminate all immunogenic epitopes.

A third method of overcoming immune responses against xenogeneic proteins is to prepare entirely human antibodies. The most common approach is to fuse human splenocytes or peripheral blood lymphocytes with HGPRT-deficient mouse myeloma cells (mouse myeloma cells are used rather than human ones because human myelomas often produce unstable hybridomas and may contain infectious tumorigenic agents). Alternatively, cell lines expressing human monoclonal antibodies can be created by immortalizing peripheral blood lymphocytes by means of Epstein-Barr virus (EBV) infection, though at the risk of contaminating the final product with infectious EBV virions. Finally, individual immunoglobulin genes can be removed from B cells and transferred to other cell lines for expression and purification.

The difficulty with each approach for preparing human monoclonal antibodies lies in the general inability to vaccinate a specific human host against a specific antigen and then easily recover antigen-specific human B cells. In spite of these difficulties, human monoclonal antibodies remain the goal because they usually do not elicit immune responses (although anti-idiotypic and anti-isotypic antibodies can arise). Patients have received multiple infusions of a single human monoclonal antibody for as long as two years without ill effect. Also, because the plasma half-life of human monoclonal antibodies approaches that of normal circulating human immunoglobulin (i.e., about 20 days), high antibody levels can be maintained by weekly infusions, increasing the potential for adequate tumor penetration and providing convenience for the patient.[13]

Although human monoclonal antibodies may offer significant advantages in the repetitive treatment of chronic disease, production difficulties and the potential for contamination by human pathogens still limit their availability. Bioengineering may again play a major role, in this case by moving specific immunoglobulin genes from human cells to xenogeneic cell lines that are more effective in generating antibodies.

Clinical Activity

Monoclonal antibodies have been studied clinically for many indications. They are administered either alone or—more frequently—with toxins attached to augment their potential for specific cell killing.

CONJUGATED ANTIBODIES

In conjugated antibodies, radioisotopes, toxins, or drugs are attached to the basic immunoglobulin structure, most often in order to visualize and treat cancer or other diseases. For diagnostic products, radioisotopes may either be covalently bound to the immunoglobulin (e.g., ^{123}I, ^{125}I, or ^{131}I), or coordinated within a chelate—such as ethylenediamine tetraacetic acid (EDTA) or diethylenetriamine pentaacetic acid (DTPA)—that is attached to

FIGURE 4

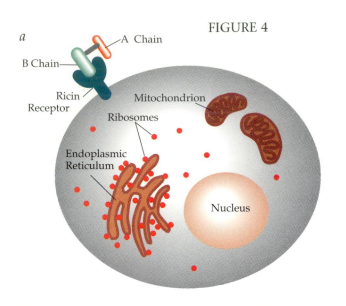

a

A Chain

B Chain

Ricin Receptor

Mitochondrion

Ribosomes

Endoplasmic Reticulum

Nucleus

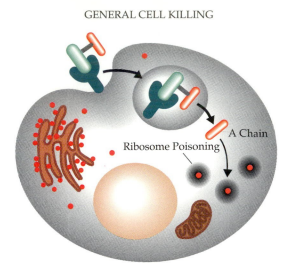

GENERAL CELL KILLING

A Chain

Ribosome Poisoning

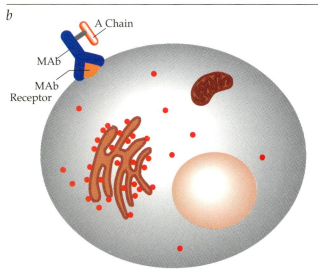

b

A Chain

MAb

MAb Receptor

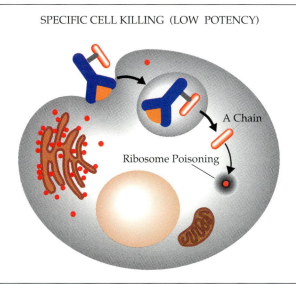

SPECIFIC CELL KILLING (LOW POTENCY)

A Chain

Ribosome Poisoning

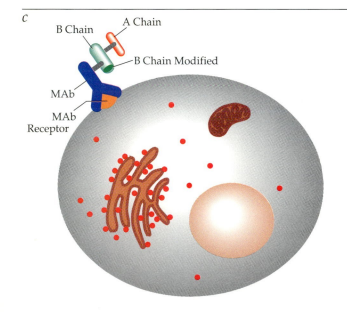

c

B Chain

A Chain

B Chain Modified

MAb

MAb Receptor

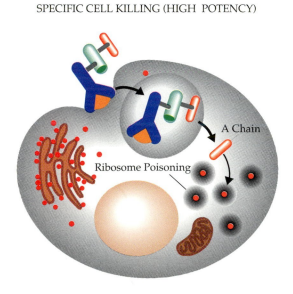

SPECIFIC CELL KILLING (HIGH POTENCY)

A Chain

Ribosome Poisoning

the protein (e.g., ^{99m}Tc, ^{111}In, or ^{67}Cu), or chelated directly by immunoglobulin amino acid residues (e.g., ^{99m}Tc). For tumor therapy, high-energy radionuclides such as ^{131}I, ^{125}I, ^{90}Y, or ^{186}Re have been attached to monoclonal antibodies by similar methods.

Originally, these so-called magic bullets were expected to have a great potential for tumor-specific imaging and treatment: they would focus large amounts of potentially lethal antibody on specific tumor cells and no other cells. Unfortunately, both physiology and stability problems have limited their efficacy in humans. First, because of metabolic processes, chemical-bond instability, or diffusion barriers, it is rare that more than 0.1 percent of the injected antibody dose reaches the target tissue. Second, hepatic enzymes that normally catabolize thyroxine rapidly dehalogenate most iodine-labeled antibodies. Third, serum proteins can literally strip technetium from immunoglobulin amino acids by trans-chelation, yielding antibodies that cannot image as well as free pertechnetate, which is rapidly taken up by the thyroid and stomach. Additionally, indium, whose chemistry is similar to that of iron, is concentrated in the liver, spleen, and marrow; radionuclides with an ionic charge radius similar to that of calcium, such as yttrium, are deposited in bone. In each case, the liberated radionuclide is highly concentrated in normal tissue, especially bone and bone marrow, and can lead to false-positive results or to significant dose-limiting toxicity.

Finally, despite earlier hopes, there does not seem to be a truly specific tumor antigen; the target antigen or cross-reacting antigens can be expressed unexpectedly on normal cells. For example, inflamed bowel cannot readily be differentiated from colon cancer by specific radiolabeled monoclonal antibodies to tumor-associated glycoprotein-72 (TAG-72) because the antigen can be expressed by both tissues.[14] Similarly, the carcinoembryonic antigen (CEA) is greatly overexpressed by colorectal adenocarcinomas, and plasma levels of CEA are considered a marker of disease activity. However, the NCA-95 epitope on the CEA tumor antigen is also present on granulocytes; early experiments in which radiolabeled anti-CEA antibody was administered to kill CEA-expressing tumors caused severe granulocytopenia.[15] (More recently, the cause of the granulocytopenia has been found and new antibodies have been bio-engineered to narrow target specificity and thereby increase the clinical utility of radiolabeled anti-CEA antibodies.)

Cytotoxic agents—chemotherapeutic drugs or protein-synthesis inhibitors such as ricin or *Pseudomonas* exotoxin—can also be delivered to target tissues by linkage to monoclonal antibodies [*see Figure 4*]. Many of these toxins have been modified so that they are relatively inactive until

Figure 4 (a) The A chain of ricin is an extremely potent poison of ribosomes, essential elements in the cell's protein-synthesizing machinery. Ricin, however, has almost no cell specificity and will kill normal cells as well as tumor cells. (b) To circumvent this problem, the ricin A chain has been linked to a monoclonal antibody that is specific for tumor cells. Although this approach greatly enhances cell specificity, it lowers the potency of ricin because the absence of the B chain affects transport of the toxic A chain across the cell membrane. (c) To overcome this limitation, a newer approach links the whole toxin (i.e., the A and B chains) to the monoclonal antibody but chemically modifies the B chain to minimize binding of the antibody-toxin conjugate to nontumor cells. This approach increases the potency of the toxic effect while retaining cell specificity.

they are freed from the antibody inside the cell. This approach makes it possible to deliver large amounts of the toxin with minimal whole-body toxicity.

Two major factors complicate therapy with toxin-conjugated antibodies. First, the linkage between the toxin and the antibody must be strong enough to withstand chemical and physical forces in the circulation and yet weak enough to allow the toxin to be freed from the antibody once the complex arrives within the cell. Second, unexpected specific or nonspecific binding of the antibody-toxin conjugate to normal tissues, especially the liver, can result in significant unwanted toxicity.

Several approaches are under investigation to improve the therapeutic index of immunotoxins: (1) elimination or chemical modification of the ricin toxin B chain to reduce undesired carbohydrate-specific receptor binding; (2) design of hindered disulfide linkers that would make the disulfide bond less susceptible to breakage and thereby decrease nonspecific dissociation of toxin and antibody; and (3) the identification of antigens that are rarely expressed on nontarget tissues and are also very rapidly internalized together with the bound antibody-toxin conjugate into target cells.

Unlabeled Antibodies

Not all antibodies need to carry a toxin or radionuclide to be effective. So-called naked or cold immunoglobulins either can direct a normal immune response, such as complement fixation or antibody-dependent cell-mediated cytotoxicity, against a target tissue or can block receptor and ligand binding. For example, OKT3, a murine IgG_{2a} antibody, lyses CD3-positive T cells in vivo, resulting in intense immunosuppression. Tumor-specific antibodies can purge bone marrow of cancer or T cells. The antibody termed 7E3 interferes with fibrinogen binding by specifically blocking the glycoprotein IIb/IIIa receptor complex on platelets, thereby inhibiting platelet aggregation.[16]

As in the case of radiolabeled and toxin-conjugated antibodies, the dose-limiting toxicity of unlabeled antibodies is most often related to normal-tissue cross-reactivity. The ganglioside G_{D2} is present on neuroblastomas, melanomas, astrocytomas, malignant gliomas, and many sarcomas, and it has therefore been the target of many antibody-based therapies. However, G_{D2} is also present on some normal central and peripheral neurons. Severe neuropathies have occurred in patients receiving unlabeled G_{D2}-specific antibodies, probably as a direct result of antibody-mediated damage.[17]

Future Developments in Monoclonal Antibodies

The detailed understanding of immunoglobulin molecules that led to chimeric antibodies is now contributing to the generation of more highly controlled chimeric fusions using murine complementarity-determining regions (CDRs) and a human immunoglobulin framework to yield a fusion protein that has greater than 95 percent homology with human immunoglobulins [*see Figure 3*]. The greater homology achieved in these so-called humanized antibodies is expected to reduce HAMA formation without affecting the flexibility and ease of production of murine antibody.

More important, the application of molecular biology and bioengineering techniques to immunoglobulin molecules has resulted in three recent advances: generation of monoclonal antibodies that do not require the cell-fusion techniques of Kohler and Milstein,[18,19] development of markedly truncated single-chain antibody-like molecules in which the variable regions of heavy and light chains are linked by a small peptide,[20] and even reduction of the antibody to a totally synthetic molecule that mimics an antigen-binding site.[21] Such products may revolutionize the approach to cell-specific targeting and at the same time make it less expensive because the genes can be expressed in transgenic animals or plants.[22]

Finally, monoclonal antibody therapy may be improved by such biotechnology-developed agents as interferon gamma, which upregulate the expression of the CEA and TAG-72 cancer antigens. Again, an antibody coupled to interleukin-2 (IL-2) has been shown to display substantially improved xenograft imaging, possibly as a result of an IL-2–induced improvement of the tumor's vascular permeability.[23] Attempts are also being made to combine several monoclonal antibodies into a so-called oligoclonal serum that has high target specificity but low normal-tissue reactivity—an interesting acknowledgment of the power of xenogeneic polyclonal sera.

The promise of monoclonal antibodies as magic bullets against disease has proved harder to fulfill than was originally predicted. Yet after 10 years of laboratory and clinical research, new understanding of monoclonal antibody structure and metabolism, coupled with major advances in molecular biology, may finally enable monoclonal antibodies to become a powerful tool in human medicine.

Cytokines

The development of bioengineered cytokines has been much more rapid than the development of monoclonal antibodies. Cytokines are small secreted or membrane-bound proteins or glycoproteins that mediate cell-to-cell interactions through specific cell-surface receptors. They regulate a broad range of biologic activities, including hematopoiesis; the immune response to microbial, parasitic, viral, or other antigens; and inflammatory responses to trauma. It should therefore be no surprise that cytokines have attracted the attention of virologists, immunologists, hematologists, cell biologists, neurologists, and especially oncologists.

Originally these protein messengers were thought to act only between lymphocytes and were called lymphokines. The proteins have since been found to act on many cell types, and so they are called cytokines, of which the lymphokines make up only a small portion. Cytokines are categorized as interferons (IFNs), interleukins (ILs), colony-stimulating factors (CSFs), or growth factors (GFs). They share several basic features, such as low molecular weight (approximately 10 to 20 kd), a structure rich in alpha-helices stabilized by disulfide bonds, and (usually) the ability to retain in vivo biologic function when deglycosylated (erythropoietin being the most notable exception). They also frequently share common biologic properties, including overlapping biologic effects (e.g., T cell proliferation has been reported to be enhanced by IL-1, IL-2, IL-4, IL-6, IL-7, IL-9, and

IL-12) and bioactivity at picomolar concentrations, which is mediated by high-affinity cell-surface receptors.

The pleiotropic nature of such responses is not unexpected. First, cytokines typically act on target cells that may in turn produce additional cytokines, generating a complex network of redundant, synergistic, and inhibitory cytokine interactions. Second, and very important, this cytokine cascade is thought to take place in cell-to-cell microenvironments. Third, there is significant homology among receptors, so that one type of receptor may be activated when an unrelated cytokine having a similar receptor is present in very high concentrations. To be sure, many of the pleiotropic effects identified in vitro may not occur normally in vivo. The fact remains that systemic administration to humans of very large quantities of cytokines may result in the stimulation of irrelevant target cells, leading to significant unexpected (and unwanted) activity and even toxicity.

The existence of secreted factors in unpurified supernatants of activated cells was appreciated for many years, but only after they were sequenced, cloned, expressed, and purified were cytokines available in quantities sufficient to permit their unique functions and activities to be studied first in vitro and then in vivo. In many cases, better understanding of the biologic actions of a new cytokine has been gained through studies of transgenic animals in which the gene for the factor is either overexpressed or suppressed or deleted and the animal is observed for normal, abnormal, or disease states. Transgenic mice have provided a model of overproduction when a foreign or exogenous gene has been transferred to the animal's inheritable genome and then expressed.[24] Alternatively, so-called knockout mice can be created by deleting, inactivating, or mutating a specific gene to determine that gene's usual role.[25]

Cytokine Receptors

Cytokines mediate their biologic effects through specific cell-surface receptors, many of which have recently been isolated, characterized, and cloned for further study. The molecular characterization of numerous receptor subunits has revealed sequence and structural homologies among receptors for different cytokines that may explain some of the redundant pleiotropic effects of cytokines.

Several cytokine-receptor superfamilies have been identified to date.[26,27] Members of the largest such gene family, the hematopoietin-receptor superfamily, share a common external domain having two conserved amino acid sequences. Members of this superfamily include the receptors for IL-2 (β-subunit), IL-3, IL-4, IL-5, IL-6, IL-7, erythropoietin, growth hormone, prolactin, granulocyte-macrophage colony-stimulating factor (GM-CSF), and granulocyte colony-stimulating factor (G-CSF). Another group, the receptors for IL-1, platelet-derived growth factor (PDGF), macrophage colony-stimulating factor (M-CSF), stem cell factor (SCF), and fibroblast growth factor (FGF), share structural homology with the immunoglobulin gene family. Other receptor families include the tumor necrosis factor (TNF) receptor family, the tyrosine kinase family, and the G protein–linked receptor family.

Naturally occurring soluble forms of the receptors for some of these factors, including IL-2α, IL-4, IL-5, IL-6, IL-7, TNF, and interferon gamma have been found. Their biologic function is still speculative, but such soluble cytokine receptors, along with monoclonal antibodies directed against the receptors and receptor antagonists, are being clinically evaluated for the treatment of many disease states and for blocking such unwanted immune reactions as graft rejection and autoimmunity.[26,27]

Advances in genetic engineering and in large-scale fermentation and purification have made possible the evaluation of cytokines in clinical trials. A brief description of some of the cytokine-related fruits of biotechnology and their broad clinical applications follows.

Interferon

Interferon was discovered in 1957 by Isaacs and Lindenmann as a soluble antiviral substance that could be produced by many different cell types in response to a variety of agents, including viruses, bacteria, and mitogens.[28] Interferon has since been classified into three major families: α, β, and γ [*see Table 2*]. Interferon alfa (IFN-α), of which there are 22 species,[29] is predominantly produced by leukocytes, interferon beta (IFN-β) by fibroblasts, and interferon gamma (IFN-γ) by T cells. In addition to its antiviral activity, interferon affects immunomodulation, growth, and differentiation; regulates cell-surface antigen and gene expression; and has antitumor activity. These broad biologic effects were appreciated for many years while it was still not possible to conduct clinical trials because of the lack of sufficient quantities of purified material. It was not until the early 1980s that subtypes of human IFN-α were cloned and expressed in *E. coli* and unlimited quantities of purified material subsequently became available for clinical trials.

Recombinant IFN-α was the first biotechnology product to be approved by the FDA. The original FDA-approved indication was for the treatment of hairy cell leukemia, in which interferon is thought to act directly on the malignant cell to bring it back under normal control. Recombinant IFN-α, IFN-β, and IFN-γ are currently being investigated in patients with a wide variety of malignancies, infections, allergies, and autoimmune diseases.[30]

Interleukins

In the early 1960s, investigators showed that T cells could be activated with mitogens or antigens to produce both a proliferative response and soluble factors capable of supporting and amplifying activated cells.[31] The term interleukin originally referred to a group of proteins produced by lymphocytes and mononuclear cells that mediated proliferative and differentiative signals among leukocytes. Later it became evident that non-lymphoid cells could produce and respond to the same factors.

As each new factor was discovered, its functional activity was described and a name was assigned by the discoverer that corresponded to the observed biologic activity; a single interleukin could be described by a long and confusing list of acronyms based on its purification, protein sequencing, and characterization history. To bring order to the field, the International Union of Immunological Societies (IUIS) Nomenclature Committee now assigns designations at periodic lymphokine workshops[32] that consider all the available biochemical, biophysical, and activity evidence before assigning simple common names. As in the case of the interferons,

Table 2 Molecular Weight and Chromosomal Location
of Genes Encoding Various Human Cytokines

	Preferred Name	Alternative Name	Molecular Weight (kd)	Chromosome Number
Interferons	Interferon alfa (IFN-α)	Leukocyte interferon	18	9
	Interferon beta (IFN-β)	Fibroblast interferon	22	9
	Interferon gamma (IFN-γ)	Immune interferon	20–25	12
Hematopoietic Growth Factors	Granulocyte colony-stimulating factor (G-CSF)	Colony-stimulating factor–β (CSF-β)	18–22	17
	Granulocyte-macrophage colony-stimulating factor (GM-CSF)	Neutrophil migration inhibitory factor from T cells (NIF-T)	15–22	5
	Macrophage colony-stimulating factor (M-CSF)	Colony-stimulating factor–1 (CSF-1)	45	5
	Erythropoietin (EPO)	—	34–39	7
	Stem cell factor (SCF)	c-*kit* Ligand (KL)	19	4
Other Growth Factors	Epidermal growth factor (EGF)	—	6	5
	Fibroblast growth factor (FGF), acidic or basic	—	17	5 (acidic FGF), 4 (basic FGF)
	Nerve growth factor–β (NGF-β)	—	13	1
	Platelet-derived growth factor (PDGF)	—	14–18	7, 22
	Transforming growth factor–β (TGF-β)	—	12	19
Interleukins	Interleukin-1α (IL-1α)	Endogenous pyrogen	17	2
	IL-1β	Lymphotoxin	17	2
	IL-2	T cell growth factor (TCGF)	15	4
	IL-3	Multi-CSF	15–28	5
	IL-4	B cell stimulating factor–1 (BSF-1)	15	5
	IL-5	Eosinophil differentiation factor (EDF)	18	5
	IL-6	BSF-2	21	7
	IL-7	Lymphopoietin-1 (LP-1)	17	8
	IL-8	Neutrophil-activating protein–1 (NAP-1)	10	4
	IL-9	TCGFp40	40	5
	IL-10	Cytokine synthesis inhibitory factor (CSIF)	30–40	Unknown
	IL-11	Adipogenesis inhibitory factor (AGIF)	23	19
	IL-12	Natural killer stimulatory factor (NKSF)	75	Unknown

the advent of recombinant DNA technology has made many more interleukins available for functional characterization and, in some cases, clinical trials. Much is now known about the biochemical properties and activities of interleukins 1 through 12 [*see Tables 2 and 3*]. IL-1, IL-2, and IL-3 will now be discussed in more detail.

INTERLEUKIN-1

IL-1 is the name given to two 17 kd polypeptides (IL-1α and IL-1β), which are products of two distinct genes.[33] Both molecular forms are synthesized as 31 kd precursors, which are cleaved to yield active mature forms. IL-1 is produced primarily by cells of the monocyte-macrophage lineage; a variety of other cells, such as fibroblasts, stromal cells, and endothelial cells, may also produce IL-1 in response to injury, infection, and inflammatory agents.

IL-1 has a wide range of hematopoietic, immunologic, metabolic, and inflammatory properties. It is known as the prototype of the so-called proinflammatory cytokines because it induces fever, acute-phase reaction proteins, and neutropenia when administered systemically. Two cell-surface receptor types have been identified, which can bind either form of IL-1 but show preference for one or the other form depending on individual tissue and cell type. IL-1α preferentially interacts with the type I receptor (80 kd) on T cells, fibroblasts, endothelial cells, chondrocytes, hepatocytes, and keratinocytes; IL-1β interacts preferentially with a type II receptor (68 kd) found on monocytes, B cells, neutrophils, and bone-marrow cells.

Unwanted production or overproduction of IL-1 is associated with many acute and chronic inflammatory disease states,[33] and therefore many therapeutic strategies have focused on inhibiting IL-1's detrimental effects by blocking its binding to its receptor. Naturally occurring IL-1 inhibitors have been found in the urine of patients with monocytic leukemia; they appear to be produced by the same cells that secrete IL-1 itself. Based on the sequence of one of these inhibitors, a recombinant IL-1 receptor antagonist (IL-1ra) has been cloned.[34] IL-1ra has been found to suppress or prevent many IL-1–induced inflammatory responses in vivo.[33] Another approach has been to develop soluble truncated IL-1 receptors to bind IL-1 and prevent its interaction with cell-associated receptors. A third approach, which would only block IL-1β (the predominant form of IL-1 in human biologic fluids), is to inhibit the IL-1β converting enzyme, which cleaves the inactive precursor to the active form.[35] Curbing the actions of IL-1 may come to play an important role in the treatment of such inflammatory disorders as septic shock, rheumatoid arthritis, and inflammatory bowel disease.

INTERLEUKIN-2

IL-2 is a 15 kd polypeptide produced by activated T cells. It is thought to play a critical role in normal immune responses by potentiating the proliferation and differentiation of T and B cells, augmenting natural killer (NK) cytolytic activity, generating lymphokine-activated killer (LAK) cells, upregulating its own receptor, and inducing a variety of other lymphokines. Individuals defective in IL-2 production develop severe combined immunodeficiencies. Hence, IL-2 has been investigated for the treatment of infectious diseases, malignancies, and defects in cell-mediated immunity.[36]

IL-2 was licensed in May 1992 for the treatment of patients with metastatic renal cell carcinoma; IL-2 is thought to augment the patient's

Table 3   Effects of Various Interleukins and Growth Factors on Target Cells

	Cytokine	Source	Target Cells	Effects
Interleukins	IL-1α	Monocytes, macrophages, fibroblasts, endothelial cells	T cells, B cells, macrophages, fibroblasts, endothelial cells, hepatocytes	Proinflammatory effect
	IL-1β	Epithelial cells, astrocytes	Neutrophils, B cells, macrophages, monocytes	Proinflammatory effect
	IL-2	T cells	T cells, B cells, monocytes, NK cells	Proliferation, differentiation, up-regulation, activation
	IL-3	T cells, mast cells, NK cells, monocytes	Hematopoietic and myelopoietic stem cells	Proliferation, differentiation
	IL-4	T cells, stromal cells	T cells, B cells, monocytes, mast cells	Differentiation, stimulation, inhibition, survival
	IL-5	T cells	Eosinophils	Proliferation, increased survival
			T cells	CD8+ T cell differentiation
	IL-6	Macrophages, fibroblasts, mast cells, T cells, hepatocytes, astrocytes, endothelial cells	B cells, neurons, megakaryocytes, hepatocytes, mesangial cells	Activation, growth, differentiation
	IL-7	Lymphoid tissue, stromal cells	B cells, T cells	B cell growth, T cell activation
	IL-8	Monocytes, macrophages, alveolar macrophages, hepatocytes	Neutrophils, T cells	Chemotaxis, proinflammatory effect
	IL-9	Activated CD4+ T cells	Mast cells, T cells	Survival and growth
			Stem cells	Growth and colony formation
	IL-10	B cells, CD4+ T cells, monocytes	B cells	Inhibition of IFN-γ and TNF-α; B cell growth and differentiation
	IL-11	Stromal cells	Plasma cells, B cells, macrophages, megakaryoctes	Proliferation and development
	IL-12	B cells	T cells, NK cells	Proliferation of activated cells; induction of IFN-γ
Growth Factors	EGF	Brain, kidney, salivary gland	Epithelial and endothelial cells, fibroblasts, keratinocytes	Proliferation, angiogenesis, wound healing
	FGF	Multiple cell sources	Mesodermal and ectodermal cells	Stimulation, angiogenesis, wound healing
	NGF-β, brain-derived neurotropic factor (BDNF), neuro-trophin-3 (NT-3), ciliary neurotropic factor (CNTF)	Brain	Sensory and sympathetic nerve cells	Development and survival
	PDGF	Platelets	Fibroblasts, endothelial cells	Wound healing, arterial injury, bone marrow fibrosis
	TGF-β	Multiple cell sources		Both immunosuppressive and immunostimulatory effects

immune response to the tumor. Because of IL-2's known effects on immune function, it is also being studied clinically in conjunction with adoptive immunotherapies employing such cells as LAK cells and tumor-infiltrating lymphocytes (TILs) to treat various cancers.[37] In each case, a patient's own lymphocytes are collected either nonselectively from the blood or directly from tumor tissue, expanded to very high numbers by exposure to IL-2, and then reinfused into the patient along with very high doses of IL-2 in the hope that tumor-specific cell-mediated cytotoxicity will occur.

This method has achieved some success. Unfortunately, high-dose IL-2 therapy has been limited by dose-dependent systemic toxicities, including widespread extravascular fluid extravasation from a vascular-leak syndrome, multiple organ dysfunction, and significant cardiac and central nervous system toxicities.[38] The administration of lower doses together with TILs is being explored; lower IL-2 doses are also being investigated in the treatment of patients with such infectious diseases as lepromatous leprosy and acquired immunodeficiency syndrome (AIDS).[39]

IL-2's effects are mediated through IL-2 receptors, which consist of at least two subunits, a 55 kd subunit and a 70 to 75 kd subunit. High-, intermediate-, and low-affinity forms of the receptor have been characterized on the basis of whether the two chains are expressed together or separately.[40] The IL-2 receptor has been favored for immunotherapy because it is expressed predominantly on activated lymphocytes and not on precursors or normal tissue. Novel approaches to anti-IL-2 receptor therapy have included toxin-conjugated IL-2 fusion proteins and radionuclide chelate–coupled monoclonal antibodies[40] in the treatment of hematologic malignancies and such unwanted immune responses as graft rejection and autoimmune diseases.

INTERLEUKIN-3

IL-3 is a 15 to 25 kd polypeptide secreted by activated T cells, mast cells, NK cells, and monocytes. It stimulates the proliferation and differentiation of hematopoietic and myelopoietic stem cells.[41] Because human IL-3 is highly species-specific and is not dependent on glycosylation for function, genetically engineered molecules produced in different expression systems should be equally effective.[42]

IL-3 binds to a single class of high-affinity receptors found on most human hematopoietic stem cells, where it stimulates proliferation and differentiation. As a result, IL-3 has potential applications in the treatment of the cytopenias associated with aplastic anemia, chemotherapy, radiotherapy, bone-marrow transplants, and other iatrogenic bone-marrow failures.[43] IL-3 may also be effective in combination with other, later-acting hematopoietic growth factors given either simultaneously or sequentially to enhance and accelerate hematopoietic cell production.

Hematopoietic Growth Factors

A number of polypeptide growth factors coordinate the growth and differentiation of hematopoietic cells. They were originally termed colony-stimulating factors for their ability to generate colonies from individual bone-marrow progenitor cells in semisoft agar cultures.[44,45] Several hematopoietic growth factors have now been cloned with recombinant DNA technology and produced on a large scale. They include G-CSF, GM-CSF, M-CSF, SCF, and (as already discussed) erythropoietin and IL-3 [*see Tables 2 and 3*]. T cells, endothelial cells, epithelial cells, fibroblasts, and monocytes often synthesize these factors in response to stress and such inflammatory stimuli as IL-1, endotoxin, and tumor necrosis factor (TNF). Clinical use of human growth factors has focused on the reversal of congenital or iatrogenic cytopenias.[46-48]

An issue that has been raised is what constitutes an appropriate end point for the clinical use of these products in various disease states. Discussion has focused on the adjuvant administration of G-CSF and GM-CSF to reverse the myelotoxic effects of chemotherapy, radiation therapy, and bone-marrow transplantation in anticancer therapy and the myelotoxic effects of AZT in patients infected with human immunodeficiency virus (HIV). Demonstration of clinical efficacy, as opposed to simply a restoration of blood-cell levels, is emphasized as a therapeutic goal. That is, to be considered effective, the product must show some direct benefit to the patient—for example, a decreased incidence of infectious episodes, fewer days of hospitalization for antibiotic therapy, or evidence of increased survival.

G-CSF was licensed in 1991 for the treatment of neutropenia after myelosuppressive anticancer drug therapy. In a single phase III study, G-CSF decreased the incidence of infection, the incidence and length of hospitalization, and intravenous antibiotic administration in granulocytopenic patients. Also in 1991, GM-CSF was licensed for patients who had not recovered adequate granulocyte function after undergoing autologous bone-marrow transplantation for non-Hodgkin's lymphoma, Hodgkin's disease, or acute lymphoblastic leukemia. The use of M-CSF to treat gynecologic malignancies and leukopenia in transplantation settings is being investigated.[48] (Caution must be exercised in treating myeloid malignancies with the CSFs because of the possibility that these agents might actually enhance cancer growth.) Several other cytokines are also being investigated [*see Tables 2 and 3*], including the nerve-growth factors, PDGF, and epidermal growth factor (EGF).

The tumor necrosis factors were originally described as factors in endotoxin-treated mice that could cause hemorrhagic necrosis and regression of tumors.[49] TNF was also termed cachectin (which causes anorexia and weight loss in chronic disease), and TNF-β was known as lymphotoxin. TNF is associated with such conditions as inflammation, acute infection, and chronic disease. TNF is a trimer, which may be important in developing approaches to neutralize or block TNF's effects with antagonists or monoclonal antibodies.[50]

Rational Drug Design and HIV

Most monoclonal antibodies and cytokines have been developed for clinical indications only after they have been found to bind certain epitopes or to perform certain functions in vitro. Rarely were products made to specification; rather, wide-ranging clinical studies were undertaken primarily to find uses for products that had been made available in large quantities by new production methods. Biotechnology is changing all that. New drug products can be rationally designed for specific indications, as best illustrated by the production of vaccines and immunotherapeutics to prevent HIV infection or delay its progression.[51,52]

As the basic virology of HIV is dissected, agents that interfere with the life cycle, the infectivity, or both aspects of the virus can be precisely designed, modified, and manufactured. Success in the generation of new antiviral agents depends on the scientist's ability to identify and characterize the cellular and molecular elements of a protective anti-HIV response. Molecular biologic techniques make it possible not only to produce essentially nonimmunogenic proteins but also to produce vaccines that express specific viral antigens in their most immunogenic format, thus providing the basis for rational vaccine development.

Vaccines

Historically, the control of viral epidemics has relied on the development of inexpensive and effective prophylactic vaccines because specific treatments for established viral infections have proved elusive. Vaccines have generally been manufactured from killed or attenuated strains of otherwise pathogenic viruses, and this traditional strategy is currently being considered in HIV vaccine development with some encouraging results.

Published findings indicate that the simian immunodeficiency virus and HIV remain immunogenic after being inactivated and that immunization with these agents can confer protection on nonhuman primates.[53-55] However, there are several potential drawbacks to whole killed or attenuated HIV viruses. The denaturing agents that can completely inactivate live virions can also destroy the three-dimensional structure of the virus, resulting in a loss of immunogenicity. And the rapid mutation rate of HIV increases the possibility that an attenuated virus might be genetically unstable and regain pathogenicity.[56] Another potential drawback to these approaches is that the many different proteins present in a whole-virus preparation may compete with one another to induce distinct immune responses; if human immune protection relies on the response to one or a very few critical epitopes, such antigenic competition might interfere with vaccine efficacy. Finally, there is a small but disturbing possibility that infectious viral DNA might persist and be transmitted in killed or attenuated preparations.

To circumvent these problems, biotechnologists are developing vaccines that selectively express only the proteins or protein subunits that are most likely to be required to generate maximally protective immune responses. For this strategy to be successful, the determinants that are critical to immune function must be accurately identified. This has not proved to be an easy task. Opinions differ on whether T-cell or B-cell epitopes are more important, whether the antigens should be expressed in native or denatured form, and whether viral capsid or nuclear proteins are the most appropriate antigens for inclusion in a vaccine.[57-60]

Specific Approaches to Therapy

Significant differences also exist in the selection of optimal immunization strategies. Some groups are employing purified recombinant viral glycoprotein or proteins. Other investigators take an approach in which genes encoding these proteins are introduced into relatively nonpathogenic viruses such as vaccinia, with which volunteers will then be infected. Still other groups are contemplating the introduction of antisense oligonucleotides into cells to interfere with HIV replication. Finally, a large number of immunotherapeutic agents designed to halt the spread of virus in patients with AIDS are under consideration.

IMMUNIZATION WITH HIV PROTEINS

Considerable evidence suggests that the envelope glycoprotein of HIV-1 moderates the binding of the virus to T cells by way of the lymphocyte's CD4 receptor.[61-63] The envelope glycoprotein, a gp120 molecule, is also a dominant target of the host's humoral and cell-mediated immune responses.[64] Considerable effort has therefore been directed toward mapping the immunogenic determinants expressed by gp120 and identifying the epitopes that elicit a protective immune response.

At least five distinct regions of the gp120 molecule are recognized by B or T cells,[65,66] and several of them elicit neutralizing antibodies.[57] The principal neutralizing determinant, known as the V3 loop region, is considered promising for vaccines.[64,67-69] However, different HIV strains express different amino acid sequences in this region, with strain-to-strain variability as high as 50 percent,[70-72] so that antibodies that neutralize one isolate of HIV may be ineffective against another.[73-75] Investigators of gp120-based vaccines are therefore considering combining proteins from different HIV isolates of inducing more generalized neutralizing responses. There is also interest in constructing multimers of the V3 loop region— multiple short stretches of peptide bound together—to form a stronger immunogen for use in vaccines.[76]

It is possible that protection against HIV infection requires immunization with viral proteins other than, or in addition to, gp120. Studies of serum antibodies from HIV-infected patients have identified multiple epitopes on different HIV proteins, including gag, pol, gp30, p17, and p41. Some of these are linear epitopes expressed on denatured virus, whereas others have an intricate three-dimensional conformation.[77-79] The relative contribution of these sites to the overall anti-HIV response and their potential for providing protection against infection when incorporated in a vaccine remain uncertain.

INDUCTION OF CELL-MEDIATED IMMUNITY

Some have argued that the humoral anti-HIV response may be irrelevant— that protection depends on T-cell lysis of infected cells.[80-84] A number of investigators have shown that cytotoxic T cells can in fact be generated against HIV envelope, core, and polymerase proteins and that some of these responses block HIV replication in vitro.[84] One of the best ways of inducing cell-mediated immunity involves the processing of viral antigens by host cells and the presentation of the resulting peptides by host major histocompatibility complex (MHC) antigens. In the case of polio vaccine, this was accomplished by immunizing with live, attenuated virus. In the case of HIV, a different, molecular approach is being taken: HIV genes are transferred into relatively nonpathogenic carrier viruses. A number of viruses could potentially serve as host to transferred HIV genes, but vaccinia has proved particularly effective. A great deal is already known about vaccinia, which can act as a carrier for large amounts of exogenous DNA,[85] and attenuated strains are available into which HIV genes can easily be introduced.[86,87] Results to date have shown that naive individuals immunized with vaccinia carrying the gene encoding gp160 develop strong primary responses to vaccinia antigens and generate secondary immune responses to HIV antigens.[88-90]

There are drawbacks to the vaccinia approach. A substantial proportion of Americans have already been immunized with this virus and may not respond to gp120-vaccinia on being reimmunized. Vaccinia virus is also contagious and can cause severe disease in immunosuppressed populations, especially those with AIDS. Still, the capacity to introduce a large number of genes from many different pathogenic viruses into a single virus carrier makes this a potentially very useful model for universal immunization.

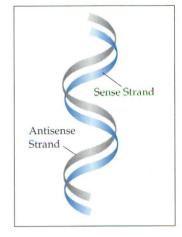

ANTISENSE OLIGONUCLEOTIDES

A more novel approach to the prevention and treatment of HIV infection involves antisense oligonucleotides [*see Figure 5*]. A strand of nucleotides whose sequence is complementary to that of HIV-1 RNA can inhibit the replication of virus in infected cells.[91] The antisense oligonucleotide combines with the so-called sense strand of viral RNA, preventing its translation into protein products. If all cells in the body contained antisense oligonucleotides complementary to HIV genes, integration or replication of the HIV virus might be prevented. There is some in vitro evidence that this technique might be feasible.[92]

There are, of course, drawbacks to the introduction of foreign DNA into human cells. The antisense DNA could unexpectedly interrupt the function of a normal regulatory gene, resulting in cell death or the development of a malignancy.[91] Moreover, there are major technical hurdles blocking the efficient introduction of antisense DNA into a large fraction of human somatic or germline cells, and the long-term sequelae of such treatment have not been investigated.[92] Even if it is unlikely to be effective as a vaccine in uninfected individuals, however, the antisense strategy might prevent or delay progression to disease in individuals already infected with HIV.

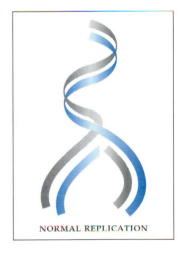

Some one million Americans are already HIV-positive, but this represents only a small fraction of those infected worldwide. Agents capable of inactivating free virus or killing virus-infected cells may be required to treat these patients; toward this end, agents that prevent the binding of HIV to host cells or that lyse cells containing HIV before they can produce more infectious virions are being developed and tested.

Figure 5 *Normal replication of the chromosomes entails the synthesis of new copies of both the sense (blue) and the complementary antisense (light gray) strands. When the system is flooded with antisense oligonucleotides (dark gray) that are complementary to the sense strand, further replication of the chromosome stops.*

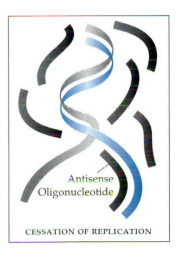

RIBOZYMES

Another possible antisense gene therapy approach is the use of site-specific ribozymes to stop DNA replication through breakage of the DNA strands. From the earliest description of ribozymes in RNA plant viruses through the seminal work of Thomas Cech,[93,94] the application of specific RNA strands that can produce catalytic scission of specific DNA has intrigued HIV researchers.[95,96] Unlike antisense RNA, which must be supplied in stoichiometrically equivalent doses to block target DNA, ribozymes, in hammerhead or hairpin configurations, can cause breakage of phosphodiester bonds in multiple molecules through their non–self-destructive catalytic activity. Unfortunately, the hypermutability of the HIV genome could be a problem for ribozymes, as it is for many other therapeutic and diagnostic modalities. However, the use of ribozymes focused on highly conserved areas of the HIV genome or the use of multiple types of ribozymes to attack several areas of the genome could result in the elimination of intracellular HIV infections.[96,97]

CD4: ALONE AND IN COMBINATION

As noted above, HIV binds to and gains access to human T cells by way of membrane-bound CD4. The CD4 molecule has been cloned, and when it is present as a humoral protein, it can bind HIV and thus inhibit viral binding to T cells. Unfortunately, free CD4 injected into patients has a short lifespan, and is therefore not therapeutically effective.[98-100] To circumvent this problem, investigators have generated a chimeric protein consisting of two CD4s attached to the heavy-chain constant region of the IgG molecule. The resultant CD4-IgG has a relatively long half-life and still inhibits the binding of HIV to human cells.[101] Clinical trials are under way to examine whether this agent can slow disease progression in HIV-positive patients. It may also be valuable for preventing maternal-fetal HIV transmission or for treating medical personnel exposed to HIV by needlestick.

The CD4 molecule can also be coupled to toxins, causing them to bind and lyse HIV-infected cells. Since gp120 appears on the surface of infected lymphocytes before intact virions are released, a toxin-CD4 conjugate might kill such cells before they liberate infectious virus. Anti-HIV antibodies coupled to toxins might also be used in this manner.

Prospects for Bioengineered Agents

Molecular biologists in industry, academia, and government are working to develop vaccines and immunotherapeutics for the prevention or treatment of HIV infection and many other diseases. Available, cutting-edge technology is being applied to design novel biologic agents that will maximize the host's ability to respond to, neutralize, and kill various pathogens. Significant strides have been taken in the past decade in identifying the immunogenic determinants expressed by the HIV virus and determining the mechanism of HIV's infection and replication. The same tools are dissecting the surface determinants of tumors to identify targets for antibodies or cytokines. It seems likely that agents currently being designed and tested through rational, step-by-step identification and engineering will successfully be applied to clinical care in the near future.

References

1. Eschbach JW: The anemia of chronic renal failure: pathophysiology and the effects of recombinant erythropoietin. *Kidney Int* 35:134, 1989

2. Lacombe C, DaSilva J, Bruneval P, et al: Peritubular cells are the site of erythropoietin synthesis in murine hypoxic kidney. *J Clin Invest* 81:620, 1988

3. Schuster SJ, Wilson JH, Erslev AJ, et al: Physiologic regulation and tissue localization of renal erythropoietin messenger RNA. *Blood* 70:316, 1987

4. Spivak JL: The mechanism of action of erythropoietin. *Int J Cell Cloning* 4:139, 1986

5. Bondurant MC, Khoury MJ: Anemia induces accumulation of erythropoietin mRNA in the kidney and liver. *Mol Cell Biol* 6:2731, 1986

6. Jacobsen LO, Goldwasser E, Fried WE, et al: Role of the kidney in erythropoiesis. *Nature* 179:633, 1957

7. Miyake T, Kung CKH, Goldwasser E: Purification of human erythropoietin. *J Biol Chem* 252:5558, 1977

8. Jacobs K, Shoemaker C, Rudersdorf R, et al: Isolation and characterization of genomic and cDNA clones of human erythropoietin. *Nature* 313:806, 1985

9. Lin FK, Suggs S, Lin CH, et al: Cloning and expression of the human erythropoietin gene. *Proc Natl Acad Sci USA* 82:7580, 1985

10. Curtis BM, Williams DE, Broxmeyer HE, et al: Enhanced hematopoietic activity of a human granulocyte/macrophage colony-stimulating factor-interleukin 3 fusion protein. *Proc Natl Acad Sci USA* 88:5809, 1991

11. Isaacs JD: The antiglobulin response to therapeutic antibodies. *Semin Immunol* 2:449, 1990

12. Milstein C: Monoclonal antibodies. *Sci Am* 243(4):56, 1980

13. Drobyski WR, Gottlieb M, Carrigan D, et al: Phase I study of safety and pharmacokinetics of a human anticytomegalovirus monoclonal antibody in allogeneic bone marrow transplant recipients. *Transplantation* 51:1190, 1991

14. Thor A, Itzkowitz SH, Schlom J, et al: Tumor-associated glycoprotein (TAG-72) expression in ulcerative colitis. *Int J Cancer* 43:810, 1989

15. Dillman RO, Beauregard JC, Sobol RE, et al: Lack of radioimmunodetection and complications associated with monoclonal anticarcinoembryonic antigen antibody cross-reactivity with antigen on circulating cells. *Cancer Res* 44:2213, 1984

16. Gold HK, Gimple LW, Yasuda T, et al: Pharmacodynamic study of F(ab')$_2$ fragments of murine monoclonal antibody 7E3 directed against human platelet glycoprotein IIb/IIIa in patients with unstable angina pectoris. *J Clin Invest* 86:651, 1990

17. Saleh MN, Khazaeli MB, Wheeler RH, et al: Phase 1 trial of the murine monoclonal anti-GD2 antibody 14G2a in metastatic melanoma. *Cancer Res* 52:4342, 1992

18. Winter G, Milstein C: Man-made antibodies. *Nature* 349:293, 1991

19. Huse WD, Sastry L, Iverson SA, et al: Generation of a large combinatorial library of the immunoglobulin repertoire in phage lambda. *Science* 246:1275, 1989

20. Pluckthun A, Pfitzinger, I: Comparison of the Fv fragments of different phosphorylcholine binding antibodies expressed in E. coli. *Ann NY Acad Sci* 646:115, 1991

21. Saragovi HU, Fitzpatrick D, Raktabutr A, et al: Design and synthesis of a mimetic from an antibody complementarity-determining region. *Science* 253:792, 1991

22. Hiatt A, Cafferkey R, Bowdish K: Production of antibodies in transgenic plants. *Nature* 342:76, 1989

23. LeBerthon B, Khawli LA, Alauddin M, et al: Enhanced tumor uptake of macromolecules induced by a novel vasoactive interleukin 2 immunoconjugate. *Cancer Res* 51:2694, 1991

24. Saffer JD: Transgenic mice in biomedical research. *Lab Anim* MAR:30, 1992

25. Rajewsky K: A phenotype or not: targeting genes in the immune system. *Science* 256:483, 1992

26. Cosman D, Lyman SD, Idzerda RL, et al: A new cytokine receptor superfamily. *TIBS* 15:265, 1990

27. Kaczmarski RS, Mufti GJ: The cytokine receptor superfamily. *Blood Rev* 5:193, 1991

28. Isaacs A: Interferon. *Sci Am* 204(5):51, 1961

29. Zoon KC, Miller D, Bekisz J, et al: Purification and characterization of multiple components of human lymphoblastoid interferon-α. *J Biol Chem* 267:15210, 1992

30. Biotechnology Medicines: 1993 Survey Report, Pharmaceutical Manufacturers Association, 1993

31. Trotta PP: Cytokines: an overview. *Am J Reprod Immunol* 25:137, 1991

32. WHO-IUIS Nomenclature Subcommittee on Interleukin Designation: Nomenclature for secreted regulatory proteins of the immune system (interleukins). *Blood* 79:1645, 1992

33. Dinarello CA: Interleukin-1 and interleukin-1 antagonism. *Blood* 77:1627, 1991

34. Eisenberg SP, Evans RJ, Arend WP, et al: Primary structure and functional expression from complementary DNA of a human interleukin-1 receptor antagonist. *Nature* 343:341, 1990

35. Cerretti DP, Kozlosky CJ, Mosley B, et al: Molecular cloning of the interleukin-1β converting enzyme. *Science* 256:97, 1992

36. Smith KA: Interleukin 2: inception, impact and implications. *Science* 240:1169, 1988

37. Rosenberg SA: Adoptive immunotherapy for cancer. *Sci Am* 262(5):62, 1990

38. Siegel JP, Puri RK: Interleukin-2 toxicity. *J Clin Oncol* 9:694, 1991

39. Kaplan G, Cohn ZA, Smith KA: Rational immunotherapy with interleukin 2. *Bio/Tech* 10:157, 1992

40. Waldmann TA: The multi-subunit interleukin-2 receptor. *Annu Rev Biochem* 58:875, 1989

41. Ihle JN, Pepersack L, Rebar L: Regulation of T cell differentiation: in vitro induction of 20α-hydroxysteroid dehydrogenase in splenic lymphocytes from athymic mice by a unique lymphokine. *J Immunol* 126:2184, 1981

42. Sunderland MC, Roodman GD: Interleukin-3: its biology and potential uses in pediatric hematology/oncology. *Am J Pediatr Hematol Oncol* 13:414, 1991

43. Kurzrock R, Estrov Z, Talpaz M, et al: Interleukin-3. *Am J Clin Oncol* 14(suppl 1):S45, 1991

44. Pluznik DH, Sachs L: The cloning of normal "mast" cells in tissue culture. *J Cell Comp Physiol* 66:319, 1965

45. Bradley TR, Metcalf D: The growth of mouse bone marrow cells in vitro. *Aust J Exp Biol Med Sci* 44:287, 1966

46. Groopman JE, Molina JM, Scadden DT: Hematopoietic growth factors: biology and clinical applications. *N Engl J Med* 321:1449, 1989

47. Niskanen E: Hematopoietic growth factors in clinical hematology. *Ann Med* 23:615, 1991

48. Herrmann F, Lindemann A, Mertelsmann R: G-CSF and M-CSF: from molecular biology to clinical application. *Biotherapy* 2:315, 1990

49. Old LJ: Tumor necrosis factor. *Sci Am* 258(5):59, 1988

50. Beutler B: The tumor necrosis factors: cachectin and lymphotoxin. *Hosp Pract* 25:45, 1990

51. Prince HE, Dermani-Arab V, Fahey JL: Depressed interleukin 2 receptor expression in acquired immunodeficiency and lymphadenopathy syndromes. *J Immunol* 133:1313, 1984

52. Lane HC, Fauci AS: Immunologic abnormalities in the acquired immunodeficiency syndrome. *Annu Rev Immunol* 3:477, 1985

53. Murphey-Corb M, Martin LN, Davison-Fairburn B, et al: A formalin-inactivated whole SIV vaccine confers protection in Macaques. *Science* 246:1293, 1989

54. Carlson JR, McGraw TP, Keddie E, et al: Vaccine protection of rhesus macaques against Simian Immunodeficiency Virus infection. *AIDS Res Hum Retroviruses* 6:1239, 1990

55. Girard M, Kieny MP, Pinter A, et al: Immunization of chimpanzees confers protection against challenge with human immunodeficiency virus. *Proc Natl Acad Sci USA* 88:542, 1991

56. Hahn BH, Shaw GM, Taylor ME, et al: Genetic variation in HTLV-III/LAV over time in patients with AIDS or at risk for AIDS. *Science* 232:1548, 1986

57. Weiss RA, Clapham PR, Weber JN, et al: Variable and conserved neutralization antigens of human immunodeficiency virus. *Nature* 324:572, 1986

58. Matthews TJ, Langlois AJ, Robey WG, et al: Restricted neutralization of divergent human T-lymphocyte virus type III isolates by antibodies to the major envelope glycoprotein. *Proc Natl Acad Sci USA* 83:9709, 1986

59. Laurence J, Saunders A, Kulkosky J: Characterization and clinical association of antibody inhibitory to HIV reverse transcriptase activity. *Science* 235:1501, 1987

60. Cullen BR: Trans-activation of human immunodeficiency virus occurs via a bimodal mechanism. *Cell* 46:973, 1986

61. Dalgleish AG, Beverley PC, Clapham PR, et al: The CD4 (T4) antigen is an essential component of the receptor for the AIDS retrovirus. *Nature* 312:763, 1984

62. McDougal JS, Nicholson JKA, Cross GD, et al: Binding of the human retrovirus HTLV-III/LAV/ARV/HIV to the CD4 (T4) molecule: conformation dependence, epitope mapping, antibody inhibition, and potential for idiotypic mimicry. *J Immunol* 137:2937, 1986

63. Sodroski J, Goh WC, Rosen C, et al: Role of the HTLV-III/LAV envelope in syncytium formation and cytopathicity. *Nature* 322:470, 1986

64. Homsy J, Steimer K, Kaslow R: Towards an AIDS vaccine: challenges and prospects. *Immunol Today* 8:193, 1987

65. Benjouad A, Gluckman J, Rochat H, et al: Influence of carbohydrate moieties on the immunogenicity of human immunodeficiency virus type 1 recombinant gp160. *J Virol* 66:2473, 1992

66. Broliden PA, Gegerfelt A, Clapham P, et al: Identification of human neutralization-inducing regions of the human immunodeficiency virus type 1 envelope glycoproteins. *Proc Natl Acad Sci USA* 89:461, 1992

67. Arthur LO, Pyle SW, Nara PL, et al: Serological responses in chimpanzees inoculated with human immunodeficiency virus glycoprotein (gp120) subunit vaccine. *Proc Natl Acad Sci USA* 84:8583, 1987

68. Putney SD, Matthews TJ, Robey WG, et al: HTLV-III/LAV neutralizing antibodies to an *E. coli* produced fragment of the virus envelope. *Science* 234:1392, 1986

69. Goudsmit J, Debouck C, Meloen RH, et al: human immunodeficiency virus type 1 neutralization epitope with conserved architecture elicits early type-specific antibodies in experimentally infected chimpanzees. *Proc Natl Acad Sci USA* 85:4478, 1988

70. Willey RL, Rutledge RA, Dias S, et al: Identification of conserved and divergent domains within the envelope gene of the acquired immunodeficiency syndrome retrovirus. *Proc Natl Acad Sci USA* 83:5038, 1986

71. Coffin JM: Genetic variation in AIDS viruses. *Cell* 46:1, 1986

72. Starcich BR, Hahn BH, Shaw GM, et al: Identification and characterization of conserved and variable regions in the envelope gene of HTLV-III/LAV, the retrovirus of AIDS. *Cell* 45:637, 1986

73. Matthews TJ, Langlois AJ, Robey WG, et al: Restricted neutralization of divergent HTLV-III/LAV isolates by antibodies to the major envelope glycoprotein. *Haematology and Blood Transfusion* 31:414, 1987

74. Hu SL, Abrams K, Barber GN, et al: Protection of macaques against SIV infection by subunit vaccines of SIV envelope glycoprotein gp160. *Science* 255:456, 1992

75. Berman PW, Gregory TJ, Riddle L, et al: Protection of chimpanzees from infection by HIV-1 after vaccination with recombinant glycoprotein gp120 but not gp160. *Nature* 345:622, 1990

76. Wang CY, Looney DJ, Li ML, et al: Long-term high-titer neutralizing activity induced by octameric synthetic HIV-1 antigen. *Science* 254:285, 1991

77. Ho DD, Fung MS, Cao Y, et al: Another discontinuous epitope on glycoprotein gp120 that is important in human immunodeficiency virus type 1 neutralization is identified by a monoclonal antibody. *Proc Natl Acad Sci USA* 88:8949, 1991

78. Hansen JES, Clausen H, Nielsen C, et al: Inhibition of human immunodeficiency virus (HIV) infection in vitro by anticarbohydrate monoclonal antibodies: peripheral glycosylation of HIV envelope glycoprotein gp120 may be a target for virus neutralization. *J Virol* 64:2833, 1990

79. Berkower I, Murphy D, Smith CC, et al: A predominant group-specific neutralizing epitope of human immunodeficiency virus type 1 maps to residues 342 to 511 of the envelope glycoprotein gp120. *J Virol* 65:5983, 1991

80. Hosmalin A, Nara PL, Zweig M, et al: Priming with T helper cell epitope peptides enhances the antibody response to the envelope glycoprotein of HIV-1 in primates. *J Immunol* 146:1667, 1991

81. Plata F, Autran B, Martins LP, et al: AIDS virus-specific cytotoxic T lymphocytes in lung disorders. *Nature* 328:348, 1987

82. Walker BD, Chakrabarti S, Moss B, et al: HIV-specific cytotoxic T lymphocytes in seropositive individuals. *Nature* 328:345, 1987

83. Tsubota H, Lord CI, Watkins DI, et al: A cytotoxic T lymphocyte inhibits acquired immunodeficiency syndrome virus replication in peripheral blood lymphocytes. *J Exp Med* 169:1421, 1989

84. Kannagi M, Chalifoux LV, Lord CI, et al: Suppression of simian immunodeficiency virus replication in vitro by CD8+ lymphocytes. *J Immunol* 140:2237, 1988

85. Smith GL, Moss B: Infectious poxvirus vectors have capacity for at least 25,000 base pairs of foreign DNA. *Gene* 25:21, 1983

86. Yilma T, Hsu D, Jones L, et al: Protection of cattle against rinderpest with vaccinia virus recombinants expressing the HA or F gene. *Science* 242:1058, 1988

87. Bennink JR, Yewdell JW, Smith GL, et al: Recombinant vaccinia virus primes and stimulates influenza haemagglutinin-specific cytotoxic T cells. *Nature* 311:578, 1984

88. Kieny MP, Rautmann G, Schmitt D, et al: AIDS virus env protein expressed from a recombinant vaccinia virus. *Biotechnology* 4:790, 1986

89. Hu SL, Kosowoski SG, Dalrymple JM: Expression of AIDS virus envelope gene in recombinant vaccinia viruses. *Nature* 320:537, 1986

90. Chakrabarti S, Robert-Guroff M, Wong-Stall F, et al: Expression of the HTLV-III envelope gene by a recombinant vaccinia virus. *Nature* 320:535, 1986

91. Lisziewicz J, Sun D, Klotman M, et al: Specific inhibition of human immunodeficiency virus type 1 replication by antisense oligonucleotides: an in vitro model for treatment. *Proc Natl Acad Sci USA* 89:11209, 1992

92. Sullenger BA, Gallardo HF, Ungers GE, et al: Overexpression of TAR sequences renders cells resistant to human immunodeficiency virus replication. *Cell* 63:601, 1990

93. Cech TR, Bass B: Biological catalysis by RNA. *Annu Rev Biochem* 55:599, 1986

94. Cech TR: The chemistry of self-splicing RNA and RNA enzymes. *Science* 236:1532, 1987

95. Sarver N, Cantin EM, Chang PS, et al: Ribozymes as potential anti–HIV-1 therapeutic agents. *Science* 247:1222, 1990

96. Rossi JJ, Elkins D, Zaia JA, et al: Ribozymes as anti–HIV-1 therapeutic agents: principles, applications, and problems. *AIDS Res Hum Retroviruses* 8:183, 1992

97. Yu M, Ojwang J, Yamada O: A hairpin ribozyme inhibits expression of diverse strains of human immunodeficiency virus type 1. *Proc Natl Acad Sci USA* 90:6340, 1993

98. Smith DH, Byrn RA, Marsters SA, et al: Blocking of HIV-1 infectivity by a soluble, secreted form of the CD4 antigen. *Science* 238:1704, 1987

99. Traunecker A, Luke W, Karjalainen K: Soluble CD4 molecules neutralize human immunodeficiency virus type 1. *Nature* 331:84, 1988

100. Fisher RA, Bertonis JM, Meier W, et al: HIV infection is blocked in vitro by recombinant soluble CD4. *Nature* 331:76, 1988

101. Traunecker A, Schneider J, Kiefer H, et al: Highly efficient neutralization of HIV with recombinant CD4-immunoglobulin molecules. *Nature* 339:68, 1989

Acknowledgments

Figures 1 through 3   Adapted from *Recombinant DNA*, 2nd ed., by J. D. Watson, J. Witkowski, M. Gilman, et al. Scientific American Books, New York, 1992. © 1992 James D. Watson, Jan Witkowski, Michael Gilman, Mark Zoller. Used with permission.

Figures 4, 5   Dana Burns.

CHAPTER 12

Gene Therapy

Curtis L. Scribner, M.D., Paul Aebersold, Ph.D.

Modifying cells to express new proteins, applied so successfully to the manufacture of human proteins in prokaryotic or xenogeneic eukaryotic cells, has long been envisioned as a means of correcting human inborn genetic defects. For example, one might cure hemophilia by modifying somatic cells to secrete the missing clotting factor. Although gene therapy is simple and elegant in concept, a number of obstacles must be overcome in the development of reliable procedures for implementing this technique.

Quite aside from the technical difficulties, the ethics of modifying human cells to express new genetic information has been intensively discussed. The Recombinant DNA Advisory Committee (RAC), formed by the National Institutes of Health to advise the Director on approval of recombinant DNA research at institutions receiving federal grant funding, created a Human Gene Therapy Subcommittee specifically to consider the ethical, medical, and legal issues related to gene-therapy protocols. Although modifying somatic cells to compensate for a genetic defect might appear straightforward, some critics have feared that gene therapy in humans could open a Pandora's box of genetic horrors. (The RAC has indicated that it will not even consider protocols for modification of germ cells.)

In 1987, the gene therapy subcommittee rejected a protocol to treat children with severe combined immunodeficiency disease by inserting the human gene for the enzyme adenosine deaminase into their bone-marrow cells by means of a retroviral gene-transfer system. In 1989, however, after extensive review, the Director of the National Institutes of Health signed the first authorization to transfer genetically modified cells into humans—

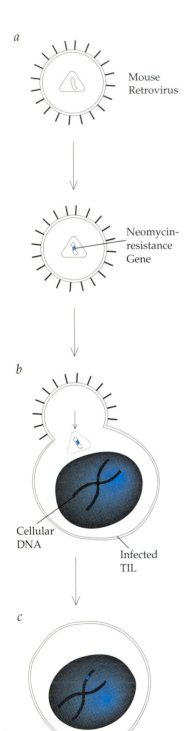

a

Mouse
Retrovirus

Neomycin-
resistance
Gene

b

Cellular
DNA

Infected
TIL

c

Gene-Altered
TIL

not as a therapeutic procedure but as a marker to evaluate one form of cancer therapy. Under the protocol, terminal cancer patients were treated with autologous tumor-infiltrating lymphocytes (TILs) that carried a bacterial gene for resistance to neomycin [*see Figure 1*]. The product of this bacterial gene permitted the modified cells to grow in the presence of a neomycin analogue that is toxic to normal cells. Data from the trial showed that the marked TILs survived for a few weeks after infusion into the patients[1] and that they could be recovered selectively from blood and tumor biopsies when grown in vitro with interleukin-2.[2]

The first therapeutic human gene transfer took place at the National Institutes of Health on September 14, 1990. Autologous T cells modified to express adenosine deaminase were infused into a child with severe combined immune deficiency. (Adenosine deaminase is critical for normal immune function, and children born without a functional gene for the enzyme accumulate intracellular levels of adenosine that are toxic to nearly all of their T cells.) The child had previously been treated with a recombinant DNA version of adenosine deaminase conjugated to polyethylene glycol but was still unable to respond immunologically to normal childhood vaccinations. On the second anniversary of her first gene therapy, after several courses of the treatment, this patient had normal levels of peripheral blood T cells, had produced antibodies and delayed-type hypersensitivity to several vaccination antigens, and had started to live the life of a normal school child after years of isolation.[3,4] Gene therapy had come of age, and several dozen clinical trials were soon in progress with marker or therapeutic genes.

The term gene therapy can be applied loosely to any clinical use of recombinant DNA technology to modify somatic cells. Alternatively, the term can be more strictly applied so that it denotes only the replacement of defective or missing genes, because neither marking cells for scientific purposes nor vaccinating healthy subjects constitutes therapy. The term gene transfer is sometimes used to distinguish these latter types of clinical applications, but the fact remains that genes that are not defective or missing in the patient are also being transferred into patients' cells to stimulate immune responses or to deliver a potentially therapeutic protein. In this chapter, the term gene therapy will therefore be applied loosely.

Technology for Gene Therapy

For the pharmaceutical production of a human protein, only a single recombinant cell that secretes copious amounts of the desired product need be identified. Such a cell can be cloned and expanded, and aliquots

Figure 1 *(a) A bacterial gene that can make cells resistant to the lethal effects of neomycin is inserted into a mouse retrovirus, replacing retroviral genes needed for viral replication. (b) The virus carrying the neomycin-resistance gene is then cultured with tumor-infiltrating lymphocytes (TILs) so that the virus can infect the cells. (c) The retrovirus then incorporates its genetic material into the cellular DNA. Because the altered TILs express the foreign gene, they are resistant to neomycin and can easily be distinguished from other cells in the body. Thus, the survival of TILs in patients treated with this modality can be evaluated.*

of the progeny can be saved in a master cell bank for initiating future production of the recombinant product; the efficiency of gene transfer at the start of the process is therefore not particularly important. For gene therapy, on the other hand, improved, radically different technologies have had to be developed to achieve the necessary high-efficiency gene transfer into large numbers of cells. At present, only constitutive systems have been used to express proteins that are not particularly toxic, such as adenosine deaminase, or proteins that are administered in controlled dose escalations. A makeshift way to prevent runaway overdosing is to include a suicide gene along with the therapeutic gene, so that the modified cells can be killed if necessary. Eventually, no doubt, more elegant regulated systems for protein expression will be developed, so that a protein such as insulin can be produced under physiologic control.

Cloned DNA has been transduced efficiently into human cells with genetically altered murine retroviruses.[5] Messenger RNA (mRNA) from these viruses is reverse transcribed in recipient cells, and the resulting DNA is incorporated into the host genome during cell replication. (Gene transduction with retroviruses does not work in cells that do not divide.) The genetically altered retroviruses are produced by cells modified to carry viral polymerase and envelope genes on one or two gene inserts and the packaging sequences and structural gene of interest on a separate insert. Consequently, these cells make complete virions, capable of infection but not of replication, by packaging the gene-therapy mRNA transcribed from one insert into virus coat proteins translated from mRNA from another insert.[6,7] The efficiency of gene transduction into host cells depends on the titer of the retroviral vector and the percentage of replicating host cells; the efficiency generally ranges from one percent to 20 percent.

Other types of viruses that are being developed or considered as gene-therapy vectors include adeno, adeno-associated, Epstein-Barr, herpes, and human immunodeficiency viruses. Adenovirus vectors carrying the cystic fibrosis transmembrane conductance regulator (CFTR) gene, which encodes a chloride ion channel, have been successfully introduced into airway epithelial cells in animals and have expressed the human protein in these cells.[8] Such vectors are now being employed in clinical trials to administer this gene directly to the airways of patients with cystic fibrosis. Adenovirus DNA does not incorporate into the infected host-cell genome, and for the cystic fibrosis indication, the cells most easily infected with adenovirus slough off over time. Thus, patients with cystic fibrosis would most likely have to be treated periodically for gene therapy to be effective.

On the other hand, DNA from adeno-associated virus, a parvovirus, integrates at a specific site in the human genome (at the telomere of chromosome 19) in the absence of helper viruses. Adeno-associated viruses thus share with retroviruses the advantage of delivering stable genetic modifications to the recipient cells.[9] Herpesvirus vectors are also attractive candidates for the genetic modification of neurons, which do not divide in adults.[10] Similarly, there is interest in using modified human immunodeficiency virus (HIV) as a vector to deliver protective genes in vivo to the very cells at risk for HIV infection.[11] Protective genes, for example, might code for antisense mRNA to viral genes, for decoy mRNA to bind viral regulatory proteins, or for ribozymes that would inactivate viral mRNA.[12]

Viruses are only one approach to the genetic modification of target cells. The efficiency of naked-DNA transfection has been increased by formulating the DNA with liposomes to facilitate cellular uptake.[13] Directed DNA transfection is being developed by binding plasmids to positively charged polylysine, which in turn can be conjugated to such human proteins as transferrin.[14] Such complexes preferentially target the plasmid genes to cells bearing transferrin receptors, where the complexes are internalized by receptor-mediated endocytosis. Receptor-mediated transformation of hepatocytes has been demonstrated with a plasmid conjugate containing asialoglycoprotein.[15] A so-called gene gun has been developed to blast plasmid DNA through cell membranes.[16] This gene gun could conceivably be used for vaccinations (e.g., of patients with the acquired immunodeficiency syndrome [AIDS]), injecting fibroblasts and muscle cells with DNA coding for viral antigen to evoke cellular rather than humoral immunity.

Clinical Indications for Gene Therapy

Conditions caused by inherited mutant genes are the most obvious candidates for management by gene therapy [see Table 1]. Familial hypercholesterolemia is caused by defects in the genes for low-density lipoprotein (LDL) receptors. Homozygotes have extraordinarily high levels of serum LDL cholesterol, develop atherosclerosis, and often suffer myocardial infarctions as children. In a preclinical study with Watanabe (heritable hyperlipidemic) rabbits in which modified hepatocytes were injected into the spleens, there was a long-term decrease of 30 to 50 percent in baseline serum cholesterol levels.[17] The clinical protocol approved by the RAC for patients with familial hypercholesterolemia, which is intended to demonstrate proof of the concept of gene therapy as well as help the patients, requires partial liver resection to obtain autologous hepatocytes. In this procedure, the patient's hepatocytes are transduced ex vivo with retroviral vectors carrying the normal LDL gene to express functional LDL receptors and then injected into the patient's portal circulation [see Figure 2]. A progress report to the RAC in December 1992 showed that the serum cholesterol level of the first patient managed according to this protocol was lower after treatment. If other patients show similar benefit, there will be impetus for developing a method for targeting the gene to the liver in vivo, both to avoid the morbidity of a partial resection and to permit repeated applications of the therapy as necessary to achieve appropriate lowering of serum LDL cholesterol.

Cystic fibrosis affects about 30,000 persons in the United States, and few individuals with the disease survive beyond 30 years of age. In December 1992, the RAC approved three protocols from different investigators to treat patients with cystic fibrosis by direct airway administration of adenovirus vectors. It is thought that transduction of five to 10 percent of airway epithelial cells to express the normal chloride ion transmembrane conductance regulator would be sufficient to prevent accumulation of mucus in the lungs and halt progression of the disease. As mentioned earlier, there is no expectation that epithelial stem cells can be transduced

Table 1 Inherited Diseases That Are Candidates for Gene Therapy

Disorder	Incidence	Normal Product of Defective Gene	Target Cells
Hemoglobin-opathies (thalassemias)	1 in 600 in certain ethnic groups	Constituents of hemoglobin	Bone marrow cells (which give rise to circulating blood)
Severe combined immuno-deficiency (SCID)	Rare	Adenosine deaminase (ADA) in about a quarter of SCID patients	Bone marrow cells or T cells
Hemophilia A Hemophilia B	1 in 10,000 males 1 in 30,000 males	Blood-clotting factor VIII Blood-clotting factor IX	Liver cells or fibroblasts
Familial hyper-cholesterolemia	1 in 500	Liver receptor for low-density lipoprotein (LDL)	Liver cells
Inherited emphysema	1 in 3,500	α_1-Antitrypsin (liver product that protects lungs from enzymatic degradation)	Lung or liver cells
Cystic fibrosis	1 in 2,500 Caucasians	Substance important for keeping air tubes in lungs free of mucus	Lung cells
Duchenne's muscular dystrophy	1 in 10,000 males	Dystrophin (structural component of muscle)	Muscle cells (particularly embryonic ones that develop into muscle fibers)
Lysosomal storage diseases	1 in 1,500 acquires some form	Enzymes that degrade complex molecules in intracellular compartments known as lysosomes	Vary, depending on disorder

by this approach, and thus the gene therapy will have to be repeated when the majority of transduced epithelial cells have sloughed off.

There has also been vigorous application of gene-transfer technology for treatment of cancer. In some cases the cells are modified to provide a novel method of drug delivery rather than to correct a defective gene. For example, TILs have been modified ex vivo to secrete tumor necrosis factor (TNF) constitutively [*see Figure 3*]. Since TILs preferentially accumulate in tumors several days after infusion,[18] it is hoped that the resulting localized concentrations of TNF may be sufficient to cause the desired hemorrhagic necrosis of the tumor, which cannot be achieved by systemic delivery of the cytokine because of its toxicity. Other cancer trials are exploring vaccinating patients with autologous tumor cells that have been modified to secrete interleukin-2 or TNF. The gene-transfer technology provides a continuous physiologic dose of cytokine as an adjuvant to the patient's own tumor antigens. The technique has produced cell-mediated immunity in mice.[19-21]

The first clinical trial to utilize in vivo gene transfection began in 1992 for the treatment of HLA-B7–negative patients with malignant melanoma. The protocol involves direct injection into tumors of plasmid DNA carrying the gene for human HLA-B7. HLA-B7 is not a common major histocompatibility antigen in individuals in the United States, so most patients with malignant melanoma will be HLA-B7–negative. The expression of allogeneic major histocompatibility complex protein is expected to provoke an immune response that will destroy transduced cells. The expectation is not that all tumor cells will be transduced to express HLA-B7 but rather that the inflammatory reaction will result in antitumor as well as allogeneic immunity. This approach has proved somewhat effective in murine models.[22]

Subsequent protocols for in vivo gene transfer were approved by the RAC in 1992. Two protocols involve treating residual non–small cell lung cancer by injecting retroviral vectors carrying either of two different genes, depending on the molecular defect in the patient's tumor, into the tumor bed. One vector will carry the p53 tumor suppressor gene and should transduce dividing cells (mostly tumor cells) to express the normal p53 protein, thereby inhibiting abnormal growth in tumor cells that have the mutant p53 gene. The other vector will cause transduced cells to

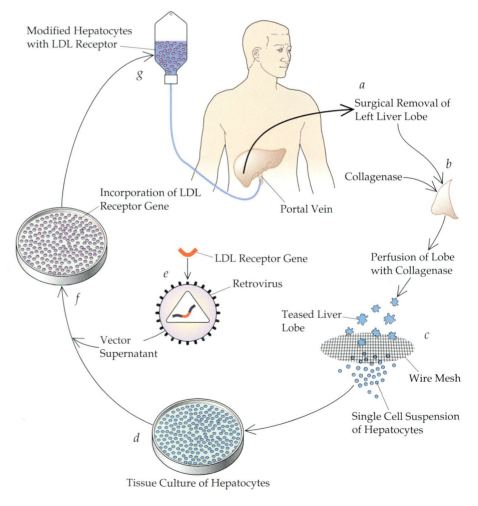

Figure 2 (a) In the gene therapy protocol approved for patients with familial hypercholesterolemia, the left liver lobe is first resected surgically to obtain autologous hepatocytes. (b) The liver lobe is perfused with collagenase, an enzyme that catalyzes the hydrolysis of peptide bonds in collagen. (c) The teased liver lobe is passed through a wire mesh, and (d) a single-cell suspension of hepatocytes is then established in tissue culture. (e) A gene encoding a normal low-density lipoprotein (LDL) receptor is inserted into a retrovirus, and (f) a supernatant containing this retroviral vector is then added to the hepatocyte tissue culture. (g) The hepatocytes, some of which take up the retroviral genetic material containing the normal LDL receptor gene, are then infused into the patient's portal circulation.

Modified Hepatocytes with LDL Receptor

Surgical Removal of Left Liver Lobe

Collagenase

Incorporation of LDL Receptor Gene

Portal Vein

Perfusion of Lobe with Collagenase

LDL Receptor Gene

Retrovirus

Teased Liver Lobe

Vector Supernatant

Wire Mesh

Single Cell Suspension of Hepatocytes

Tissue Culture of Hepatocytes

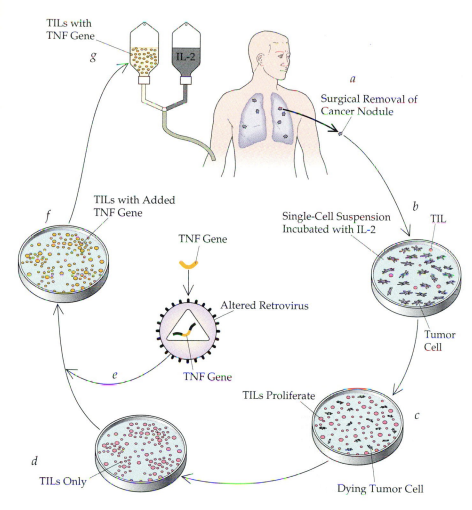

Figure 3 *In a form of cancer therapy based on gene-transfer technology, a patient's tumor-infiltrating lymphocytes (TILs) are modified ex vivo to secrete tumor necrosis factor (TNF) and then reinfused. (a) In this procedure, a nodule of cancerous tissue is first removed from a patient. (b) The cells in the nodule are separated from one another by enzymes and then cultured with interleukin-2. (c) The TILs (color), stimulated by interleukin-2, begin to proliferate rapidly and to attack the cancer cells. (d) After 30 to 45 days, the lymphocytes in the culture completely replace the tumor cells. (e) A retrovirus that has been transfected with the TNF gene is then added to the culture containing TILs. (f) Some of the TILs incorporate the TNF gene and secrete TNF constitutively. (g) TILs containing the TNF gene are then infused into the patient along with additional interleukin-2.*

express antisense mRNA for K-*ras*. By binding to K-*ras* mRNA, the antisense mRNA should inhibit translation of the mutant K-*ras* oncogenic protein, thereby bringing transduced cells under normal growth control. Even though it is unlikely that all tumor cells will be transduced by this approach, it is thought that cells whose growth control has been returned to normal will exert a normalizing influence on neighboring nontransduced tumor cells. These approaches have had some effect in preclinical in vitro systems.[23,24]

In vivo gene transfer has also been approved for the treatment of recurrent brain cancer [*see Figure 4*]. Since most brain cells do not divide, retroviruses injected into brain tumors should transduce tumor cells to a vastly greater extent than normal brain cells. The novelty of the protocol is that the murine producer cells that secrete the retrovirus vectors are themselves injected into the tumor, so that transduction of tumor cells can take place continuously over a period of days. The transduced tumor cells, as well as the murine producer cells, will express viral thymidine kinase, which renders them sensitive to killing by the antiviral base analogue ganciclovir. In preclinical studies in rats with transplantable brain tumors, total rejection of tumors occurred in some cases even when all the tumor cells were not transduced; this effect was termed a bystander

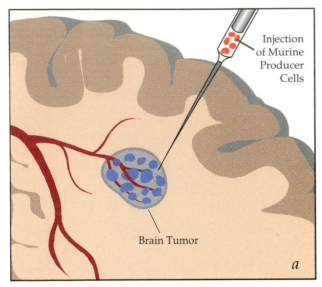

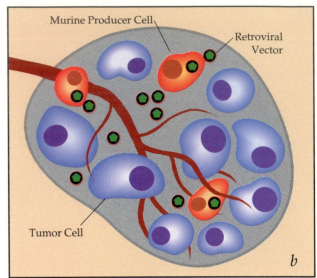

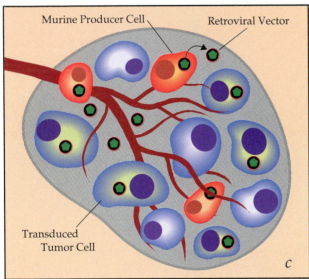

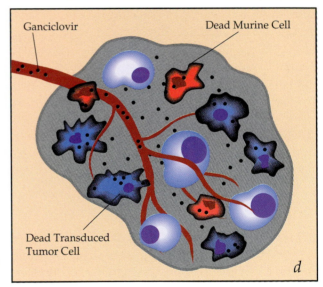

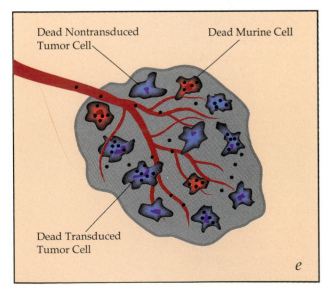

Figure 4 *(a) In a form of gene therapy that is being employed for recurrent brain cancer, murine producer cells are injected into the tumor. These cells produce a retroviral vector into which the viral thymidine kinase gene has been inserted. (b) The retroviral vector is then secreted into the surrounding tissue. (c) The vector transduces some neighboring tumor cells, which are thereby modified to express the thymidine kinase gene. (d) Systemic administration of the antiviral agent ganciclovir kills both the murine producer cells and the transduced tumor cells. (e) The death of nontransduced tumor cells may occur by a process that has been termed the bystander effect.*

effect.[25] The first patient on this protocol was injected with murine producer cells in December 1992.

Gene transfer technology has also been used to label cells so that their in vivo distribution and survival can be studied.[26] Gene marking is not intended to provide therapeutic benefit for patients, but it offers significant advantages over conventional labeling techniques and may lead to greater understanding of certain therapies. When the marker gene integrates into and replicates with the host cell genome, the cells or their progeny are marked as long as they survive. Further, the polymerase chain reaction (PCR) methodology provides an extraordinarily sensitive means for detecting the marked cells: a single cell carrying a single copy of xenogeneic DNA can be detected in a sample containing 100,000 normal cells.

Autologous bone-marrow cells are being marked before transplantation to study hematopoietic reconstitution, although very few of the marked cells are likely to be regenerating stem cells. For cancer patients treated with ablative systemic therapy and autologous bone-marrow transplants, there has always been a question as to whether relapses are caused by residual or transplanted tumor cells. Retroviral gene transfer can mark a percentage of any cancer cells remaining in the marrow, so that if patients relapse in whole or in part from the transplanted marrow, a portion of the tumor cells causing the relapse might carry the marker gene. In a limited number of patients whose infused marrow contained no acute myelogenous leukemic cells detectable by current techniques, relapse blasts have in fact been marked.[27] Gene marking appears to be a sensitive detection system for tumor cells and may be useful for investigating the efficacy of various bone-marrow purging techniques.

Safety Considerations

Gene therapy is not without risk. The introduction of retrovirus vectors results in the random integration of reverse-transcribed viral DNA into host-cell genomes. It is expected that random integration will cause insertional mutagenesis that could result in disruption of a host growth-control gene or overexpression of a host proto-oncogene, either of which might cause or predispose to malignancy. The magnitude of this risk in humans is difficult to evaluate from standard toxicology studies in mice. Consequently, all investigators using retroviral vectors must plan long-term follow-up of patients. Insertional mutagenesis is also a risk for direct DNA transfection technologies, although not particularly for those employing either adeno-associated virus, which incorporates at a specific site in the host genome, or adenovirus, which does not integrate into the host genome.

The risk of germ-line modification with retroviral gene-therapy vectors has been avoided in early in vivo protocols by treating only infertile patients, an approach that finesses the problem for initial trials but would not be appropriate if gene therapy becomes a standard treatment for certain diseases. Protocols in which patients' cells are genetically modified ex vivo eliminates the risk of accidental germ-line modification; reliance on vector viruses such as adenovirus all but eliminates the risk. (The RAC, in approving protocols for the treatment of cystic fibrosis, insisted that fertile patients be included if they practice appropriate birth control.)

The cells in which replication-incompetent viral vectors are produced must contain all the genetic information necessary to produce replication-competent viruses. Even though the information required for viral replication is carried on separate DNA inserts, recombination events can occur and lead to the production of replication-competent viruses. Sensitive quality-control tests have been developed to assure that clinical lots of gene-therapy vectors are free of any replication-competent viruses.

Before the first human gene transfer in 1989, a number of primates, some of them immunosuppressed, were challenged with high titers of replication-competent murine retroviruses without any evidence of pathological changes.[28,29] In 1991, however, in an experiment with high-titer vector preparations known to be contaminated with replication-competent viruses, three of eight irradiated monkeys infused with autologous transduced bone marrow developed T-cell lymphomas about 200 days after treatment.[30] These three monkeys had not developed antibodies to the murine viruses. Their lymphoma cells each contained 10 to 50 inserts of replication-competent viral genomes. This experimental result confirmed the necessity of quality-control testing for replication-competent viruses but also raised concerns as to whether current testing procedures were sensitive enough to warrant the use of retroviral vectors in immunosuppressed patients.

If the gene-therapy vector is a virus that normally infects humans, such as adenovirus, there is some risk that unforeseen recombination events could take place between a wild-type virus and the gene-therapy vector. Conceivably, the wild-type virus could acquire a therapeutic vector gene and introduce it into the general population. In approving adenovirus vectors for treatment of patients with cystic fibrosis, the RAC weighed expert testimony that wild-type viruses had outcompeted every modified laboratory strain constructed and that constitutive overexpression of the cystic fibrosis transmembrane conductance regulator in transgenic mice produced absolutely no pathological changes. The RAC concluded that even if there were recombination between the vector and wild-type adenovirus, there would be minimal risk to patients and to the public health. As of November 1993, the RAC had not been presented with protocols involving herpesvirus or HIV as gene-therapy vectors.

Prospects and Problems

The medical community has not been idle in developing modalities other than gene transfer for the treatment of genetic diseases. Patients with hemophilia have been treated with clotting factors from human plasma or recombinant sources. Patients with cystic fibrosis have been treated with recombinant DNAse to reduce the viscosity of fluid in the lungs. Although gene therapy may provide more effective and durable treatments for some patients with inherited genetic diseases, it may fail entirely or create new medical problems for other patients. For example, if the cells of a hemophilic patient were permanently modified to secrete clotting factor VIII, the usual option of withholding dosing if antibody complexes became problematic would be eliminated. Likewise, expression of LDL receptors on autologous liver cells may render them antigenic in patients with gene deletions, leading to immune rejection and treatment failure. It is a common assumption that gene therapy in patients carrying inherited point mutations is not likely to provoke an immune response against modified cells expressing the normal protein. In patients carrying gene deletions, however, certain peptide sequences of the normal protein will be novel to the immune system and may provoke rejection of the modified cells.

Predictions about the prospects of gene therapy for the treatment of cancer also cannot be reliable at this early stage of development. Certainly gene therapists face the same problem as traditional oncologists, namely that of eliminating every cancer cell from the body. Only time will tell whether a bystander effect can eradicate all malignant cells in a localized brain tumor when only a portion of those cells have been genetically sensitized to an antiviral agent. For cancers with micrometastases, it may not be possible to direct gene-therapy vectors preferentially to tumor cells, because it has been difficult to identify cell-surface differences between tumor cells and normal cells on the basis of antigenicity. Malignant melanoma is the only human tumor for which there is strong evidence of cellular immunity,[31] and so immunization of patients with genetically modified malignant melanoma cells may indeed lead to systemic immunity and tumor rejection. For most human cancers there is very little evidence for the existence of cellular immunity, and one should not expect gene therapy immunization strategies to be significantly more effective than other autologous cancer vaccines have been.

Predictions about the prospects for gene therapy for AIDS are equally premature at this time. It is technically feasible to modify human CD4$^+$ cells to express antisense mRNA to HIV transcripts that protect them from cellular toxicity in vitro.[32] Whether infusion of protected CD4$^+$ cells into patients will alter the complicated course of the disease remains to be seen. The destruction of dendritic cells in lymph nodes by HIV and the consequent reduction in antigen presentation might be more damaging to a patient's immunity than the destruction of CD4$^+$ cells. At present, it is not clear whether gene therapy vectors can be designed to deliver protective genes to these dendritic cells in vivo. Gene-transfer technology can also be applied to modify autologous cells to express HIV proteins for purposes of therapeutic vaccination, but it remains to be seen whether raising antibody titers to HIV proteins will benefit the patient.

When recombinant DNA technology was first applied to the production of previously scarce human proteins such as interferon, there was a general belief that miracle cures for disease were at hand. As is all too evident, cancer and infectious diseases still claim millions of lives every year. Today gene therapy technology is new, and optimism abounds; it would be a disservice to the ingenuity of the human mind to predict limitations on its future. The dream of gene therapists is to take a vial off the pharmacy shelf, inject the contents into a patient with a genetic defect, have the vector target the appropriate cells, have the defective gene replaced with a good copy, and send the patient home to live a normal life. As is the case for monoclonal antibody, recombinant cytokine, and vaccine technologies, only time and clinical testing will tell whether such hopes are realistic.

References

1. Rosenberg SA, Aebersold P, Cornetta K, et al: Gene transfer into humans—immunotherapy of patients with advanced melanoma, using tumor-infiltrating lymphocytes modified by retroviral gene transduction. *N Engl J Med* 323:570, 1990

2. Aebersold P, Kasid A, Rosenberg SA: Selection of gene-marked tumor infiltrating lymphocytes from post-treatment biopsies: a case study. *Hum Gene Ther* 1:373, 1990

3. Culver KW, Anderson WF, Blaese RM: Lymphocyte gene therapy. *Hum Gene Ther* 2:107, 1991

4. Culver KW, Berger M, Miller AD, et al: Lymphocyte gene therapy for adenosine deaminase deficiency. *Pediatr Res* 31:149A, 1992

5. Miller AD, Rosman GJ: Improved retroviral vectors for gene transfer and expression. *Biotechniques* 7:980, 1989

6. Miller AD, Buttimore C: Redesign of retrovirus packaging cell lines to avoid recombination leading to helper virus production. *Mol Cell Biol* 6:2895, 1986

7. Danos O, Mulligan RC: Safe and efficient generation of recombinant retroviruses with amphotropic and ecotropic host ranges. *Proc Natl Acad Sci USA* 85:6460, 1988

8. Rosenfeld MA, Yoshimura K, Trapnell DC, et al: In vivo transfer of the human cystic fibrosis transmembrane conductance regulator gene to the airway epithelium. *Cell* 68:143, 1992

9. Flotte TR, Solow R, Owens RA, et al: Gene expression from adeno-associated virus vectors in airway epithelial cells. *Am J Respir Cell Mol Biol* 7:349, 1992

10. Breakefield XO, DeLuca NA: Herpes simplex virus for gene delivery to neurons. *New Biol* 3:203, 1991

11. Poznansky M, Lever A, Bergeron L, et al: Gene transfer into human lymphocytes by a defective human immunodeficiency virus type 1 vector. *J Virol* 65:532, 1991

12. Sarver N, Cantin EM, Chang PS, et al: Ribozymes as potential anti-HIV-1 therapeutic agents. *Science* 247:1222, 1990

13. Wang C-Y, Huang L: Highly efficient DNA delivery mediated by pH-sensitive immunoliposomes. *Biochemistry* 28:9508, 1989

14. Wagner E, Zenke M, Cotten M, et al: Transferrin-polycation conjugates as carriers for DNA uptake into cells. *Proc Natl Acad Sci USA* 87:3410, 1990

15. Wu GY, Wu CH: Receptor-mediated in vitro gene transformation by a soluble DNA carrier system. *J Biol Chem* 262:4429, 1987

16. Yang N-S, Burkholder J, Roberts B, et al: In vivo and in vitro gene transfer to mammalian somatic cells by particle bombardment. *Proc Natl Acad Sci USA* 87:9568, 1990

17. Chowdhury JR, Grossman M, Gupta S, et al: Long-term improvement of hypercholesterolemia after ex vivo gene therapy in LDLR-deficient rabbits. *Science* 254:1802, 1991

18. Griffith KD, Read EJ, Carrasquillo JA, et al: In vivo distribution of adoptively transferred indium-111-labeled tumor infiltrating lymphocytes and peripheral blood lymphocytes in patients with metastatic melanoma. *J Natl Cancer Inst* 81:1709, 1989

19. Gansbacher B, Zier K, Daniels B, et al: Interleukin-2 gene transfer into tumor cells abrogates tumorigenicity and induces protective immunity. *J Exp Med* 172:1217, 1990

20. Fearon ER, Pardoll DM, Itaya T, et al: Interleukin-2 production by tumor cells bypasses T helper function in the generation of an antitumor response. *Cell* 60:397, 1990

21. Asher AL, Mulé JJ, Kasid A, et al: Murine tumor cells transduced with the gene for tumor necrosis factor-alpha: evidence for paracrine immune effects of tumor necrosis factor against tumors. *J Immunol* 146:3227, 1991

22. Plautz GE, Yang ZY, Wu BY, et al: Immunotherapy of malignancy by in vivo gene transfer into tumors. *Proc Natl Acad Sci USA* 90:4645, 1993

23. Mukhopadhyay T, Cavender A, Tainski M, et al: Expression of antisense K-ras message in a human lung cancer cell line with a spontaneous activated K-ras oncogene alters the transformed phenotype. *Proc Amer Assoc Cancer Res* 31:304, 1990

24. Mukhopadhyay T, Cavender AC, Branch CD, et al: Expression and regulation of wild type p53 gene in human non-small cell lung cancer cell lines carrying normal or mutated p53 gene. *J Cell Biochem* 15F(suppl):22, 1991

25. Culver KW, Ram Z, Wallbridge S, et al: In vivo gene transfer with retroviral vector-producer cells for treatment of experimental brain tumors. *Science* 256:1550, 1992

26. Morgan RA, Cornetta K, Anderson WF: Applications of the polymerase chain reaction in retroviral-mediated gene transfer and the analysis of gene-marked human TIL cells. *Hum Gen Ther* 1:135, 1990

27. Brenner MK, Rill DR, Moen RC, et al: Gene-marking to trace origin of relapse after autologous bone marrow transplantation. *Lancet* 341:85, 1993

28. Cornetta K, Moen RC, Culver K, et al: Amphotropic murine leukemia retrovirus is not an acute pathogen for primates. *Hum Gene Ther* 1:15, 1990

29. Cornetta K, Morgan RA, Gillio A, et al: No retroviremia or pathology in long-term follow-up of monkeys exposed to a murine amphotropic retrovirus. *Hum Gene Ther* 2:215, 1991

30. Donahue RE, Kessler SW, Bodine D, et al: Helper virus induced T cell lymphoma in nonhuman primates after retroviral mediated gene transfer. *J Exp Med* 176:1125, 1992

31. Hom SS, Topalian SL, Simonis T, et al: Common expression of melanoma tumor-associated antigens recognized by human tumor infiltrating lymphocytes: analysis by human lymphocyte antigen restriction. *J Immunother* 10:153, 1991

32. Chatterjee S, Johnson PR, Wong KK, Jr: Dual-target inhibition of HIV-1 in vitro by means of an adeno-associated virus antisense vector. *Science* 258:1485, 1992

Acknowledgments

Figures 1, 3   Adapted from "Adoptive Immunotherapy for Cancer," by S. A. Rosenberg, in *Scientific American* 262(5):62, 1990. © 1990 Scientific American, Inc. All rights reserved. Used by permission.

Figure 1   Talar Agasyan.

Figures 2, 3   Tom Moore.

Figure 4   Dana Burns.

Index

A